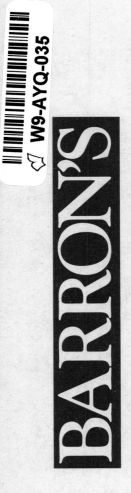
BARRON'S

HOW TO PREPARE FOR THE

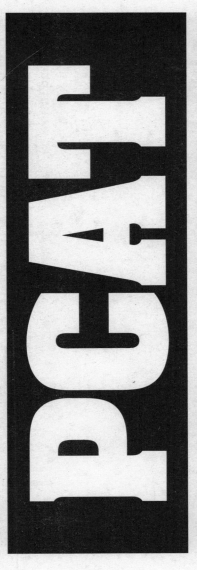

PCAT

PHARMACY COLLEGE ADMISSION TEST

2ND EDITION

Marie A. Chisholm, Pharm.D., R.Ph.

CONTRIBUTING AUTHORS

Marie A. Chisholm, Pharm.D., R.Ph.
Associate Professor of Pharmacy
and Associate Professor of Medicine
University of Georgia College of Pharmacy
Athens, Georgia
Medical College of Georgia
Augusta, Georgia

Kenneth M. Duke, M.B.A., R.Ph.
Clinical Assistant Professor of Pharmacy
and Assistant to the Dean
University of Georgia College of Pharmacy
Athens, Georgia

Monica McCarthy Ali, Ph.D., R.Ph.
Associate Professor of Chemistry
Oxford College of Emory University
Oxford, Georgia

Jeanne Prine, Ph.D.
University of Georgia College of Pharmacy
Athens, Georgia

Flynn W. Warren, M.S., R.Ph.
Assistant Dean for Student Affairs
and Clinical Professor
University of Georgia College of Pharmacy
Athens, Georgia

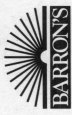

BARRON'S

Acknowledgments

The authors would like to thank their families and colleagues for their support, and to dedicate this book to them and to the authors' students past and future.

All inquiries should be addressed to:
Barron's Educational Series, Inc.
250 Wireless Boulevard
Hauppauge, NY 11788
www.barronseduc.com

International Standard Book No. 0-7641-1713-0

Library of Congress Catalog Card No. 2002018429

Library of Congress Cataloging-in-Publication Data
Chisholm, Marie A.
    Barron's PCAT: how to prepare for the Pharmacy college admission test /
Marie A. Chisholm.—2nd ed.
        p.   cm.
    Previous ed. published as: How to prepare for the PCAT, Pharmacy
college admission test. Hauppauge, NY: Barron's Educational Series, c1998.
    ISBN 0-7641-1713-0
    1. Pharmacy colleges—United States—Entrance examinations—Study
guides.   2. Pharmacy—Examinations, questions, etc.   3. Pharmacy—
Vocational guidance.   I. Title: PCAT   II. Chisholm, Marie A. How to
prepare for the PCAT, Pharmacy college admission test.   III. Title.
    RS105 .C47 2002
    615'.1'076—dc21
                                                                    2002018429

PRINTED IN THE UNITED STATES OF AMERICA

9 8 7 6 5

Contents

iii

Introduction to the Guide

PURPOSE OF THIS BOOK

The Pharmacy College Admission Test (PCAT) was developed to provide college admission committees with comparable information about the academic abilities of applicants in designated areas. For many colleges and schools of pharmacy, grades achieved in college pre-pharmacy courses and PCAT scores are the two most important objective criteria used to evaluate students for admission. Therefore, it is very important for you to perform your very best on the PCAT.

This study guide can be very useful in preparing you for the PCAT and for pharmacy education. When used properly and in combination with other materials, this guide will enhance your chances in the applicant pool of a college or school of pharmacy. All chapters are written by practicing pharmacists and/or pharmacist-educators (professors or instructors) with extensive experience in the admission procedures of U.S. pharmacy schools. In addition, each chapter author has special expertise in the designated subject to help you do your best on the PCAT.

This guide should help to focus your review by outlining and reviewing subjects that are currently included on the PCAT. In addition, this guide can be very useful in the early stages of your pre-pharmacy education by pointing out the areas that will be covered on the PCAT. Thus, you will be able to prioritize topics for studying, a step that will aid you in achieving your desired score.

Remember, your pre-pharmacy courses are designed to serve as the foundation for your pharmacy education, and the PCAT is intended to determine your grasp of this material and your ability to apply it toward your continued education. To be successful on the PCAT, it is important not only that you understand the material in a particular course, but also that you can apply it to your future program of higher education. If you take your pre-pharmacy courses with this fact in mind, the PCAT should be less of a problem.

Use this and any other study guide as just that—a guide to what and how to study. The chance that the same questions contained in this text will be on the exam you take is remote; however, the likelihood that the same material will be covered is great. When reviewing a particular question, don't just look for the sentence or phrase that "answers the question"; study that topic and refresh your understanding of the material. Pay particular attention to facts that are related but differ in a "testable" way. For example, do you remember the terms *mitosis* and *meiosis*? Probably you remember these words and perhaps know that they have something to do with cell propagation, but that isn't enough. If the multiple-choice answers to a question on the PCAT include descriptions of both mitosis and meiosis, you must be able to distinguish between the terms to select the correct answer, or risk receiving no more credit than someone who never took a biology course.

This book reviews ALL sections of the PCAT and therefore serves as a good focal point to begin studying for the exam. Please keep in mind however, that this is a guide, and its purpose is not to review all required pre-pharmacy courses, but rather to aid you in studying for the PCAT.

FORMAT AND USE OF THIS BOOK

The format of this book is very simple. Chapter 1 covers general information about the profession of pharmacy, pharmacy school admissions, and pharmacy education. In Chapters 2 and 3 general information on the PCAT and specific test-taking strategies and tactics are presented. Five chapters of review in verbal ability, biology, chemistry, quantitative ability, and reading comprehension follow. After the subject review, each chapter has a set of questions with full explanatory answers to test, review, and enhance your knowledge of the various subjects. Finally, so you can practice taking the exam and evaluate your skills, two sample PCATs with full explanatory answers are provided in Chapters 9 and 10.

Planning for a Career in Pharmacy

IMPORTANT CONSIDERATIONS IN PLANNING YOUR PHARMACY EDUCATION

On the following page is a flowchart that displays some general guidelines to help you in planning your pharmacy education, from your first college course, to completing the admission process at a U.S. college/school of pharmacy. For additional information, refer to the pre-pharmacy advisor at the institution where you are taking your pre-pharmacy required courses, and to the college/school of pharmacy you wish to attend. The information given in this chapter should not replace or supersede information obtained from your pre-pharmacy advisor or the college/school of pharmacy in which you would like to continue your education.

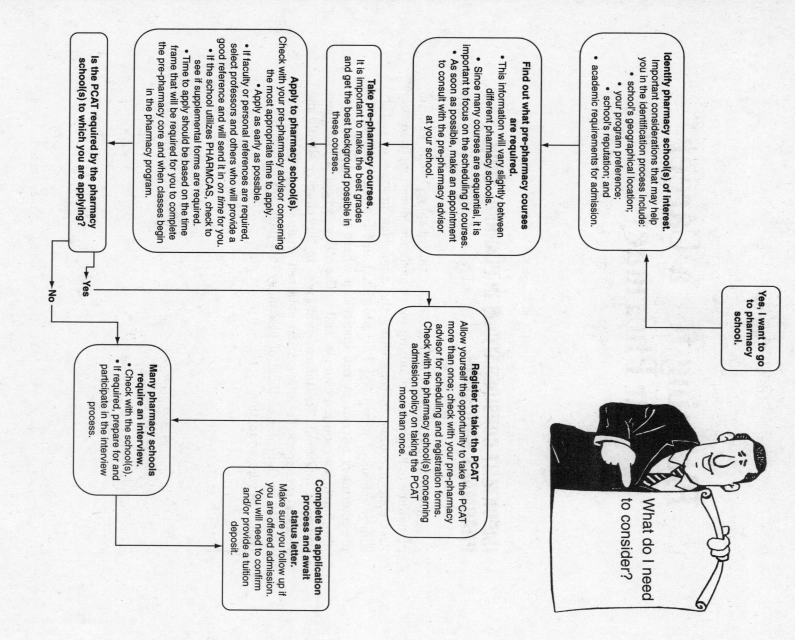

Yes, I want to go to pharmacy school.

What do I need to consider?

Identify pharmacy school(s) of interest.
Important considerations that may help you in the identification process include:
- school's geographical location;
- your program preference;
- school's reputation; and
- academic requirements for admission.

Find out what pre-pharmacy courses are required.
- This information will vary slightly between different pharmacy schools.
- Since many courses are sequential, it is important to focus on the scheduling of courses.
- As soon as possible, make an appointment to consult with the pre-pharmacy advisor at your school.

Take pre-pharmacy courses.
It is important to make the best grades and get the best background possible in these courses.

Apply to pharmacy school(s).
Check with your pre-pharmacy advisor concerning the most appropriate time to apply.
- Apply as early as possible.
- If faculty or personal references are required, select professors and others who will provide a good reference and will send it in *on time* for you.
- If the school utilizes PHARMCAS, check to see if supplemental forms are required.
- Time to apply should be based on the time frame that will be required for you to complete the pre-pharmacy core and when classes begin in the pharmacy program.

Is the PCAT required by the pharmacy school(s) to which you are applying?

No / **Yes**

Register to take the PCAT
Allow yourself the opportunity to take the PCAT more than once; check with your pre-pharmacy advisor for scheduling and registration forms. Check with the pharmacy school(s) concerning admission policy on taking the PCAT more than once.

Many pharmacy schools require an interview.
- Check with the school(s).
- If required, prepare for and participate in the interview process.

Complete the application process and await status letter.
Make sure you follow up if you are offered admission. You will need to confirm and/or provide a tuition deposit.

PRE-PHARMACY CURRICULUMS

You should be familiar with the requirements of each of the institutions you wish to apply. Although many students who apply to pharmacy school have more than the minimum pre-pharmacy course requirements, and have attended college for more than two years, the pre-pharmacy required coursework can usually be completed within two years. Pre-pharmacy curricula at each school may vary, but there are similarities that will give the student an idea of the type of courses that are required. Below is an outline detailing the subject areas covered by most pre-pharmacy curriculum.

Pre-Pharmacy Curriculum Outline

Humanities and Fine Arts Courses

English—Two courses to one year.
Literature—One course.
Speech—One course.

Social Science Courses

History—One or more courses.
Political Science—One course. This course may be covered with an additional History course.
Economics—One course.
Other Social Science elective—One course (e.g., Sociology, Psychology, Anthropology, or additional History courses).

Math and Science Courses

Pre-Calculus—One course. Some programs may only require Calculus courses, but prerequisites may be required of some post-secondary applicants.
Calculus—One or two courses.
Statistics—One course.
Biological Sciences—Two courses or one year with labs. Some programs may require Anatomy and Physiology as a pre-pharmacy course.
Chemistry—Four courses to two years. These courses include General Chemistry and Organic Chemistry with labs.
Physics—up to two courses or one year. Physics is not required by some programs.

Each program will have its own pre-pharmacy course requirements and you should obtain this information directly from the desired school. Many colleges and universities offer pre-professional advising programs to assist students in course selection. Utilize these advisors and the recruitment and admission staff of your desired pharmacy program as important resources. Since many programs only accept students once a year, if you do not complete the pre-pharmacy curriculum by the designated time, it may delay acceptance by an entire academic year. If you have previously completed coursework that you expect to receive credit for, in lieu of some specific pre-pharmacy prerequisites, verify whether the course will satisfy requirements early in your application process.

DOCTORAL OF PHARMACY DEGREE CURRICULUMS

Doctoral of Pharmacy Degree—"2+4" Program

Each school or college of pharmacy has a list of courses which are considered as prerequisites to the pharmacy professional program. The prerequisites for a pre-pharmacy curriculum will take approximately two years to complete. This pre-pharmacy curriculum, along with the four year professional curriculum compose what is called a "2+4" professional doctor of pharmacy degree program. There are at least two variations to this model (see below).

Doctoral of Pharmacy Degree—"0+6 Program"

One of the variations to the "2+4" program is the "0+6" program. This program allows students to be accepted directly into the school or college of pharmacy where they will complete the pre-pharmacy core as part of a six-year academic program. Most of these programs also consider applicants to the professional program; however, if the student is accepted, the student will enter at the beginning of the third year of the program. These students complete their pre-pharmacy requirements partially or completely at other institutions.

Doctoral of Pharmacy Degree—"Year-Round Classes"

In this variation, the institution offers "year-round" classes. The student completes the entire professional program in three calendar years. These students also must complete a pre-pharmacy curriculum of approximately two years of prerequisite coursework prior to entering the professional curriculum.

PHARMCAS—PHARMACY COLLEGE APPLICATION SERVICE

Pharmacy College Application Service (PharmCAS) is a centralized service designed to assemble, process, and distribute information for pharmacy applicants. It is being developed with the assistance of the American Association of Colleges of Pharmacy (AACP). It will allow you to apply online and submit application materials to one or more of the participating institutions. Not all schools and colleges of pharmacy will utilize this service to process applications. You should contact the school(s) or college(s) of your choice directly to determine whether PharmCAS will be involved in the application process for that program. The first year of operation for PharmCAS is scheduled to be for students planning to enter a pharmacy program in 2003.

As of July 2001, there are three possible scenarios of how an application for admission might be processed once the PharmCAS service is operational:

- The institution provides their own application materials only and does not receive or require that application materials be submitted via PharmCAS.
- The institution requires application via PharmCAS, but also requires additional application materials to be filed directly with the institution.
- The institution accepts applications and materials from PharmCAS only.

Most institutions will fall into one of these scenarios. Again, you need to contact the school or college of pharmacy in which you are interested to make sure you know to whom you must apply, what materials are required to be submitted, and by which route. Due dates for application materials vary widely, contact the institutions and APPLY EARLY.

PharmCAS has developed a website for the application service which contains information regarding application procedures, costs, lists of participating institutions, additional information and links regarding careers in pharmacy. Currently, you may "register" and go through the online application process on a trial basis at no charge, but NO APPLICATION MATERIALS WILL BE SUBMITTED via PharmCAS until the 2003 application cycle begins.

The website address is: www.pharmcas.org. PharmCAS applicants will complete the application online. The information required includes biographical data, academic course history for all post secondary institutions attended, work experience, extracurricular activities, and a personal statement.

When functional, PharmCAS is designed to allow students to submit application materials online directly to the service for processing and distribution to participating institutions. Through PharmCAS a student may be able to apply to a number of participating institutions by submitting materials only once. Students will pay a base fee to apply via PharmCAS and have their materials submitted to a single participating institution. PharmCas will charge an additional fee to have materials submitted to other participating institutions.

Please refer to the PharmCAS website (www.pharmcas.org) for up-to-date listings of participating institutions.

U.S. COLLEGES AND SCHOOLS OF PHARMACY ADMISSION REQUIREMENTS

Applications for admission to schools and colleges of pharmacy have increased significantly during the 1990s. For example, the American Association of Colleges of Pharmacy (AACP) reported an average application-to-enrollment ratio of approximately 3:1 for U.S. schools of pharmacy in 1990, and an average applicant-to-enrollment ratio of 6:1 in 1994. The increased number of applicants can be interpreted in many ways in terms of pharmacy practice and education, but what it means to the student applicant is certain—increased competition for acceptance into a pharmacy school.

All schools of pharmacy utilize the college pre-pharmacy grade-point average (GPA) in evaluating candidates for admission. In addition to the GPA, approximately 50 percent of pharmacy schools utilize the PCAT in selecting students. Therefore, the two main selection criteria for admission are the PCAT scores and the pre-pharmacy GPA. Some schools also conduct interviews to evaluate students for acceptance; however, whether a candidate is selected for an interview is often dependent on his or her GPA and PCAT performance.

Since acceptance into pharmacy school is very competitive and the two most commonly used criteria for selection are the GPA and the PCAT scores, it is extremely important for you to perform your best in both areas: required pre-pharmacy courses and the PCAT.

PHARMACY PROFESSIONAL DEGREES: BACCALAUREATE IN PHARMACY AND DOCTOR OF PHARMACY DEGREES

There are 83 colleges and schools of pharmacy in the United States as of July 2001. A couple of these institutions offer both professional degrees, the Bachelor of Science (B.S.) and the Doctor of Pharmacy (Pharm.D.); however, most schools offer only one professional degree (see the following section, entitled "Professional Degrees Offered by U.S. Colleges and Schools of Pharmacy"). The minimum length of time to obtain the B.S. degree is fairly consistent from institution to institution and generally is five years, including an average of two years for completing the pre-pharmacy requirements and three years in the professional program.

Schools of pharmacy may offer the Pharm.D. degree in a "tracking" program, an entry-level program, and/or a post-B.S. program. In a pharmacy school that offers a "tracking" program, a B.S. student may decide to "track" into the Pharm.D. program, generally after the student has successfully completed two years of pharmacy school. The entry-level Pharm.D. program is generally a four-year program undertaken after completing the pre-pharmacy requirements. In the post-B.S. program, the student has already graduated from pharmacy school with a B.S. in pharmacy (hence, the name "post-B.S."). The post-B.S. program and the tracking program may fluctuate in duration depending on the specific institution.

The Pharm.D. curriculum is generally more clinically orientated than the B.S. curriculum and includes additional didactic courses. The Pharm.D. curriculum also provides students with several additional experiential rotations (approximately 1500 clerkship hours) in many different pharmacy environments, compared to the B.S. program, which provides approximately 600 hours of experiential training. It is evident by the following pages that most colleges/schools offer the Pharm.D. as the only professional degree.

PROFESSIONAL DEGREES OFFERED BY U.S. COLLEGES AND SCHOOLS OF PHARMACY

The following information represents the 83 U.S. colleges and schools of pharmacy as reported by each school in July 2001. To obtain the most current information, contact the specific college or school of pharmacy in which you are interested.

Colleges and Schools That Offer Both Professional Degrees, B.S. and Pharm.D.

Massachusetts College of Pharmacy—Boston

Texas Southern University

Colleges and Schools that Offer the Pharm.D. as the Only Professional Degree

Auburn University
Butler University
Ferris State University
Florida A & M University
Campbell University
Creighton University
Drake University
Duquesne University
Hampton University
Howard University
Idaho State University
Long Island University
Massachusetts College of
 Pharmacy—Worcester
Medical University of South Carolina
Mercer University
Midwestern University—Chicago
Midwestern University—Glendale
North Dakota State University
Northeastern University
Nova Southeastern University
Ohio Northern University
Ohio State University
Oregon State University
Palm Beach Atlantic College
Philadelphia College of
 Pharmacy and Science
Purdue University
Rutgers University
Samford University
State University of NY—Buffalo
St. John's University
St. Louis College of Pharmacy
Shenandoah University
South Dakota State University
Southwestern Oklahoma State
Temple University
Texas Tech University
Union University
University of Arizona

University of Arkansas
University of California
University of Cincinnati
University of Colorado
University of Connecticut
University of Georgia
University of Florida
University of Houston
University of Illinois
University of Iowa
University of Kansas
University of Kentucky
University of Louisiana
University of Maryland
University of Michigan
University of Minnesota
University of Mississippi
University of Missouri
University of Montana
University of Nebraska
University of New Mexico
University of North Carolina
University of Oklahoma
University of the Pacific
University of Pittsburgh
University of Puerto Rico
University of Rhode Island
University of South Carolina
University of Southern
 California
University of Tennessee
University of Texas
University of Toledo
University of Utah
University of Washington
University of Wisconsin
University of Wyoming
Virginia Commonwealth
 University
Washington State University

Wayne State University
Western Univ. of Health
West Virginia University
Wilkes University
Xavier University

DIRECTORY OF U.S. COLLEGES AND SCHOOLS OF PHARMACY

Alabama

School of Pharmacy
Auburn University
217 Pharmacy Building
Auburn University, AL 36849-5501
(334) 844-8348
http://pharmacy.auburn.edu/
Professional Degree Offered:
Doctor of Pharmacy

McWhorter School of Pharmacy
Samford University
800 Lakeshore Drive
Birmingham, AL 35229-7027
(205) 726-2820
www.samford.edu/schools/pharmacy.html
Professional Degree Offered:
Doctor of Pharmacy

Arizona

College of Pharmacy—Glendale
Midwestern University
19555 North 59th Avenue
Glendale, AZ 85308
(623) 572-3500
www.midwestern.edu/Pages/CPG.html
Professional Degree Offered:
Doctor of Pharmacy

College of Pharmacy
University of Arizona
1703 East Mabel, P.O. Box 210207
Tucson, AZ 85721-0207
(520) 626-1427
www.pharmacy.arizona.edu
Professional Degree Offered:
  Doctor of Pharmacy

Arkansas

College of Pharmacy
University of Arkansas for Medical Sciences
4301 West Markham Street, Slot 522
Little Rock, AR 72205-7122
(501) 686-5557
www.uams.edu/cop
Professional Degree Offered:
  Doctor of Pharmacy

California

School of Pharmacy
University of California
UCSF Box 0446
San Francisco, CA 94143-0446
(415) 476-1225
www.sop.ucsf.edu
Professional Degree Offered:
  Doctor of Pharmacy

School of Pharmacy & Health Sciences
University of the Pacific
3601 Pacific Avenue
Stockton, CA 95211
(209) 946-2561
www1.uop.edu/pharmacy/index.html
Professional Degree Offered:
  Doctor of Pharmacy

School of Pharmacy
University of Southern California
1985 Zonal Avenue
Los Angeles, CA 90089-9121
(323) 442-1369
http://pharmacy.usc.edu
Professional Degree Offered:
   Doctor of Pharmacy

College of Pharmacy
Western University of Health Sciences
College Plaza, 309 East Second Street
Pomona, CA 91766-1854
909-623-6116
www.westernu.edu/cp.html
Professional Degree Offered:
   Doctor of Pharmacy

Colorado

School of Pharmacy
University of Colorado Health Sciences Center
4200 East Ninth Avenue, C238
Denver, CO 80262-0238
(303) 315-6100
www.uchsc.edu/sp/sp/
Professional Degree Offered:
   Doctor of Pharmacy

Connecticut

School of Pharmacy
University of Connecticut
372 Fairfield Road; Unit 2092
Storrs, CT 06269-2092
(860) 486-4066
http://pharmacy.uconn.edu
Professional Degree Offered:
   Doctor of Pharmacy

District of Columbia

School of Pharmacy
Howard University
2300 4th Street, N.W.
Washington, DC 20059
(202) 806-6530
www.cpnahs.howard.edu/Pharmacy/index.htm
Professional Degree Offered:
  Doctor of Pharmacy

Florida

College of Pharmacy and Pharmaceutical Sciences
Florida Agricultural and Mechanical University
Room 201 Dyson Pharmacy Building
Tallahassee, FL 32307-3800
(850) 599-3593
http://168.223.36.3/acad/colleges/copps/
Professional Degree Offered:
  Doctor of Pharmacy

College of Pharmacy
Nova Southeastern University
Health Professions Division
3200 S. University Dr.
Ft. Lauderdale, FL 33328
(954) 262-1300
http://pharmacy.nova.edu
Professional Degree Offered:
  Doctor of Pharmacy

College of Pharmacy
Palm Beach Atlantic College
P.O. Box 24708
West Palm Beach, FL 33416
(561) 803-2000
www.pbac.edu/academic/pharmacy/grant.htm
Professional Degree Offered:
  Doctor of Pharmacy

College of Pharmacy
University of Florida
P.O. Box 100484, JHMHC
1600 SW Archer Rd. M-454
Gainesville, FL 32610-0484
(904) 392-9713 ext.3
www.cop.ufl.edu
Professional Degree Offered:
Doctor of Pharmacy

Georgia

Southern School of Pharmacy
Mercer University
3001 Mercer University Drive
Atlanta, GA 30341-4415
(678) 547-6232
www.mercer.edu/pharmacy/
Professional Degree Offered:
Doctor of Pharmacy

College of Pharmacy
University of Georgia
D.W. Brooks Drive
Athens, GA 30602-2351
(706) 542-1911
www.rx.uga.edu
Professional Degrees Offered:
Doctor of Pharmacy

Idaho

College of Pharmacy
Idaho State University
Campus Box 8288
Pocatello, ID 83209-8288
(208) 282-2175
http://rx.isu.edu
Professional Degree Offered:
Doctor of Pharmacy

Illinois

College of Pharmacy
Midwestern University—Chicago
555 31st Street
Downers Grove, IL 60515-1235
(630) 971-6417
www.midwestern.edu/pages/ccp.html
Professional Degree Offered:
    Doctor of Pharmacy

College of Pharmacy
University of Illinois—Chicago
833 South Wood Street; M/C 874
Chicago, IL 60612-7230
(312) 996-7242
www.uic.edu/pharmacy
Professional Degree Offered:
    Doctor of Pharmacy

Indiana

College of Pharmacy and Health Sciences
Butler University
4600 Sunset Avenue
Indianapolis, IN 46208-3485
(317) 940-9969
http://butler.edu/cophs
Professional Degree Offered:
    Doctor of Pharmacy

School of Pharmacy and Pharmacal Science
Purdue University
1330 Heine Pharmacy Building
West Lafayette, IN 47907-1330
(765) 494-1357
www.pharmacy.purdue.edu
Professional Degrees Offered:
    Doctor of Pharmacy

Iowa

College of Pharmacy and Health Sciences
Drake University
2507 University Avenue
Des Moines, IA 50311-4505
(515) 271-3018
http://pharmacy.drake.edu
Professional Degree Offered:
Doctor of Pharmacy

College of Pharmacy
University of Iowa
115 South Grand Avenue
Iowa City, IA 52242
(319) 335-8794
www.uiowa.edu/~pharmacy/
Professional Degree Offered:
Doctor of Pharmacy

Kansas

School of Pharmacy
University of Kansas
Malott Hall
1251 Wescoe Hall Drive, Rm. 2056
Lawrence, KS 66045-2500
(785) 864-3591
www.pharm.ukans.edu/dean/index.htm
Professional Degree Offered:
Doctor of Pharmacy

Kentucky

College of Pharmacy
University of Kentucky
Rose Street—Pharmacy Building
Lexington, KY 40536-0082
(859) 323-5761
www.uky.edu/pharmacy/
Professional Degree Offered:
Doctor of Pharmacy

Louisiana

University of Louisiana at Monroe
College of Pharmacy
700 University Avenue
Monroe, LA 71209-0400
(318) 342-1600
http://rxweb.ulm.edu/pharmacy
Professional Degrees Offered:
 Doctor of Pharmacy

College of Pharmacy
Xavier University of Louisiana
1 Drexal Drive
New Orleans, LA 70125-1098
(504) 483-7424
www.xula.edu/Pharmacy.html
Professional Degree Offered:
 Doctor of Pharmacy

Maryland

School of Pharmacy
University of Maryland
20 North Pine Street
Baltimore, MD 21201-1180
(410) 706-7650
www.pharmacy.umaryland.edu/
Professional Degree Offered:
 Doctor of Pharmacy

Massachusetts

Massachusetts College of Pharmacy and Health Sciences—Boston
179 Longwood Avenue
Boston, MA 02115-5896
(617) 732-2825
www.mcp.edu
Professional Degrees Offered:
 Doctor of Pharmacy/Baccalaureate in Pharmacy

Massachusetts College of Pharmacy and Health
  Sciences—Worcester
19 Foster Street
Worcester, MA 01608
(508) 890-8855
www.mcp.edu
Professional Degrees Offered:
Doctor of Pharmacy

Bouve College of Pharmacy and Health Sciences
Northeastern University
206 Muger Hall
Boston, MA 02115-5000
(617) 373-8917
www.bouve.neu.edu/pharma.html
Professional Degree Offered:
Doctor of Pharmacy

Michigan

College of Pharmacy
Ferris State University
220 Ferris Drive
Big Rapids, MI 49307-2740
(231) 591-3780
www.pharmacy.ferris.edu
Professional Degree Offered:
Doctor of Pharmacy

College of Pharmacy
University of Michigan
428 Church Street
Ann Arbor, MI 48109-1065
(734) 764-7312
www.umich.edu/~pharmacy/
Professional Degree Offered:
Doctor of Pharmacy

Wayne State University
College of Pharmacy and Allied Health Professions
139 Shapero Hall
Detroit, MI 48202-3489
(313) 577-1716
http://wizard.pharm.wayne.edu/
Professional Degrees Offered:
    Doctor of Pharmacy

Minnesota

College of Pharmacy
University of Minnesota
308 Harvard Street SE
5-110 Weaver-Densford Hall
Minneapolis, MN 55455-0343
(612) 624-9490
www.pharmacy.umn.edu
Professional Degree Offered:
    Doctor of Pharmacy

Mississippi

School of Pharmacy
University of Mississippi
P.O. Box 1848
University, MS 38677
(662) 915-7265
www.olemiss.edu/depts/pharm_school/
Professional Degree Offered:
    Doctor of Pharmacy

Missouri

St. Louis College of Pharmacy
4588 Parkview Place
St. Louis, MO 63110-1088
(314) 367-8700
www.stlcop.edu
Professional Degree Offered:
    Doctor of Pharmacy

School of Pharmacy
University of Missouri—Kansas City
5005 Rockhill Road
Kansas City, MO 64110-2499
(816) 235-1608
www.umkc.edu/pharm
Professional Degree Offered:
Doctor of Pharmacy

Montana

School of Pharmacy and Allied Health Sciences
University of Montana
340 Skaggs Building
Missoula, MT 59812-1512
(406) 243-4621
www.umt.edu/pharmacy
Professional Degrees Offered:
Doctor of Pharmacy

Nebraska

School of Pharmacy and Allied Health Professions
Creighton University
2500 California Plaza
Omaha, NE 68178-0401
(402) 280-2662
www.spahp.creighton.edu/
Professional Degree Offered:
Doctor of Pharmacy

College of Pharmacy
University of Nebraska
986000 Nebraska Medical Center
Omaha, NE 68198-6000
(402) 559-4333
www.unmc.edu/Pharmacy
Professional Degree Offered:
Doctor of Pharmacy

New Jersey

College of Pharmacy
Rutgers University
State University of New Jersey
160 Frelinghuysen Road
Piscataway, NJ 08854-8020
(908) 445-2675
http://pharmacy.rutgers.edu/
Professional Degree Offered:
Doctor of Pharmacy

New Mexico

College of Pharmacy
University of New Mexico
2502 Marble NE
Albuquerque, NM 87131-5691
(505) 272-3241
http://hsc.unm.edu/pharmacy/
Professional Degree Offered:
Doctor of Pharmacy

New York

Arnold and Marie Schwartz College of Pharmacy and
    Health Sciences
Long Island University
75 DeKalb Avenue at University Plaza
Brooklyn, NY 11201-5497
(718) 488-1004
www.liu.edu/cwis/pharmacy/pharmacy.html
Professional Degree Offered:
Doctor of Pharmacy

School of Pharmacy
University at Buffalo—State University of New York
126 Cooke Hall
Buffalo, NY 14260-1200
(716) 645-2823
www.pharmacy.buffalo.edu
Professional Degree Offered:
Doctor of Pharmacy

St. John's University
College of Pharmacy and Allied Health Professions
8000 Utopia Parkway
Jamaica, NY 11439
(718) 990-6275
www.stjohns.edu/academics/pahp
Professional Degree Offered:
Doctor of Pharmacy

Albany College of Pharmacy
Union University
106 New Scotland Avenue
Albany, NY 12208-3492
(518) 445-7202
www.acp.edu/welcome.html
Professional Degree Offered:
Doctor of Pharmacy

North Carolina

School of Pharmacy
Campbell University
P.O. Box 1090
Buies Creek, NC 27506
(910) 893-1200
www.campbell.edu/pharmacy/
Professional Degree Offered:
Doctor of Pharmacy

School of Pharmacy
University of North Carolina at Chapel Hill
Beard Hall, CB #7360
Chapel Hill, NC 27599-7360
(919) 966-1121
www.pharmacy.unc.edu
Professional Degree Offered:
Doctor of Pharmacy

North Dakota

North Dakota State University
College of Pharmacy
123 Sudro Hall
Fargo, ND 58105-5055
(701) 231-7456
www.ndsu.nodak.edu/pharmacy/
Professional Degree Offered:
  Doctor of Pharmacy

Ohio

College of Pharmacy
Ohio Northern University
525 South Main
Ada, OH 45810
(419) 772-2278
www.onu.edu/pharmacy
Professional Degree Offered:
  Doctor of Pharmacy

College of Pharmacy
Ohio State University
500 West 12th Avenue
Columbus, OH 43210-1291
(614) 292-2266
www.pharmacy.ohio-state.edu
Professional Degree Offered:
  Doctor of Pharmacy

College of Pharmacy
University of Cincinnati
P.O. Box 670004
Cincinnati, OH 45267-0004
(513) 558-3784
www.pharmacy.uc.edu
Professional Degree Offered:
  Doctor of Pharmacy

College of Pharmacy
University of Toledo
2801 West Bancroft Street
Toledo, OH 43606-3390
(419) 530-1904
www.utpharmacy.org
Professional Degree Offered:
Doctor of Pharmacy

Oklahoma

School of Pharmacy
Southwestern Oklahoma State University
100 Campus Drive
Weatherford, OK 73096-3098
(580) 774-3105
www.swosu.edu/depts/pharmacy/index.htm
Professional Degree Offered:
Doctor of Pharmacy

College of Pharmacy
University of Oklahoma
P.O. Box 26901
1110 N.Stonewall
Oklahoma City, OK 73190
(405) 271-6484
www.oupharmacy.com
Professional Degree Offered:
Doctor of Pharmacy

Oregon

College of Pharmacy
Oregon State University
Pharmacy Building 203
Corvallis, OR 97331-3507
(541) 737-3424
http://pharmacy.orst.edu
Professional Degree Offered:
Doctor of Pharmacy

Pennsylvania

Mylan School of Pharmacy
Duquesne University
600 Forbes Ave
Pittsburgh, PA 15282
(412) 396-6380
www.pharmacy.duq.edu/
Professional Degree Offered:
    Doctor of Pharmacy

Philadelphia College of Pharmacy and Science
University of the Sciences in Philadelphia
600 South 43rd Street
Philadelphia, PA 19104-4495
(215) 596-8800
www.usip.edu/academics/pharmacy.html
Professional Degree Offered:
    Doctor of Pharmacy

School of Pharmacy
Temple University
3307 North Broad Street
Philadelphia, PA 19140
(215) 707-4990
www.temple.edu/pharmacy
Professional Degree Offered:
    Doctor of Pharmacy

School of Pharmacy
University of Pittsburgh
1104 Salk Hall
Pittsburgh, PA 15261-1911
(412) 648-8579
www.pharmacy.pitt.edu
Professional Degrees Offered:
    Doctor of Pharmacy

Nesbitt School of Pharmacy
Wilkes University
P.O. Box 111
Wilkes-Barre, PA 18766
(570) 408-4280
http://pharmacy.wilkes.edu
Professional Degree Offered:
    Doctor of Pharmacy

Puerto Rico

School of Pharmacy
University of Puerto Rico
P.O. Box 365067
San Juan, PR 00936-5067
(787) 758-2525 ext. 5407
www.rcm.upr.edu/academics.html
Professional Degree Offered:
Doctor of Pharmacy

Rhode Island

College of Pharmacy
University of Rhode Island
Fogarty Hall, 41 Lower College Road
Kingston, RI 02881-0809
(401) 874-5842
www.uri.edu/pharmacy/
Professional Degree Offered:
Doctor of Pharmacy

South Carolina

College of Pharmacy
Medical University of South Carolina
P.O. Box 250141; 280 Calhoun St.
Charleston, SC 29425-2301
(843) 792-3115
www.musc.edu/pharmacy/
Professional Degree Offered:
Doctor of Pharmacy

College of Pharmacy
University of South Carolina
700 Sumter Street
Columbia, SC 29208
(803) 777-4151
www.pharm.sc.edu
Professional Degree Offered:
Doctor of Pharmacy

South Dakota

College of Pharmacy
South Dakota State University
Box 2202C
Brookings, SD 57007-0099
(605) 688-6197
www.sdstate.edu/Academics/CollegeOfPharmacy/
Professional Degree Offered:
  Doctor of Pharmacy

Tennessee

College of Pharmacy
University of Tennessee
847 Monroe Avenue, 226 Johnson Building
Memphis, TN 38163
(901) 448-6036
http://pharmacy.utmem.edu/
Professional Degree Offered:
  Doctor of Pharmacy

Texas

College of Pharmacy and Health Sciences
Texas Southern University
3100 Cleburne Street
Houston, TX 77004
(713) 313-7574
www.tsu.edu/pharmacy/default.htm
Professional Degrees Offered:
  Doctor of Pharmacy/Baccalaureate in Pharmacy

School of Pharmacy
Texas Tech University
University Health Sciences Center
1300 South Coulter Street
Amarillo, TX 79106
(806) 354-5463
http://ismo.ama.ttuhsc.edu/
Professional Degree Offered:
  Doctor of Pharmacy

College of Pharmacy
University of Houston
4800 Calhoun Boulevard
Houston, TX 77204-5511
(713) 743-1300
www.uh.edu/pharmacy/index2.html
Professional Degree Offered:
Doctor of Pharmacy

College of Pharmacy
University of Texas—Austin
2409 University Avenue
Austin, TX 78712-1074
(512) 471-1737
www.utexas.edu/pharmacy
Professional Degree Offered:
Doctor of Pharmacy

Utah

College of Pharmacy
University of Utah
30 South 2000 East, Room 201
Salt Lake City, UT 84112-5820
(801) 581-6731
www.pharmacy.utah.edu/
Professional Degrees Offered:
Doctor of Pharmacy

Virginia

School of Pharmacy
Hampton University
Kittrell Hall
Hampton, VA 23668
(757) 727-5071
http://www.hamptonu.edu/pharm/index.htm
Professional Degree Offered:
Doctor of Pharmacy

Bernard J. Dunn School of Pharmacy
Shenandoah University
1460 University Drive
Winchester, VA 22601
(540) 678-4340
http://pharmacy.su.edu
Professional Degree Offered:
    Doctor of Pharmacy

School of Pharmacy
Virginia Commonwealth University
410 North 12th Street
MCV Campus-Box 980581
Richmond, VA 23219
(804) 828-3000
www.pharmacy.vcu.edu/
Professional Degree Offered:
    Doctor of Pharmacy

Washington

School of Pharmacy
University of Washington
Box 357631
Seattle, WA 98195-7631
(206) 685-2715
www.depts.washington.edu/pharminf/index.htm
Professional Degree Offered:
    Doctor of Pharmacy

College of Pharmacy
Washington State University
P.O Box 646510
Pullman, WA 99164-6510
(509) 335-8664
www.pharmacy.wsu.edu/
Professional Degree Offered:
    Doctor of Pharmacy

West Virginia

School of Pharmacy
West Virginia University Health Sciences Center
PO Box 9500; 1136 HSCN
Morgantown, WV 26506-9500
(304) 293-5101
www.hsc.wvu.edu./sop/
Professional Degree Offered:
Doctor of Pharmacy

Wisconsin

School of Pharmacy
University of Wisconsin—Madison
777 Highland Avenue
Madison, WI 53705
(608) 262-1414
www.pharmacy.wisc.edu/
Professional Degree Offered:
Doctor of Pharmacy

Wyoming

School of Pharmacy
University of Wyoming
P.O. Box 3375
Laramie, WY 82071-3375
(307) 766-6120
www.uwyo.edu/pharmacy/pharmacy.htm
Professional Degree Offered:
Doctor of Pharmacy

PHARMACY GRADUATE DEGREES OFFERED BY U.S. COLLEGES AND SCHOOLS OF PHARMACY

Master of Science (M.S.) and Doctor of Philosophy (Ph.D.) degrees are available for pharmacy disciplines including, but not limited to, medicinal chemistry, pharmaceutics, pharmacology, pharmacy care administration, and toxicology. For more information regarding graduate programs, you should contact the specific college or school of pharmacy in which you are interested.

POSTGRADUATE TRAINING: RESIDENCIES AND FELLOWSHIPS

A graduate of a college or school of pharmacy may decide to pursue postgraduate training in a specific area of pharmacy practice or pharmacy research. (See the following section, entitled "Residency and Fellowship programs: Areas of Pharmacy Practice and Research.") Residencies and fellowships are two distinct types of postgraduate training programs. General requirements for an applicant seeking a residency or fellowship include graduation from an accredited college or school of pharmacy and an interest in and aptitude for advanced training in pharmacy. A resident or fellow receives a stipend plus benefits (insurance, vacation, etc.). The amount of the stipend and the specific benefits vary according to the individual program.

Residencies

A residency is an organized, directed, postgraduate training program in a defined area of pharmacy practice. Residencies are typically one year in duration; however, some may be longer. The primary goal of a residency is to train pharmacists in a specific area of pharmacy practice. The objective of a residency is to develop competent practitioners who are able to provide such pharmacy services as the following: clinical, drug information, pharmacotherapeutic dosing and monitoring, and administration.

A pharmacy practice residency is a general residency in pharmacy practice and is most often affiliated with a hospital. In addition to pharmacy practice residencies, a host of specialized residencies exists. A specialized residency focuses on a particular niche of pharmacy practice; pediatric pharmacy, psychiatric pharmacy, and nuclear pharmacy are all examples of specialized residencies. Whether the residency is a pharmacy practice residency or a specialty residency, training typically involves structured rotations within the pharmacy department as well as medical rotations with physicians and other health care professionals. The practice experiences of residents are closely directed and evaluated by qualified practitioner-preceptors who are trained in particular areas of pharmacy practice.

The American Society of Health-System Pharmacists is the accrediting body for residencies. To obtain a list of postgraduate pharmacy practice residency programs, write to the society at the address below:

American Society of Health-System Pharmacists
4630 Montgomery Avenue
Bethesda, MD 20814

Fellowships

A fellowship is a directed, highly individualized, postgraduate program, typically two years in duration, that is designed to prepare the participant to become an independent researcher. The primary goal of a fellowship is to develop competency in scientific pharmacy research. A fellow works under the close direction and instruction of a qualified researcher-preceptor. Many fellowships are affiliated with a college or school of pharmacy. To obtain a list of postgraduate fellowship programs, you can write to the American College of Clinical Pharmacy at the address below:

American College of Clinical Pharmacy
3101 Broadway, Suite 380
Kansas City, MO 64111

Residency and Fellowship Programs: Areas of Pharmacy Practice and Research

Administration	Immunology
Ambulatory Care	Infectious Disease
Biotechnology	Internal Medicine
Cardiology	Managed Care
Clinical Pharmacology	Neonatology
Critical Care	Nephrology
Drug Development	Neurology
Drug Information	Nuclear Pharmacy
Emergency Medicine	Nutrition
Family Medicine	Oncology
Geriatrics	Outcomes Research
Home Health Care	Pain Management
Hospital Pharmacy	Pediatrics

Pharmaceutical Care
Pharmacoeconomics
Pharmacoepidemiology
Pharmacokinetics
Pharmacy Practice

Psychopharmacy
Pulmonary
Rheumatology
Toxicology
Transplantation

ADMISSION COMMITTEES

The individuals who wrote the "Admission Committees" and the "Interview Process" sections of this book have served on pharmacy school admissions committees for several years. Based on their experiences, they have summarized their observations of students who were successful in being accepted into a college/school of pharmacy. The following describes the purpose of the admission committee and provides tips to successfully guide you through the admission process.

The purpose of the admission committee for a pharmacy school is to select the most qualified students to enter the program. The phrase "most qualified student" will have a slightly different interpretation by each committee and may vary slightly within an institution from year to year. As soon as possible, contact the institutions in which you are interested and request materials regarding application requirements. It is also important to review materials most schools make available on the internet. By reviewing these materials you should be able to determine not only the requirements for the institution, but, which factors are utilized to select students for admission.

The committees will use various sources of information and mechanisms to compare students to make selection decisions. You should make sure that the information requested is provided for the committee. You may provide additional information that you think is important for the committee to understand your interest in pharmacy and their program in particular. If you have a special interest, ability, or experience that you think would be helpful in your application, include a letter or other supporting documentation in the materials you submit to the institution(s) for the committee to consider.

As important as it is for you to do well academically and to take the required courses, the practice of pharmacy requires various skills and talents which you may develop and enhance prior to attending a pharmacy school. Some of these areas include:

- Work Experience
- Communication Skills
- Community Involvement
- Entrepreneurial Ability

Some institutions will request information regarding the activities listed above as part of the applications, others may rely on recommendations to provide this information. More and more institutions are utilizing a personal interview as part of the application process to give the student a chance to present information regarding their personal and academic background. You should determine how to best develop and exhibit your skills in these areas, and also, how to communicate this information to the pharmacy college(s)/school(s).

Work experience provides the student with a background about the workplace in general. It also gives students a chance to develop good work habits and communication skills. Work experience in the profession of pharmacy will be an excellent way for you to understand what pharmacy is about and whether your interests and skills are compatible. Also, you will be able to find out more information about the variety of career opportunities that exist in the practice of pharmacy. Work experience in pharmacy is great, but other jobs can also be supportive and provide information about a student's interests and abilities. Work in a doctor's office, a health clinic, or hospital setting should provide the student with a knowledge of health care issues, contact with patients, and a chance to see various health care professionals in action. Additionally, seemingly unrelated jobs in retail or food services still provide a medium for the student to develop good work skills, communication skills, and the ability to work with people. No matter what work experience you have, try to see what aspects of that job might apply to your activities as a pharmacist or pharmacy student. Make sure to communicate this effectively to the admissions committee.

Communication skills are important in all aspects of a pharmacy. Students and pharmacists must be able to communicate effectively with a wide range of people. Also, they must be able to communicate about potentially complex subject matter in a manner that is effective for their audience, whether it be a patient, another student, a professor or other health care professional. Additionally, the ability to listen effectively is just as important as the ability to communicate.

Community involvement is a way for the admissions committee to determine more about the character of an applicant. The practice of pharmacy requires that a person be empathetic to the needs of the patient or other professional contact. This means that a pharmacist can be most effective when they can "put themselves in the other's shoes." By showing a history of participation in organizations that show compassion by assisting others, you may be more likely to have the desired character to practice effectively and ethically. It is suggested that you show a history of participation in these types of activities, not just a recent participation in one or two events just to have something to place on an application or state in an interview. Make sure that you can talk about the type of activities or events you have been involved in, not just list organizations or events.

Entrepreneurship is the interest in new opportunities, not only business ventures, but also professional development and new ways of doing things. Pharmacy, like most professions, will go through various changes throughout one's career and the ability and interest to pursue new avenues of practice assures that one will continue to be competent and competitive in practice. A committee might assess an applicant's entrepreneurial abilities through questions in the interview such as "tell me about a project you instituted or carried out with others." By asking such a question, the committee might be looking for creativity, leadership skills, and motivation.

It is important to realize the composition of the admissions committee. Committees may consist of any combination of faculty members, pharmacists, non-pharmacists, alumni members, and administrative members. Be sure to think in terms of what that type of individual would want to know about you that will help them realize you will be a good pharmacy student and practitioner.

Not all students will have experience or strong backgrounds in each of the areas mentioned; however, you want to have a good mixture of skills and talents. Don't go out and try to "check-off all the blocks" just to satisfy the committee. It is important that you represent yourself completely and honestly to the committee so that your interest can best be served and the committee can assess not only what you bring to the program, but how their program will benefit your development as a pharmacist.

THE INTERVIEW PROCESS

Some schools require an interview as part of the admission process. The structure and goals of this process will vary between programs. This general information regarding interviews is meant to help you have a better idea of what to expect and therefore be more effective in communicating your abilities and desires to the interviewers. Even if a program does not require an interview, you may have the opportunity in your contact with an institution to utilize these points to enhance your application. Either way, one of the most positive benefits of preparing yourself for an interview is that it gives you a structured assessment of your strengths, weaknesses, and professional goals. By quantifying these at this critical time in your career, you will be sure of your goals and motivation for your chosen career path.

There are many texts providing copious information on how interviews are structured and how to prepare yourself for this event. Most of these address the pursuit of a job in your chosen field. This fact makes their recommendations a bit more structured than might be appropriate for an academic interview for a position in a professional program. Overall, the committee or interviewer is not looking for one right person for the job. They look for a wide range of backgrounds and interests that will not only assure the students success in a rigorous academic program, but will also provide support for a variety of practice settings. Not everyone will work in a direct patient care environment for his or her whole career. As important as patient empathy is to a health care professional, some are going to be better than others and some will work in an area where this skill is not the most important one required on a case-by-case basis. There is room for diversity in pharmacy programs in every sense of the word. Just as interviewees will vary, so will the interviewers. Some will be more skilled than others and some may look at the applicant in terms of their own career choices. It is important for you to try and listen to the interviewer and determine what is meant by the question being asked and how you should best relate your own feelings while being sensitive to the setting and the audience. One thing that comes through in the interview texts reviewed is that honesty is the best policy. If you feel that you have to compromise your interests to say what the interviewer wants to hear, you should review your choice of this institution or career pursuit.

Overall, the greatest benefit to be gained by the interview is for the committee to see the sincerity of the interest you have in the program and a career in pharmacy. Also, it is important that you receive positive reinforcement of your goals and helpful information from the institution administering the interview. Try to get as much information as possible about the program and have some good questions ready (for example, a question or two about points that were brought up by the committee members). This shows the committee that you are "thinking on your feet."

Based on our experience, here are three of the most common topics discussed during a pharmacy program interview:

Professional Background
Academic Background
Personal Background

Professional Background

Basically, you have been preparing all of your life for the interview. However, you should spend some significant time before the interview making an "inventory" of your answer to the question "why pharmacy?". Here are some questions of self-assessment to help you prepare for this type of discussion.

When did you first consider pharmacy as a career?
What other careers did you consider?
Who influenced your choice of career, and how (actively or through example)?
Who would you consider to be your mentor? Why?
What type of jobs have you held? What have been your likes and dislikes about those jobs?
What other career or academic pursuits interest you?
What type of career in pharmacy interests you most?

Any student can come up with answers to these types of questions. Ideally, there is no right or wrong answer. What the committee should be looking for is the background information that you relate to support your answers. Avoid yes or no answers to questions posed to you. Additionally, avoid one-liner answers. Understand that any answers to the questions, such as the ones above, should include an implicit explanation of why or how did you arrive at that decision. This is the best way to relate to the committee the maturity of your decision-making process and career interest. It also helps minimize the problem with a difficult interviewer who may be looking for your answer to match their choices. If you have a good explanation of how you arrived at that decision, it validates your answer.

Be aware of the professional questions being posed to you as an applicant. The interviewers have been in their profession a long time and often can only relate to subject matter that they have come to accept as common knowledge. An example of a question being asked about a professional setting scenario is—"What would you do if a patient comes in and needs a refill for so and so and you have no refills indicated on the prescription?" The possible answers are myriad, and often the question is asked of a student who has retail pharmacy experience and has observed a pharmacist handle this situation many times. If you do not have any experience or any idea of how to answer this question, consider explaining your lack of experience in that area and that this is the type of thing you know training in the professional program will provide. Then, try to relate the question to something you are more familiar with. For example, you might respond, "It sounds like this is a question that deals with utilizing appropriate people skills and ethical behavior on the part of the pharmacist; let me tell you about a situation that I dealt with in a job where we had an employee who was involved in stealing. . . ." This allows you to put the question on your own terms and to talk about something about which you are familiar. Follow-up your description with a question as to whether that scenario related sufficiently to the professional question posed by the interviewer(s).

Ideally, you will have some professional pharmacy or related experiences to utilize in the interview. This not only shows your competency in areas that you have been trained, but also, that you are making your decision regarding a career choice based on personal experience. Pharmacy jobs for pre-pharmacy students can be difficult to obtain, particularly if you are in an area with a high concentration of pharmacy students. Often, students first think of retail because this practice option is so visible, but don't neglect opportunities in hospitals, clinics, long-term care facilities and many other areas where pharmacists or other healthcare professionals have the opportunity to work with interested students. Hopefully you started working in a related area as early as high school. In doing this, you may have had the opportunity to advance to a position which provides direct contact with the operation of a pharmacy.

Academic Background

The nature of academic performance reported to the institution you are applying is very quantitative. All require that transcripts be provided and often calculate a single grade point average (GPA) for ranking the applicant pool. Some interviews may be conducted "blind" in that the interviewers have no opportunity to view the student's credentials prior to the interview. In this case, you may still bring this information into the process if they refer to your performance or discuss this as part of the interview. If academics is a strong point in your background, by all means, include it in your discussions. Most interviewers will have had the chance to review a student's admission file before and during the interview. It is important that all available materials, transcripts, and other required information have been provided and that your application is as complete as possible. Also, the committee may ask specific questions regarding courses that you did especially well in or faced challenges. Don't try to ignore bad academic events or specific grades. Address them honestly to the committee and explain any extenuating circumstances which may have adversely affected performance on a short term. Point out improvements or trends which show improved effort or understanding of vital material. Talk about additional courses that you may have taken which, even though not required, might provide a benefit during the pharmacy program or in professional practice. Even courses in business, psychology, writing or education can be very applicable and helpful in one's career pursuit. Usually, high school grades or performance are not an issue, but if you had a particularly good experience in a class or with a teacher which was pivotal in your career choice or academic performance, it would be good to include this in your discussion.

Be aware of the pre-pharmacy requirements for the program and discuss how you plan to complete any remaining courses in time to begin the professional program in the desired term. If you have courses for which you hope to receive credit toward pharmacy prerequisites, check that out with the admission office before the interview. Often the interviewers are faculty who, though familiar with the requirements of the program, are not the ones to make transfer credit decisions. Putting them in this spot can make them feel less comfortable about your preparation for the program and commitment to their program in particular.

Often you will be asked if you have applied to other pharmacy or academic programs. Again, be honest and discuss other plans you have or pursuits you have considered. Considering other programs or even other academic pursuits, which are based on the interests you have stated in the interview, should be a positive factor and show that you are a serious and mature student. However, if you detect that the interviewers feel some competitiveness toward another pharmacy program which you are considering, tell them that this shows how serious you are about your pursuit of a career in pharmacy. We believe it is a good idea to consider and apply to any program you feel you could attend and get the education that will allow you to pursue your career goals.

Personal Background

The interview is a chance to put some "personality" into your application. The process, up to this point is very quantitative, with GPAs and PCAT scores often being the primary consideration that allowed you an interview. It's your responsibility to make the impression on the interviewers that you will do well in their institution and will be the type of pharmacist that they want to produce. Talk not only about the experiences in your background that led you to pharmacy, but also talk about the experiences that helped you to develop a personality that will support you through the academic program and as a pharmacist. Include information about outside activities, sports, and hobbies. Include involvement in organizations in addition to academic pursuits, such as membership in service groups. Don't just state that you were a member of so-and-so, but discuss what you did in the organization which exhibits your leadership abilities or interest in providing service to the community. Membership in honor societies should be mentioned, discuss activities or opportunities that were provided by your eligibility for membership, not just that you were a member because of your grades or other academic qualities.

As you can see the three background areas (academic, professional and personal) overlap. Since they are all so important in relaying how you got to where you are and what type of student and person you are, it is natural that the dividing line between academics, your professional pursuit, and your personality may be extensions of each other.

Tips for successful interviewing:

- Arrive on time for the interview. Arriving late may send the message that the interview is not a priority to you.
- Try to not appear to be nervous. Arriving to the interview early may give you the opportunity to adjust to the environment which may decrease your anxiety.
- Dress professionally.
- Be courteous.
- Be positive, friendly, and smile.
- Answer all questions as completely as possible.
- Speak clearly.
- Make eye contact with the interviewers.
- Don't exhibit unnecessary movements.
- Educate yourself on the institution.
- If you have questions, ask if there is enough time to ask your questions. If so, ask questions.
- If you have any materials that you want the committee to review, bring them with you to the interview.
- Listen attentively and learn from the interview. The information exchange should be a two-way process.
- Bring a pen and notebook to the interview. Have a list of questions that you may have and make notes as appropriate.
- Don't limit yourself to one or two word answers.

Conclusion of the Interview

At the end of the interview make sure you summarize your interest in the program and "wrap-up" any issues regarding remaining coursework. State your plans for future academic terms, and make sure you know what the next step will be and when you can expect to hear from the committee regarding the results of your application.

A CAREER IN PHARMACY

Over the last few decades, pharmacy practice has undergone significant changes. Since the 1960s the pharmacy profession has branched out in many directions other than traditional pharmacy settings (community and hospital). Once you have graduated from pharmacy school and have successfully passed a pharmacy state board licensure examination, career opportunities in pharmacy are great. These opportunities include, but are not limited to, community pharmacy (chain and independent), hospital pharmacy, pharmaceutical industry, government agencies, geriatric pharmacy, clinical pharmacy, pharmacy services, managed-care pharmacy, pharmaceutical research, pharmacy and medical education, nuclear pharmacy, and other specialty areas.

Job opportunities in pharmacy are immense for a person who receives either a bachelor of science (B.S.) or a doctor of pharmacy (Pharm.D.) degree. In addition, postgraduate training or graduate education provides an excellent opportunity for continuing your pharmacy education and thereby enhancing your career opportunities in this field. Although career counseling is done best in a pharmacy program, the purpose of this section is to familiarize you with several pharmacy careers (see the list that follows). Once accepted into a pharmacy school, you should inquire further about career opportunities in pharmacy.

Career Opportunities in Pharmacy

Academia

Administration
Biological Science
Clinical Pharmacy
Continuing Education
Experimental Education
Medicinal Chemistry
Pharmaceutics
Pharmacy Administration
Pharmacy Practice

Administration

Continuing Education
Professional Relations

Business

Administration
Management
Marketing
Sales

Chain (Community)

Apothecary
Franchise
Long-term Care
Home Health Care

Clinical

Adult Medicine
Ambulatory Care
Clinical Coordinator
Clinical Manager
Critical Care
Drug Information
Family Medicine
Geriatrics
Infectious Disease
Internal Medicine

Clinical (Continued)

Nutrition
Oncology
Pain Management
Pediatrics
Pharmacokinetics
Poison Control
Psychiatry
Surgery
Transplantation

Computer Technology

Consultants

Clinical Pharmacy
Home Health Care
Long-term Care

Drug Information

Federal

Alcohol, Drug Abuse, and
    Mental Health
Armed Services
Clinical Pharmacy
Drug Enforcement
    Administration
Food and Drug Administration
Health Administration
Health Care Financing
Indian Health Services

Hospital

Administration
Clinical Pharmacy
Inventory Control
Staff

Independent

Clinical Pharmacy
Franchise
Home Health Care
Long-term Care

Mail-order Pharmacy

Managed Care Pharmacy

Nuclear Pharmacy

Pharmacy Associations

Research and Development

Basic Research
Biological Sciences
Clinical Outcomes
Medicinal Chemistry
Pharmaceutics

Research and Development (Continued)

Pharmacognosy
Pharmacology
Pharmacy Administration
Pharmacy Practice

State

Board of Pharmacy
Clinical Outcomes
Department of Consumer
Affairs
Department of Health

Technical/Scientific

Drug Information
Manufacturing
Postmarketing Surveillance
Product Control

Veterans Administration Facilities

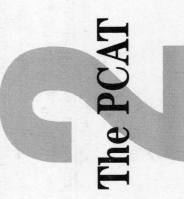

2 The PCAT

WHAT IS THE PCAT?

The Pharmacy College Admission Test (PCAT) is a national examination developed and sponsored by The Psychological Corporation and the American Association of Colleges of Pharmacy. The PCAT was developed to provide the admission committees of pharmacy schools with comparable information about the academic abilities of applicants in verbal ability, reading comprehension, chemistry, biology, and quantitative ability.

PCAT CONTENTS

Currently, the PCAT covers five content areas:

Verbal Ability. General word knowledge, measured by using analogies and antonyms.

Quantitative Ability. A combination of skills in arithmetic including fractions, percentages, decimals, reasoning ability (concepts and relationships), and algebra.

Biology. Principles and concepts of basic biology, human anatomy, and human physiology.

Chemistry. Principles and concepts of inorganic and organic chemistry. Questions may include basic chemistry knowledge, chemistry problems, application of formulas, and interpretation of results.

Reading Comprehension. Ability to comprehend, analyze, and interpret reading passages on scientific topics.

Toward the end of the exam an additional section may be included to test new question items. However, this section will not be graded or incorporated to determine your PCAT scores.

THE EXAM

You will be given approximately 3 hours and 45 minutes (including a rest break) to take the PCAT. The test consists of multiple-choice questions, each of which has only one correct answer. Each of the five sections of the PCAT is timed separately, and during the time allowed you may work only on that section.

The approximate number of questions in each section of the PCAT is shown below:

PCAT Section Area	Approximate Number of Questions
Verbal Ability	50
Quantitative Ability	65
Biology	50
Chemistry	60
Reading Comprehension	45

PCAT SCORING

Scores on the PCAT are based on the number of correct responses, and there is no penalty for guessing. A scaled and percentile score for each individual section and a composite percentile and scaled score for the test as a whole are also reported. Usually within four weeks of taking the exam, your test results are mailed to you and to the schools that you requested.

WHEN IS THE PCAT OFFERED?

The PCAT is generally offered three times a year—Fall, Winter, and Spring (usually in October, January or February, and April).

PCAT FEE

The cost, as of February 2002, of taking the PCAT at a scheduled center is $52.00. The fee also includes registration for the test, receiving your score report, and having official score reports sent to as many as three colleges/schools of pharmacy of your choice. Additional fees may apply, depending on special requests by the test taker.

PCAT INFORMATION

For more information concerning the PCAT, contact The Psychological Corporation at the address or phone number below:

The Psychological Corporation
PSE Customer Relations—PCAT
555 Academic Court
San Antonio, TX 78204–2498
1-800-622-3231

WHEN SHOULD YOU TAKE THE PCAT?

Many considerations are involved in the decision of when and how often to take the PCAT. Since many colleges/schools of pharmacy do not penalize applicants for taking the test more than once and often use the highest scores (practice differs from institution to institution, so check with the college/school that you are interested in attending), it is strongly recommended that you take the PCAT no later than the fall of the year prior to the time when you want to start pharmacy school. This strategy will allow you to retake the PCAT in the winter if desired or necessary. Also, if you follow this strategy, most schools of pharmacy will be able to consider both sets of scores before the application dead-line date.

The ultimate decision of when and how often to take the PCAT is highly individualized and depends on many circumstances, such as when you feel most comfortable taking the test (this may depend on the number of pre-pharmacy courses you have taken.) Other factors that may affect your decision are the admissions policy of the pharmacy col-lege or school you wish to attend, and your previous PCAT scores.

3

Strategies to Increase Your Score on the PCAT

PCAT SCORING

Students receive two scores in each section of the PCAT, the scaled score and the percentile score. Additionally, a scaled score and percentile score are computed and reported as a composite score.

The scaled score is computed from the number of correct answers a student provides on a particular section of the test. This is similar to standard scoring mechanisms, which indicate the number or value of correct answers versus the total possible. This differs significantly from the interpretation of the percentile score.

The percentile score represents the placement of the student's scaled score in the total pool of test takers. This pool represents other students who took the test at the same time and also factors in results from previous test administrations. It does not factor in previous attempts by the individual student, only previous pools of test takers. By definition, a 50 in the percentile column indicates that the student did better than 50 percent of the other students on that section and scored in the 50th percentile. In other words, percentile score indicates the percentage of applicants throughout the United States whose scores were lower than yours. For example, an individual who achieves a percentile score of 70 scored higher than 70 percent of other individuals who took the test.

The relationship between the scaled score and the percentile score is not linear (e.g., if a scaled score of 150 represents a 30th percentile, a scaled score of 300 does not translate to a 60th percentile). In most cases a small increase in scaled score produces a much larger movement in percentile score. For example, in order to improve a percentile score from 50 to 75, a 25% increase, a student may need only to

49

improve the scaled score by 10%. This is definitely something students should consider when trying to improve their scores. It should be an encouragement to students eager to improve their score and be more competitive.

The composite score is calculated from the five area scores. The composite scaled scores is the numeric average of the scaled score from each of the five subject areas. This average is affected like any numeric average, in that low scores in various sections pull the average down. Likewise, stronger scores in sections will pull the composite scaled score to a higher level. It is important for a student retaking the test to maintain high scores on areas in which they scored well on previous attempts, while spending extra effort to improve in areas with the lowest scores. This will more likely result in an increase in the composite scaled score, which is then assigned a percentile score based on where the score ranks in the overall pool. Just as with the individual section scores, a relatively small increase in composite scaled score may represent a significantly higher increase in the percentile score.

The composite percentile score is the best overall indicator of how a student performed on the test in comparison with the pool of PCAT test takers. Some schools require minimum levels of performance in each area of the test. Students should contact the schools in which they are interested and determine first, if the PCAT is required, find out how the PCAT score is interpreted in considering applicants for admission and how they will evaluate repeat exams. Also, determine which PCAT testing sessions will allow scores to be reported for the admission year cycle. For example, if the due date for admission materials is March 1, the April exam scores for that year will not be received in time for consideration for that admission cycle.

PCAT STRATEGIES

In taking the PCAT, work at a comfortable pace, but keep in mind that there is a time limit for each section. Be sure to answer every question. Your total PCAT score and the scores you receive on each section of the test reflect the number of correct answers only. Some tests penalize for guessing by subtracting the number of wrong answers from the number of correct answers; with the PCAT, however, this is *not* the case. Although guesses are not likely to make much difference in your scores, you shouldn't ignore this chance to avoid the total loss of points from unanswered questions. If you are able to eliminate some answers to a question, cross them out on your test booklet and then pick the *best* answer from the remaining choices.

If you finish a section before the time limit, don't go back over questions and make changes in your answers unless you are sure that an answer you have chosen is incorrect. In most cases, your first answer is likely to be correct. You may confuse yourself by dwelling on similar or related answers if you go back over questions.

The PCAT is divided into five sections. Three sections are specifically related to course work covered in the pre-pharmacy curriculum: chemistry, biology, and mathematics. Two sections are more comprehensive in nature and measure skills acquired through lifelong learning: verbal ability and reading comprehension. Because the verbal ability and reading comprehension sections assess skills acquired over a long period of time, they tend to be more difficult to study for in advance.

When you take the practice PCAT tests in this book and the actual PCAT, make sure to keep track of the time allotted for each test section. Pace yourself and work quickly but calmly through all the questions, skipping any you don't know or aren't sure of the first time around. Your aim is to complete all the questions you DO know—and to get credit for them—first. Then, as time permits, go back through each section and work on the questions with which you had difficulty. Finally, as the end of the allotted time approaches, go back through the entire section to be sure that you have entered an answer for every question. Although you may be forced to guess on some questions, there is a chance that some of your guesses will be correct. Remember, on the PCAT, your score is computed from the number of correct answers only. You are NOT penalized for guessing.

TWENTY PRESCRIPTIONS TO INCREASE YOUR SCORE ON THE PCAT

The first section of this chapter discussed general PCAT strategies. In this section you are given twenty prescriptions to improve your PCAT scores. Students who have taken the PCAT and employed these test-taking tactics have found them most useful:

Rx 1. Get an adequate amount of sleep the night before the test.
Rx 2. Allow yourself plenty of time to get to the testing site.
Rx 3. Bring at least four sharpened number 2 pencils.
Rx 4. Bring an accurate watch.
Rx 5. Bring proper identification (e.g., driver's license).

Rx 6.   Wear comfortable clothes.

Rx 7.   Know what to expect. After studying this preparation manual, you will be familiar with the types of questions that may appear on the PCAT.

Rx 8.   Read and memorize the directions for each question type (or section).

Rx 9.   Pace yourself. Work within the time restriction.

Rx 10. Answer questions to which you know the answer first.

Rx 11. Look at all the possible answers before making your final choice.

Rx 12. Eliminate as many wrong answers as possible.

Rx 13. Answer every question.

Rx 14. Remember that you are allowed to write on the test booklet. However, only the answers marked on the answer sheet will count in calculating your scores.

Rx 15. Do not make any stray marks on the answer sheet.

Rx 16. If you erase on the answer sheet, make sure you completely erase the mark you want to change.

Rx 17. Check frequently to make sure that you are marking the answer to each question next to the correct number on the answer sheet.

Rx 18. In preparing for the verbal ability section, consider reviewing a vocabulary study manual.

Rx 19. In the reading comprehension section, when asked to find the main idea, be sure to check the opening and summary sentences of the passage.

Rx 20. You cannot use a calculator on the PCAT, therefore, rounding numbers to do the math problems accurately and quickly may be beneficial.

Verbal Ability Review and Practice

TIPS FOR THE VERBAL ABILITY SECTION

The verbal ability section of the PCAT is designed to test your knowledge of words (vocabulary) and the relationships between them (antonyms and analogies). It consists of approximately 50 questions, with about half involving antonyms and the other half involving analogies. To study for the verbal ability section, you can use texts designed to help you increase your "word power" or vocabulary. Studying material on the roots of words and on prefixes and suffixes may also help you prepare for this section of the PCAT.

It is important that you understand what antonyms and analogies are before you take the PCAT. You should also be able to recognize the basic types of analogies.

Antonyms are pairs of words that are opposite or nearly opposite in meaning: *wealth* and *poverty*, *rejoice* and *mourn*, *dominant* and *submissive*, *then* and *now*. When you are trying to find the correct antonym of a word, it is helpful to consider several factors. First, what part of speech is the word? If it is a noun, look for a noun among the answer selections; if it is a verb, adjective, or adverb, search accordingly. Second, if you know the meaning of the word, rule out any choices with similar meanings; you are looking for an antonym, not a synonym. Third, be sure to read ALL the answers before making your selection. Fine shades of meaning may be represented, and you want to make the *best* choice. Finally, don't "second-guess" yourself. It usually pays to go with your first or intuitive response.

Analogies are words whose relationship to each other can be expressed as A : B :: C : D.

In words, A is to B as C is to D; for example, *meow* is to *cat* as *bark* is to *dog*. The notion of a proportion should be familiar to you from mathematics. In an analogy, however, the proportion is a logical or verbal one.

There are a number of different kinds of analogies, including cause and effect, part to whole, part to part, action to object, and analogies based on antonyms or synonyms (words with the same or nearly the same meaning), purpose or use, place, association, sequence or time, characteristic, degree, and measurement; there are even grammatical analogies. It is not necessary for you to memorize all the types of analogies, but becoming familiar with some of the main types can help you to identify them and to answer the questions on the analogy section more quickly. You should first identify the part of speech represented by the words in the analogy; then look for that part of speech among the answer selections. The practice questions and answers in this chapter will demonstrate and explain the different types of analogies and provide insight into formulating a correct answer. For a complete survey of analogies, you may wish to consult a guide to the Miller Analogies Test.

Once you have spent some time preparing yourself by studying vocabulary reviews and "word power" exercises and you feel confident that you understand what antonyms and analogies are, complete the verbal ability questions in this book. Since the explanatory answers are designed to help you become familiar with the various types of analogies, you should read them carefully.

VERBAL ABILITY ANSWER SHEET

1 Ⓐ Ⓑ Ⓒ Ⓓ	21 Ⓐ Ⓑ Ⓒ Ⓓ	41 Ⓐ Ⓑ Ⓒ Ⓓ	61 Ⓐ Ⓑ Ⓒ Ⓓ	81 Ⓐ Ⓑ Ⓒ Ⓓ
2 Ⓐ Ⓑ Ⓒ Ⓓ	22 Ⓐ Ⓑ Ⓒ Ⓓ	42 Ⓐ Ⓑ Ⓒ Ⓓ	62 Ⓐ Ⓑ Ⓒ Ⓓ	82 Ⓐ Ⓑ Ⓒ Ⓓ
3 Ⓐ Ⓑ Ⓒ Ⓓ	23 Ⓐ Ⓑ Ⓒ Ⓓ	43 Ⓐ Ⓑ Ⓒ Ⓓ	63 Ⓐ Ⓑ Ⓒ Ⓓ	83 Ⓐ Ⓑ Ⓒ Ⓓ
4 Ⓐ Ⓑ Ⓒ Ⓓ	24 Ⓐ Ⓑ Ⓒ Ⓓ	44 Ⓐ Ⓑ Ⓒ Ⓓ	64 Ⓐ Ⓑ Ⓒ Ⓓ	84 Ⓐ Ⓑ Ⓒ Ⓓ
5 Ⓐ Ⓑ Ⓒ Ⓓ	25 Ⓐ Ⓑ Ⓒ Ⓓ	45 Ⓐ Ⓑ Ⓒ Ⓓ	65 Ⓐ Ⓑ Ⓒ Ⓓ	85 Ⓐ Ⓑ Ⓒ Ⓓ
6 Ⓐ Ⓑ Ⓒ Ⓓ	26 Ⓐ Ⓑ Ⓒ Ⓓ	46 Ⓐ Ⓑ Ⓒ Ⓓ	66 Ⓐ Ⓑ Ⓒ Ⓓ	86 Ⓐ Ⓑ Ⓒ Ⓓ
7 Ⓐ Ⓑ Ⓒ Ⓓ	27 Ⓐ Ⓑ Ⓒ Ⓓ	47 Ⓐ Ⓑ Ⓒ Ⓓ	67 Ⓐ Ⓑ Ⓒ Ⓓ	87 Ⓐ Ⓑ Ⓒ Ⓓ
8 Ⓐ Ⓑ Ⓒ Ⓓ	28 Ⓐ Ⓑ Ⓒ Ⓓ	48 Ⓐ Ⓑ Ⓒ Ⓓ	68 Ⓐ Ⓑ Ⓒ Ⓓ	88 Ⓐ Ⓑ Ⓒ Ⓓ
9 Ⓐ Ⓑ Ⓒ Ⓓ	29 Ⓐ Ⓑ Ⓒ Ⓓ	49 Ⓐ Ⓑ Ⓒ Ⓓ	69 Ⓐ Ⓑ Ⓒ Ⓓ	89 Ⓐ Ⓑ Ⓒ Ⓓ
10 Ⓐ Ⓑ Ⓒ Ⓓ	30 Ⓐ Ⓑ Ⓒ Ⓓ	50 Ⓐ Ⓑ Ⓒ Ⓓ	70 Ⓐ Ⓑ Ⓒ Ⓓ	90 Ⓐ Ⓑ Ⓒ Ⓓ
11 Ⓐ Ⓑ Ⓒ Ⓓ	31 Ⓐ Ⓑ Ⓒ Ⓓ	51 Ⓐ Ⓑ Ⓒ Ⓓ	71 Ⓐ Ⓑ Ⓒ Ⓓ	91 Ⓐ Ⓑ Ⓒ Ⓓ
12 Ⓐ Ⓑ Ⓒ Ⓓ	32 Ⓐ Ⓑ Ⓒ Ⓓ	52 Ⓐ Ⓑ Ⓒ Ⓓ	72 Ⓐ Ⓑ Ⓒ Ⓓ	92 Ⓐ Ⓑ Ⓒ Ⓓ
13 Ⓐ Ⓑ Ⓒ Ⓓ	33 Ⓐ Ⓑ Ⓒ Ⓓ	53 Ⓐ Ⓑ Ⓒ Ⓓ	73 Ⓐ Ⓑ Ⓒ Ⓓ	93 Ⓐ Ⓑ Ⓒ Ⓓ
14 Ⓐ Ⓑ Ⓒ Ⓓ	34 Ⓐ Ⓑ Ⓒ Ⓓ	54 Ⓐ Ⓑ Ⓒ Ⓓ	74 Ⓐ Ⓑ Ⓒ Ⓓ	94 Ⓐ Ⓑ Ⓒ Ⓓ
15 Ⓐ Ⓑ Ⓒ Ⓓ	35 Ⓐ Ⓑ Ⓒ Ⓓ	55 Ⓐ Ⓑ Ⓒ Ⓓ	75 Ⓐ Ⓑ Ⓒ Ⓓ	95 Ⓐ Ⓑ Ⓒ Ⓓ
16 Ⓐ Ⓑ Ⓒ Ⓓ	36 Ⓐ Ⓑ Ⓒ Ⓓ	56 Ⓐ Ⓑ Ⓒ Ⓓ	76 Ⓐ Ⓑ Ⓒ Ⓓ	96 Ⓐ Ⓑ Ⓒ Ⓓ
17 Ⓐ Ⓑ Ⓒ Ⓓ	37 Ⓐ Ⓑ Ⓒ Ⓓ	57 Ⓐ Ⓑ Ⓒ Ⓓ	77 Ⓐ Ⓑ Ⓒ Ⓓ	97 Ⓐ Ⓑ Ⓒ Ⓓ
18 Ⓐ Ⓑ Ⓒ Ⓓ	38 Ⓐ Ⓑ Ⓒ Ⓓ	58 Ⓐ Ⓑ Ⓒ Ⓓ	78 Ⓐ Ⓑ Ⓒ Ⓓ	98 Ⓐ Ⓑ Ⓒ Ⓓ
19 Ⓐ Ⓑ Ⓒ Ⓓ	39 Ⓐ Ⓑ Ⓒ Ⓓ	59 Ⓐ Ⓑ Ⓒ Ⓓ	79 Ⓐ Ⓑ Ⓒ Ⓓ	99 Ⓐ Ⓑ Ⓒ Ⓓ
20 Ⓐ Ⓑ Ⓒ Ⓓ	40 Ⓐ Ⓑ Ⓒ Ⓓ	60 Ⓐ Ⓑ Ⓒ Ⓓ	80 Ⓐ Ⓑ Ⓒ Ⓓ	100 Ⓐ Ⓑ Ⓒ Ⓓ

VERBAL ABILITY PRACTICE QUESTIONS

100 Questions

Antonyms (50 Questions)

<u>Directions</u>: Select the word that is **opposite** or nearly opposite in meaning to the given word.

1. DEPRESSION

A. Void
B. Apathy
C. Elation
D. Caring

2. CONTRARY

A. Sullen
B. Complaisant
C. Large
D. Mean

3. ACKNOWLEDGE

A. Redeem
B. Sign
C. Deny
D. Stupefy

4. EASILY

A. Openly
B. Cowardly
C. Graciously
D. Laboriously

5. APPRECIATIVE

A. Ungrateful
B. Withholding
C. Stern
D. Yielding

6. FLOUT

A. Revere
B. Flaunt
C. Enjoy
D. Abjure

7. DENSE

A. Thick
B. Heavy
C. Sparse
D. Solid

8. FIRST

A. Infinite
B. Final
C. Superior
D. Inferior

9. CHOICE

A. Selection
B. Mediocre
C. Crude
D. Above average

10. ALPHA

A. Omega
B. Zero
C. Zenith
D. Omicron

11. CONFIRM

A. Revoke
B. Admit
C. Fraternize
D. Join

12. CIRCUITOUS

A. Square
B. Solid
C. Straight
D. Dense

13. VIGOR

A. Growth
B. Lethargy
C. Striving
D. Slack

14. ELUCIDATION

A. Obfuscation
B. Obviation
C. Elimination
D. Emanation

15. EGOISTIC

A. Competitive
B. Altruistic
C. Self-aggrandizing
D. Self-contained

16. FIRM

A. Solid
B. Robust
C. Level
D. Flabby

17. SPURN

A. Insulate
B. Isolate
C. Embrace
D. Scorn

18. CONFIDENTIALLY

A. Openly
B. Feverishly
C. Secretively
D. Happily

19. RETURN

A. Gain
B. Remove
C. Margin
D. Yield

20. SUCCINCTLY

A. Tough
B. Discursively
C. Waxen
D. Loudly

21. FLOW

A. Chaos
B. Order
C. Bank
D. Ebb

22. MODEST

A. Boastful
B. Shy
C. Discreet
D. Somber

29. RESERVED

A. Outgoing
B. Quotient
C. Saved
D. Restrained

30. YOUTH

A. Wisdom
B. Demographic
C. Age
D. Fleeting

31. ACQUIT

A. Acquire
B. Familiar
C. Convict
D. Reveal

32. SMOOTH

A. Restore
B. Crumple
C. Sonorous
D. Tactile

33. IMPERCEPTIBLE

A. Tiny
B. Inaudible
C. Immeasurable
D. Visible

34. CHOOSE

A. Select
B. Random
C. Reject
D. Incorporate

23. CONTEMPT

A. Spite
B. Neutral
C. Befriend
D. Regard

24. EFFORT

A. Gain
B. Ease
C. Pain
D. Result

25. CONCENTRIC

A. Eccentric
B. Conforming
C. Average
D. Coaxial

26. AVERSE

A. Avoid
B. Avid
C. Yielding
D. Relaxed

27. FACE

A. Countenance
B. Confront
C. Fault
D. Avoid

28. IMPEDIMENT

A. Aid
B. Surface
C. Boundary
D. Remove

35. SUBDUE

A. Involute
B. Dissolve
C. Folly
D. Enliven

36. BOGUS

A. Authentic
B. Popular
C. False
D. Finesse

37. MICROCOSM

A. Magnify
B. Macrocosm
C. Miniature
D. Scope

38. STERILE

A. Profound
B. Harsh
C. Fecund
D. Clean

39. INEXPERIENCED

A. Timely
B. Expert
C. Retired
D. Fictional

40. IMAGINARY

A. Actual
B. Comical
C. Practical
D. Large

41. SUBJECT

A. Text
B. Variety
C. Focused
D. Sovereign

42. DOWDY

A. Young
B. Energetic
C. Stylish
D. Dour

43. VIOLATE

A. Offend
B. Persuade
C. Observe
D. Assure

44. ACTUAL

A. Considerable
B. Virtual
C. Limited
D. Unconsidered

45. VOID

A. Empty
B. Disorder
C. Release
D. Full

46. ZEALOUS

A. Apathetic
B. Heretic
C. Timely
D. Spirited

47. LIGHT

A. Dutiful
B. Dreary
C. Extinguish
D. Intensify

48. AUTHORITARIAN

A. Expert
B. Liberal
C. Dictator
D. Trader

49. PROLOGUE

A. Premise
B. Epilogue
C. Apology
D. Grievance

50. STERN

A. Senatorial
B. Empower
C. Lenient
D. Rear

Analogies (50 Questions)

Directions: Select the word that **best** completes the analogy.

51. SPIDER : WEB :: BIRD :

A. Deck
B. Wood
C. Nest
D. Wing

52. PHARMACIST : PATIENT :: TEACHER :

A. Student
B. Prescription
C. Education
D. Textbook

53. POLYPS : CORAL :: BEES :

A. Flowers
B. Colony
C. Hive
D. Honey

54. HYPNOSIS : TRANCE :: STROKE :

A. Embolism
B. Paralysis
C. Speech
D. Rehabilitation

55. HUMIDITY : SWAMP :: ARIDITY :

A. Ocean
B. Air conditioning
C. Sea level
D. Desert

56. RIND : ORANGE :: BARK :

A. Tree
B. Dog
C. Forest
D. Leaves

57. BIKINI : MARSHALL ::
SAINT THOMAS :

A. Virgin
B. Atlantic
C. Tourism
D. Haiti

58. DENTIST : DRILL ::
ASTRONOMER :

A. Milky Way
B. Galaxies
C. Telescope
D. Magnification

59. RED : RUDDY :: METAL :

A. Element
B. Metallic
C. Strength
D. Gray

60. BOTANIST : PLANTS ::
NEUROBIOLOGIST :

A. Neurotes
B. Experiment
C. Data
D. Neurotransmitter

61. MILK : CASEIN :: WHEAT :

A. Bread
B. Carbohydrate
C. Gluten
D. Grain

62. GANGES : INDIA ::
MISSISSIPPI :

A. United States
B. Continent
C. State
D. Delta

63. TRANSPARENT : CLEAR ::
OPAQUE :

A. White
B. Heavy
C. Muddy
D. Translucent

64. ABSTAIN : INDULGE ::
LOOSEN :

A. Find
B. Tighten
C. Yield
D. Corrupt

65. AIRPLANE : HANGAR ::
AUTOMOBILE :

A. Garage
B. Travel
C. Flight
D. Passenger

66. GRAIN : WOOD ::
LUSTER :

A. Surface
B. Value
C. Diamond
D. Shine

67. VIOLINS : ORCHESTRA ::
PUPILS :

  A. Symphony
  B. Chorus
  C. Conductor
  D. Class

68. ANACONDA : BOA ::
TENNIS :

  A. Racquet
  B. Sport
  C. Court
  D. Serve

69. LENS : MICROSCOPE ::
HELMET :

  A. Weapon
  B. Battle
  C. Armor
  D. Head

70. BERMUDA : WEST
ATLANTIC ::
MADAGASCAR :

  A. Strait of Gibraltar
  B. Outer Hebrides
  C. Pacific
  D. West Indian

71. HAS FLOWN : WILL FLY ::
HAS SHOWN :

  A. Will show
  B. Has been shown
  C. Will be shown
  D. Has fled

72. SINGER : MICROPHONE ::
PHYSICIAN :

  A. Hippocratic Oath
  B. Stethoscope
  C. Nurse
  D. Surgery

73. BANYAN : TREE ::
CHRYSANTHEMUM :

  A. Stem
  B. India
  C. Japan
  D. Flower

74. BOOLEAN : ALGEBRA ::
EUCLIDEAN :

  A. Smorgasbord
  B. Geometry
  C. Ghost
  D. Gambling

75. MUZZLE : DOG ::
CEREBELLUM :

  A. Brain
  B. Reticular activating
     system
  C. Amygdala
  D. Electrode

76. DRUMS : BAND ::
GOALIE :

  A. Position
  B. Team
  C. Puck
  D. Fans

77. DROPLETS : WATER ::
GRAINS :

A. Pool
B. Precipitation
C. Moisture
D. Sand

78. SHOPPER : CALCULATOR ::
STATISTICIAN :

A. Price
B. Statistics
C. Computer
D. Savings

79. PROVIDENCE : RHODE
ISLAND :: BOISE :

A. New England
B. Arizona
C. Idaho
D. Capital

80. AREN'T : ARE NOT ::
HAVEN'T :

A. Have not
B. Has not
C. Is not
D. Are

81. LIABLE : RESPONSIBLE ::
LIBERAL :

A. Litigious
B. Generous
C. Free
D. Absolved

82. LIBRETTO : OPERA ::
SCREENPLAY :

A. Director
B. Film
C. Operetta
D. Script

83. ANDES : SOUTH
AMERICA :: ALPS :

A. Mountains
B. Europe
C. Switzerland
D. Mont Blanc

84. TIE : BIND :: ARM :

A. Hand
B. Elbow
C. Weapon
D. Prepare

85. STAND : POSITION ::
BOOK :

A. Volume
B. Title
C. Author
D. Opinion

86. EBB : FLOW :: REGRESS :

A. Advance
B. Retard
C. Shrink
D. Backslide

87. THERMOMETER :
TEMPERATURE ::
ODOMETER :

A. Time elapsed
B. Odor produced
C. Distance traveled
D. Force exerted

88. OEDIPUS COMPLEX :
FREUD :: UNCERTAINTY
PRINCIPLE :

A. Hindenberg
B. Heisenberg
C. Jung
D. Newton

89. HINDENBERG : BLIMPS ::
TITANIC :

A. Tragedies
B. Oceans
C. Icebergs
D. Ocean liners

90. TIMBUKTU : MALI ::
OSAKA :

A. Japan
B. China
C. Formosa
D. California

91. SPHYGMOMANOMETER :
BLOOD PRESSURE ::
THERMOMETER :

A. Degree
B. Ampere
C. Temperature
D. Air

92. ANTHROPOMORPHIC :
HUMAN ::
THERIOMORPHIC :

A. Inhuman
B. Evolution
C. Egypt
D. Animal

93. BLUES : MISSISSIPPI ::
BLUEGRASS :

A. Kentucky
B. Appalachia
C. Folk
D. Country

94. NUCLEAR MEMBRANE :
CELL :: HYPOTENUSE :

A. Algebra
B. Hippocrates
C. Triangle
D. Pythagoras

95. BASS : TREBLE :: ACME :

A. Pitch
B. Rhythm
C. Peak
D. Nadir

96. IMPERCEPTIBLE :
TANGIBLE :: MILD :

A. Tiny
B. Severe
C. Bland
D. Magnified

97. SEEMINGLY :
OSTENSIBLY ::
THOROUGHLY :

A. Completely
B. Openly
C. Divisively
D. Ruinously

98. MECHANIC : WRENCH ::
GARDENER :

A. Lawn
B. Grass seed
C. Annuals
D. Trowel

99. INDEPENDENCE DAY :
UNITED STATES ::
BASTILLE DAY :

A. Basque
B. France
C. Canada
D. Holland

100. SURFACE : INTERIOR ::
SUMMIT :

A. Nadir
B. Meeting
C. Diplomacy
D. Exterior

VERBAL ABILITY ANSWER KEY

1. C	21. D	41. D	61. C	81. B
2. B	22. A	42. C	62. A	82. B
3. C	23. D	43. D	63. C	83. B
4. D	24. B	44. B	64. B	84. D
5. A	25. A	45. D	65. A	85. A
6. A	26. B	46. A	66. C	86. A
7. C	27. D	47. C	67. D	87. C
8. B	28. A	48. B	68. B	88. B
9. B	29. A	49. B	69. C	89. D
10. A	30. C	50. C	70. D	90. A
11. A	31. C	51. C	71. A	91. C
12. C	32. B	52. A	72. B	92. D
13. B	33. D	53. D	73. D	93. A
14. A	34. C	54. B	74. B	94. C
15. B	35. D	55. D	75. A	95. D
16. D	36. A	56. A	76. B	96. B
17. C	37. B	57. A	77. D	97. A
18. A	38. C	58. C	78. C	98. D
19. B	39. B	59. B	79. C	99. B
20. B	40. A	60. D	80. A	100. A

VERBAL ABILITY EXPLANATORY ANSWERS

Antonyms

1. **Answer is C.** *Depression* means sadness or dejection; the opposite is *elation*, which means happiness or euphoria.

2. **Answer is B.** *Contrary* means oppositional or cranky; the opposite is *complaisant*, which means amiable or desiring to please.

3. **Answer is C.** To *acknowledge* is to recognize or admit; the opposite is to *deny*.

4. **Answer is D.** *Laboriously* means accomplished with difficulty or great effort; it is the opposite of the adverb *easily*.

5. **Answer is A.** *Appreciate* means to value, so it is the opposite of *ungrateful*.

6. **Answer is A.** To *flout* means to disregard or scoff; the opposite is to *revere*, which means to honor and respect.

7. **Answer is C.** The opposite of *dense*, which means compact, is *sparse*, which means scattered, dispersed, or meager.

8. **Answer is B.** The opposite of *first* is *final*, or last.

9. **Answer is B.** The adjective *choice* means superior, the best, worthy of being chosen; the opposite is *mediocre*, which means undistinguished.

10. **Answer is A.** *Alpha* is the first letter of the Greek alphabet, and *omega* is the last letter. These opposites denote the first and the last of a group of items.

11. **Answer is A.** To *confirm* means to ratify, consent, or validate; the opposite is to *revoke*, which means to take back, cancel, or nullify.

12. **Answer is C.** *Circuitous* means circular or winding; the opposite is *straight*.

13. **Answer is B.** *Lethargy* means drowsiness or aversion to activity; the opposite is *vigor*, which means active bodily or mental strength or force.

14. Answer is **A**. *Elucidation* clarifies or explains; *obfuscation* obscures or confuses.

15. Answer is **B**. *Egoistic* means self-concerned or self-centered; the opposite, *altruistic*, means concerned for others.

16. Answer is **D**. The opposite of *firm*, which means solid and hard, is *flabby*.

17. Answer is **C**. To *spurn* means to scorn or reject with contempt; the opposite is to *embrace*, which means to take up gladly and cherish.

18. Answer is **A**. *Confidentially* means secretly; the opposite is *openly*.

19. Answer is **B**. To *remove* something is to take it away; this is the opposite of to *return* or replace something.

20. Answer is **B**. *Succinctly* means precisely, tersely, without wasted words; the opposite is *discursively*, which means in a rambling way.

21. Answer is **D**. To *ebb* means to recede or decline; to *flow* means to rise (as applied, e.g., to a tide).

22. Answer is **A**. *Modest* means shy, not self-assertive or bold; the opposite is *boastful*, which means speaking with excessive pride or self-assertion.

23. Answer is **D**. *Regard*, which means esteem or respect, is the opposite of *contempt*, which means disdain or scorn.

24. Answer is **B**. *Effort* means the exertion of hard work or labor; its opposite, *ease*, means freedom from labor or difficulty.

25. Answer is **A**. *Concentric* means having a common center; the opposite is *eccentric*, which means lacking the same center.

26. Answer is **B**. *Averse* means disinclined; the opposite is *avid*, which means eager and enthusiastic.

27. Answer is **D**. To *face* means to confront, so the opposite is to *avoid*.

28. Answer is **A**. An *impediment* is an obstruction or hindrance; the opposite is an *aid*, that which helps or gives assistance.

29. Answer is **A**. *Reserved* means restrained or withdrawn; the opposite is *outgoing*, which means friendly and talkative.

30. Answer is **C**. The opposite of *youth* is *age*, or maturity.

31. Answer is **C**. To *acquit* is to free from (e.g., to acquit someone of a criminal charge); the opposite is to *convict*, to find guilty.

32. Answer is **B**. The opposite of to *smooth* (as applied, e.g., to a wrinkled object) is to *crumple*.

33. Answer is **D**. Since *imperceptible* means incapable of being perceived, the opposite is *visible*.

34. Answer is **C**. To *choose* means to select or prefer; the opposite is to *reject*, which means to avoid or shun.

35. Answer is **D**. To *subdue* means to tone down or reduce in intensity; the opposite is to *enliven*, which means to animate or make lively.

36. Answer is **A**. *Bogus* means counterfeit, not genuine; the opposite is *authentic*, real, trustworthy.

37. Answer is **B**. *Microcosm* means little world (usually the epitome of a larger world); the opposite is *macrocosm*, a great or large world.

38. Answer is **C**. *Sterile*, which means incapable of germinating or reproducing, is the opposite of *fecund*, which means fruitful or productive.

39. Answer is **B**. The opposite of *inexperienced* is *expert*, displaying special knowledge or skill derived from experience.

40. Answer is **A**. The opposite of *imaginary*, which means lacking factual reality, is *actual*, that is, real (existing in reality).

41. Answer is **D**. The opposite of *subject*, which means one who is under the control of another, is *sovereign*, one who is a leader, or authority, or who possesses supreme power.

42. Answer is **C**. Since *dowdy* means shabby, lacking in smartness or taste, the opposite is *stylish*, conforming to fashion.

43. <u>Answer is **D**</u>. To *violate* means to do harm to, desecrate, or disturb; the opposite is *assure*, which means to reassure or give confidence to (make feel secure).

44. <u>Answer is **B**</u>. The opposite of *actual*, which means real or existing in fact, is *virtual*, which means existing only in effect or in essence.

45. <u>Answer is **D**</u>. Since the adjective *void* means empty, its opposite is *full*.

46. <u>Answer is **A**</u>. *Zealous* is defined as full of passion or fervor; the opposite is *apathetic*, which means indifferent.

47. <u>Answer is **C**</u>. The opposite of to *light* (as applied, e.g., to a fire) is to *extinguish*, or to cause to stop burning.

48. <u>Answer is **B**</u>. *Authoritarian* means oppressive, dictatorial, or preferring complete submission to authority; the opposite is *liberal*, which means generous, broad-minded, or preferring individual freedom.

49. <u>Answer is **B**</u>. A *prologue* is a preface or an introduction (as in a literary work); its opposite is an *epilogue*, a concluding selection of a book or play.

50. <u>Answer is **C**</u>. The adjective *stern* means grim or severe, the opposite is *lenient*, which means mild, tolerant, or soothing in disposition.

Analogies

51. <u>Answer is **C**</u>. This is an analogy of association. A spider is housed in its web just as a bird uses a nest for housing.

52. <u>Answer is **A**</u>. A pharmacist cares for and instructs a patient just as a teacher instructs a student. This is an analogy of association.

53. <u>Answer is **D**</u>. In this analogy of cause and effect, bees produce honey just as polyps cause or produce coral.

54. <u>Answer is **B**</u>. This is an analogy of cause and effect. Just as hypnosis brings about a trance, a stroke may cause paralysis. (If you chose A by mistake, you identified a cause of stroke but did not complete the analogy. Be careful to match the terms appropriately.)

55. Answer is **D**. Humidity is associated with a swamp, and aridity with a desert. This may also be considered an analogy of description or characteristic.

56. Answer is **A**. In this part to whole analogy, the rind is the outer part of an orange, and the bark is the analogous (or corresponding) outer part of a tree. (If you mistakenly chose B, you made a common error by assuming that *bark* was a verb rather than a noun.

57. Answer is **A**. This is a geographical and also a part to whole analogy. Just as the island of Bikini is part of the Marshall Islands, so Saint Thomas is part of the Virgin Islands.

58. Answer is **C**. The analogy is worker to tool. An astronomer uses a telescope just as a dentist uses a drill.

59. Answer is **B**. In this grammatical analogy each noun is paired with an adjective derived from it. *Ruddy* means reddish in color, and <u>metallic</u> means made from metal or metal-like.

60. Answer is **D**. This analogy is one of association rather than worker to tool. Botanists are associated with the study of plants and neurobiologists with the study of neurotransmitters. (If you chose either C or B, your answer is too general to complete the analogy.)

61. Answer is **C**. This is a whole to part analogy. Casein is a protein occurring in milk, and gluten is a protein occurring in wheat. In each case, the protein is part of the composition of the whole.

62. Answer is **A**. This geographical analogy must be completed with the name of a country. The Ganges is a river in India, and the Mississippi is a river in the United States.

63. Answer is **C**. This analogy is based on synonyms. Just as *transparent* and *clear* are synonymous, *opaque* and *muddy* also have the same or nearly the same meaning.

64. Answer is **B**. This analogy is based on antonyms. Just as *abstain* and *indulge* have opposite meanings, so *loosen* and *tighten* are antonyms.

65. Answer is **A**. In this analogy of association, an airplane is kept in a hangar and an automobile is kept in a garage.

66. <u>Answer is **C**</u>. This is an analogy of characteristic or description. Grain is a characteristic of wood, and luster is a characteristic of a diamond.

67. <u>Answer is **D**</u>. In this part to whole analogy, violins form part of an orchestra, and a pupil is part of a class.

68. <u>Answer is **B**</u>. This is a part to whole analogy, since an anaconda is one type of boa, and tennis is one type of sport. To help clarify this kind of analogy, think of the group of all boas and the group of all sports as "wholes," of which the anaconda and tennis are merely parts.

69. <u>Answer is **C**</u>. This is a part to whole analogy. Just as a lens is part of a microscope, a helmet is part of a suit of armor.

70. <u>Answer is **D**</u>. In this geographical analogy, Bermuda is an island lying in the West Atlantic Ocean, and Madagascar is an island lying in the West Indian Ocean.

71. <u>Answer is **A**</u>. In this grammatical analogy, *will fly* and *will show* are verbs in the future tense and the active voice. (When you are working with grammatical analogies, take care to be precise. If you chose C, the tense is right but the passive voice is wrong.)

72. <u>Answer is **B**</u>. This is a worker to tool analogy. Just as a singer uses a microphone, a physician uses a stethoscope.

73. <u>Answer is **D**</u>. Although the names of two countries are included in the answer selections, this is not a geographical analogy. In this analogy of part to whole, a banyan is one kind of tree; a chrysanthemum is one kind of flower.

74. <u>Answer is **B**</u>. In this part to whole analogy, Boolean is a kind of algebra, and Euclidean is a kind of geometry.

75. <u>Answer is **A**</u>. In this part to whole analogy, the muzzle is part of a dog, and the cerebellum is part of the brain.

76. <u>Answer is **B**</u>. Drums are part of a band; a goalie is part of a team. This is an analogy of part to whole.

77. <u>Answer is **D**</u>. Droplets are a characteristic of water, and grains are an analogous characteristic of sand in this analogy of description or characteristic.

78. Answer is <u>C</u>. Since a shopper is not actually a worker, you can consider this to be an analogy of association rather than worker to tool. We associate the use of a calculator with a shopper or consumer and the use of a computer with a statistician.

79. Answer is <u>C</u>. In this geographical analogy, Providence is the capital of Rhode Island, and Boise is the capital of Idaho. (Always ask yourself how the first two terms are related, and then look for an analogous relationship between the second two terms.)

80. Answer is <u>A</u>. In this grammatical analogy, *are not* and *have not* are the plural verbs and the adverbs from which the contractions are formed. (Remember to take all the relevant factors into account. If you chose B, your answer is incorrect because *has* is third person singular, not plural).

81. Answer is <u>B</u>. This is an analogy based on synonyms. Just as *liable* and *responsible* are synonyms, *liberal* and *generous* have the same or nearly the same meaning.

82. Answer is <u>B</u>. In this analogy of purpose or use, a libretto is the text for an opera, while a screenplay is the "text" for a film.

83. Answer is <u>B</u>. In this geographical analogy, the Andes are a mountain chain in South America, and the Alps are a mountain chain in Europe. (If you chose C, your answer is incorrect because here you need to select a continent rather than a country. D is incorrect because it is the name of a single mountain in the Alps.)

84. Answer is <u>D</u>. This is an analogy based on synonyms. To *arm* and to *prepare* have the same or nearly the same meaning, just as to *tie* and to *bind* are synonymous. (Be careful to select a verb, not a noun, here.)

85. Answer is <u>A</u>. This is an analogy based on synonyms. *Stand* and *position* have the same meaning, and *book* and *volume* are likewise synonymous.

86. Answer is <u>A</u>. In this is analogy of antonyms, *ebb* and *flow* have opposite meanings, and the opposite of *regress* is *advance*.

87. Answer is <u>C</u>. In this analogy of purpose or use, a thermometer is used to measure temperature, and an odometer is used to measure distance traveled.

88. <u>Answer is **B**</u>. This is an analogy of association. The Oedipus complex is associated with Freud, and the uncertainty principle is associated with the physicist Heisenberg.

89. <u>Answer is **D**</u>. In this part to whole analogy, the Hindenberg is an example of a blimp, and the Titanic is an example of an ocean liner. (The fact that both met tragic fates is not relevant here.)

90. <u>Answer is **A**</u>. In this geographical analogy, Timbuktu is a city in Mali, and Osaka is a city in Japan.

91. <u>Answer is **C**</u>. This is an analogy of purpose or use. A sphygmomanometer is used to measure blood pressure, and a thermometer is used to measure temperature.

92. <u>Answer is **D**</u>. The word *anthropomorphic* means having human shape or human characteristics, *theriomorphic* means having an animal shape or animal characteristics. This analogy is based on the definitions of words.

93. <u>Answer is **A**</u>. This is an analogy of association. The blues are associated with Mississippi, and bluegrass music is associated with Kentucky.

94. <u>Answer is **C**</u>. In this analogy of part to whole, the nuclear membrane is part of a cell, and the hypotenuse is part of a triangle.

95. <u>Answer is **D**</u>. Since bass and treble represent opposite ends of a spectrum of sound, this can be considered either an analogy of antonyms or an analogy of degree. Acme and nadir also represent opposites.

96. <u>Answer is **B**</u>. This analogy may be considered one of antonyms or of degree, since the pairs of terms (*imperceptible* and *tangible*, *mild* and *severe*) represent opposite extremes.

97. <u>Answer is **A**</u>. This grammatical analogy involves pairs of adverbs (*seemingly* and *ostensibly*, *thoroughly* and *completely*) with the same or nearly the same meaning. This example may also be considered an analogy of synonyms.

98. <u>Answer is **D**</u>. In this worker to tool analogy, the gardener uses a trowel just as the mechanic uses a wrench. (If you chose A, you may have mistaken this for an analogy of association, but you need to select the name of a specific tool instead.)

99. <u>Answer is **B**</u>. In this analogy of association, Independence Day is a holiday associated with the United States, and Bastille Day is a holiday associated with France.

100. <u>Answer is **A**</u>. This is an analogy of antonyms. *Surface* is the opposite of *interior*, and the opposite of *summit* is *nadir*.

5
Biology Review and Practice

TIPS FOR THE BIOLOGY SECTION

The biology section of the PCAT measures your knowledge and understanding of principles and concepts in basic biology and human anatomy and physiology. Human anatomy and physiology may not be covered in general pre-pharmacy required biology courses. If you do not feel confident in this area, you can probably improve your PCAT biology scores by reviewing these subjects independently or by taking a course in human anatomy and physiology.

The biology section of the PCAT consists of approximately 50 questions. Be sure to answer all questions.

BIOLOGY REVIEW OUTLINE

I. **Molecular biology**
    A. Enzymes
    B. Energy
    C. Nucleic acids
    D. DNA
    E. RNA

II. **Cell biology**
    A. Structure
    B. Components
    C. Properties

D. Eukaryotic cell structure
E. Prokaryotic cell structure
F. Energy (Krebs cycle)
G. Cellular reproduction and division
    1. Mitosis
    2. Meiosis
H. Membrane transport
I. Cellular metabolism
    1. Respiration
        a. Aerobic
        b. Anaerobic
    2. Photosynthesis
    3. Autotrophs
    4. Heterotrophs

III. **Kingdom of life**
A. Taxonomy
B. Five kingdom classification system
    1. Monera
    2. Protista
    3. Fungi
    4. Plants
    5. Animals

IV. **Ecology**
V. **Human anatomy and physiology**
A. Cells
B. Tissues
C. Organs
D. Organ systems (anatomy and primary functions)
    1. Skeletal system
        a. Axial skeleton
        b. Appendicular skeleton
        c. Bones
        d. Joints
    2. Muscular system
    3. Circulatory system
        a. Blood
        b. Circulation
        c. Blood vessels
        d. Heart
    4. Respiratory system
        a. Ventilation
        b. Inspiration and expiration
        c. Gas exchange

5. Urinary System
   a. Anatomy of kidney
   b. Role of kidney
6. Liver
   a. Anatomy of liver
   b. Role of liver
7. Integumentary system
   a. Skin
   b. Glands
   c. Hair
   d. Nails
   e. Role of integumentary system
8. Digestive system
   a. Functions of digestive organs
   b. Digestive tract
   c. Digestive enzymes
   d. Digestive hormones
9. Sensory organs
   a. Eye
   b. Ear
   c. Nose
   d. Tongue
10. Nervous system
    a. Neuron
    b. Central nervous system
    c. Peripheral nervous system
11. Brain
    a. Parts
    b. Functions
12. Endocrine system
    a. Pancreas
    b. Thyroid gland
    c. Pituitary gland
    d. Parathyroid glands
    e. Adrenal glands
13. Reproductive system
    a. Reproductive organs (male and female)
    b. Hormones (hormonal regulation)
14. Immune system

VI. Nutrition

   A. Protein

   B. Glucose—energy

   C. Vitamins

      1. Water soluble

      2. Fat soluble

VII. Genetics

   A. Chromosomes

   B. Genes

   C. Traits

   D. Genetic diseases

BIOLOGY ANSWER SHEET

1 Ⓐ Ⓑ Ⓒ Ⓓ
2 Ⓐ Ⓑ Ⓒ Ⓓ
3 Ⓐ Ⓑ Ⓒ Ⓓ
4 Ⓐ Ⓑ Ⓒ Ⓓ
5 Ⓐ Ⓑ Ⓒ Ⓓ
6 Ⓐ Ⓑ Ⓒ Ⓓ
7 Ⓐ Ⓑ Ⓒ Ⓓ
8 Ⓐ Ⓑ Ⓒ Ⓓ
9 Ⓐ Ⓑ Ⓒ Ⓓ
10 Ⓐ Ⓑ Ⓒ Ⓓ
11 Ⓐ Ⓑ Ⓒ Ⓓ
12 Ⓐ Ⓑ Ⓒ Ⓓ
13 Ⓐ Ⓑ Ⓒ Ⓓ
14 Ⓐ Ⓑ Ⓒ Ⓓ
15 Ⓐ Ⓑ Ⓒ Ⓓ
16 Ⓐ Ⓑ Ⓒ Ⓓ
17 Ⓐ Ⓑ Ⓒ Ⓓ
18 Ⓐ Ⓑ Ⓒ Ⓓ
19 Ⓐ Ⓑ Ⓒ Ⓓ
20 Ⓐ Ⓑ Ⓒ Ⓓ

21 Ⓐ Ⓑ Ⓒ Ⓓ
22 Ⓐ Ⓑ Ⓒ Ⓓ
23 Ⓐ Ⓑ Ⓒ Ⓓ
24 Ⓐ Ⓑ Ⓒ Ⓓ
25 Ⓐ Ⓑ Ⓒ Ⓓ
26 Ⓐ Ⓑ Ⓒ Ⓓ
27 Ⓐ Ⓑ Ⓒ Ⓓ
28 Ⓐ Ⓑ Ⓒ Ⓓ
29 Ⓐ Ⓑ Ⓒ Ⓓ
30 Ⓐ Ⓑ Ⓒ Ⓓ
31 Ⓐ Ⓑ Ⓒ Ⓓ
32 Ⓐ Ⓑ Ⓒ Ⓓ
33 Ⓐ Ⓑ Ⓒ Ⓓ
34 Ⓐ Ⓑ Ⓒ Ⓓ
35 Ⓐ Ⓑ Ⓒ Ⓓ
36 Ⓐ Ⓑ Ⓒ Ⓓ
37 Ⓐ Ⓑ Ⓒ Ⓓ
38 Ⓐ Ⓑ Ⓒ Ⓓ
39 Ⓐ Ⓑ Ⓒ Ⓓ
40 Ⓐ Ⓑ Ⓒ Ⓓ

41 Ⓐ Ⓑ Ⓒ Ⓓ
42 Ⓐ Ⓑ Ⓒ Ⓓ
43 Ⓐ Ⓑ Ⓒ Ⓓ
44 Ⓐ Ⓑ Ⓒ Ⓓ
45 Ⓐ Ⓑ Ⓒ Ⓓ
46 Ⓐ Ⓑ Ⓒ Ⓓ
47 Ⓐ Ⓑ Ⓒ Ⓓ
48 Ⓐ Ⓑ Ⓒ Ⓓ
49 Ⓐ Ⓑ Ⓒ Ⓓ
50 Ⓐ Ⓑ Ⓒ Ⓓ
51 Ⓐ Ⓑ Ⓒ Ⓓ
52 Ⓐ Ⓑ Ⓒ Ⓓ
53 Ⓐ Ⓑ Ⓒ Ⓓ
54 Ⓐ Ⓑ Ⓒ Ⓓ
55 Ⓐ Ⓑ Ⓒ Ⓓ
56 Ⓐ Ⓑ Ⓒ Ⓓ
57 Ⓐ Ⓑ Ⓒ Ⓓ
58 Ⓐ Ⓑ Ⓒ Ⓓ
59 Ⓐ Ⓑ Ⓒ Ⓓ
60 Ⓐ Ⓑ Ⓒ Ⓓ

61 Ⓐ Ⓑ Ⓒ Ⓓ
62 Ⓐ Ⓑ Ⓒ Ⓓ
63 Ⓐ Ⓑ Ⓒ Ⓓ
64 Ⓐ Ⓑ Ⓒ Ⓓ
65 Ⓐ Ⓑ Ⓒ Ⓓ
66 Ⓐ Ⓑ Ⓒ Ⓓ
67 Ⓐ Ⓑ Ⓒ Ⓓ
68 Ⓐ Ⓑ Ⓒ Ⓓ
69 Ⓐ Ⓑ Ⓒ Ⓓ
70 Ⓐ Ⓑ Ⓒ Ⓓ
71 Ⓐ Ⓑ Ⓒ Ⓓ
72 Ⓐ Ⓑ Ⓒ Ⓓ
73 Ⓐ Ⓑ Ⓒ Ⓓ
74 Ⓐ Ⓑ Ⓒ Ⓓ
75 Ⓐ Ⓑ Ⓒ Ⓓ
76 Ⓐ Ⓑ Ⓒ Ⓓ
77 Ⓐ Ⓑ Ⓒ Ⓓ
78 Ⓐ Ⓑ Ⓒ Ⓓ
79 Ⓐ Ⓑ Ⓒ Ⓓ
80 Ⓐ Ⓑ Ⓒ Ⓓ

81 Ⓐ Ⓑ Ⓒ Ⓓ
82 Ⓐ Ⓑ Ⓒ Ⓓ
83 Ⓐ Ⓑ Ⓒ Ⓓ
84 Ⓐ Ⓑ Ⓒ Ⓓ
85 Ⓐ Ⓑ Ⓒ Ⓓ
86 Ⓐ Ⓑ Ⓒ Ⓓ
87 Ⓐ Ⓑ Ⓒ Ⓓ
88 Ⓐ Ⓑ Ⓒ Ⓓ
89 Ⓐ Ⓑ Ⓒ Ⓓ
90 Ⓐ Ⓑ Ⓒ Ⓓ
91 Ⓐ Ⓑ Ⓒ Ⓓ
92 Ⓐ Ⓑ Ⓒ Ⓓ
93 Ⓐ Ⓑ Ⓒ Ⓓ
94 Ⓐ Ⓑ Ⓒ Ⓓ
95 Ⓐ Ⓑ Ⓒ Ⓓ
96 Ⓐ Ⓑ Ⓒ Ⓓ
97 Ⓐ Ⓑ Ⓒ Ⓓ
98 Ⓐ Ⓑ Ⓒ Ⓓ
99 Ⓐ Ⓑ Ⓒ Ⓓ
100 Ⓐ Ⓑ Ⓒ Ⓓ

BIOLOGY PRACTICE QUESTIONS

100 Questions

Directions: Select the best answer to each of the following questions.

1. An animal cell has a

   A. cell wall.
   B. plasma membrane.
   C. nucleus.
   D. B and C

2. Which of the following is (are) true of a prokaryotic cell?

   A. These cells existed roughly 3.5 billion years ago and were the first life-forms.
   B. These cells are limited in size (ranging from 1 to 10 μm in diameter) and in complexity of chemical activities.
   C. A and B
   D. Neither A nor B

3. Which of the following is (are) characteristic of an eukaryotic cell?

   A. These cells constitute all organisms other than bacteria and cyanobacteria.
   B. Cell diameter is approximately 10–100 μm.
   C. A and B
   D. Neither A nor B

4. Mitochondria are sites of cellular

   A. respiration.
   B. elimination.
   C. protection.
   D. movement.

5. Which of the following contain(s) the genetic instructions within the cell?

A. Nuclear envelope
B. Chromosomes
C. Nucleoplasm
D. Nucleolus

6. Human sperm cells are mobile because of

A. mitochondria.
B. cilia.
C. flagella.
D. the plasma membrane.

7. Green pigments that are capable of capturing energy from sunlight are located within the

A. mitochondria.
B. chlorcasts.
C. cell wall.
D. chloroplast.

8. Which part of the cell produces ribonucleoprotein?

A. Nuclear envelope
B. Chromosomes
C. Nucleoplasm
D. Nucleolus

9. Which of the following form(s) a boundary between the nucleus and cytoplasm?

A. Nuclear envelope
B. Chromosomes
C. Nucleoplasm
D. Nucleolus

10. Which of the following is the fluid medium of the nucleus?

   A. Chloroplasm
   B. Golgi complex
   C. Nucleoplasm
   D. Nucleolus

Figure 1 is needed to answer questions 11–14.

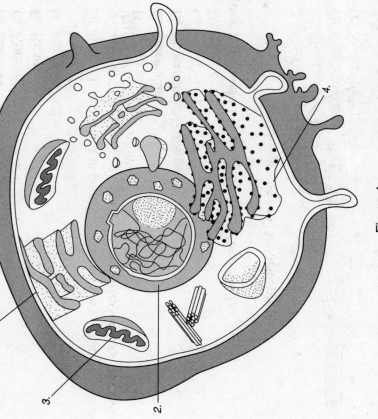

Figure 1.

11. In Figure 1, number 1 is pointing to what part of the animal cell?

   A. Rough endoplasmic reticulum
   B. Nucleus
   C. Nucleolus
   D. Plasma membrane

12. In Figure 1, number 2 is pointing to what part of the animal cell?

A. Golgi complex
B. Nucleus
C. Nucleolus
D. Plasma membrane

13. In Figure 1, number 3 is pointing to what part of the animal cell?

A. Mitochondrion
B. Nucleus
C. Nucleolus
D. Ribosomes

14. In Figure 1, number 4 is pointing to what part of the animal cell?

A. Rough endoplasmic reticulum
B. Golgi complex
C. Nucleolus
D. Plasma membrane

Figure 2 is needed to answer questions 15–18.

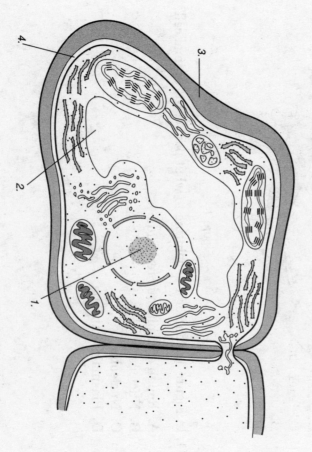

Figure 2.

15. In Figure 2, number 1 is pointing to what part of the plant cell?

 A. Mitochondrion
 B. Nucleolus
 C. Golgi complex
 D. Rough endoplasmic reticulum

16. In Figure 2, number 2 is pointing to what part of the plant cell?

 A. Nucleus
 B. Golgi complex
 C. Chloroplast
 D. Vacuole

17. In Figure 2, number 3 is pointing to what part of the plant cell?

 A. Nucleus
 B. Cell membrane
 C. Cell wall
 D. Golgi complex

18. In Figure 2, number 4 is pointing to what part of the plant cell?

 A. Golgi complex
 B. Chloroplast
 C. Leucoplast
 D. Cell membrane

Figure 3 is needed to answer questions 19–21.

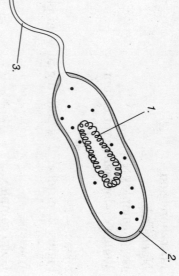

Figure 3.

19. In Figure 3, number 1 is pointing to what part of the bacterium?

A. DNA
B. Cell wall
C. Cell membrane
D. Ribosome

20. In Figure 3, number 2 is pointing to what part of the bacterium?

A. Cell wall
B. Cell membrane
C. Chloroplast
D. RNA

21. In Figure 3, number 3 is pointing to what part of the bacterium?

A. Cell membrane
B. Nucleus
C. Flagellum
D. Ribosome

22. Which of the following organelles is (are) associated with the release of energy?

A. Chloroplast
B. Mitochondria
C. Flagella
D. Endoplasmic reticulum

23. The nucleus of the cell is responsible for

A. energy production.
B. restitution.
C. synthesizing RNA and DNA.
D. mobility.

24. Diffusion is the

A. movement of molecules of one substance through the molecules of another substance from regions of lower concentration to regions of higher concentration by means of an outside energy source.

B. movement of molecules of one substance through the molecules of another substance from regions of higher concentration to regions of lower concentration by means of an outside energy source.

C. movement of molecules of one substance through the molecules of another substance from regions of lower concentration to regions of higher concentration by means of the molecules' own kinetic energy.

D. movement of molecules of one substance through the molecules of another substance from regions of higher concentration to regions of lower concentration by means of the molecules' own kinetic energy.

25. Which of the following has cell walls?

A. Animal
B. Plant
C. Neither A nor B
D. Both A and B

26. Which statement is TRUE regarding enzymes?

A. An enzyme is a protein that acts as a catalyst.
B. An enzyme is temperature dependent.
C. An enzyme is pH dependent.
D. A, B, and C

27. Transmitting genetic information from the DNA molecule in the nucleus to the cytoplasm is the responsibility of

A. transfer RNA.
B. messenger RNA.
C. Both A and B
D. Neither A nor B

28. The sugar found in DNA has _____ carbons.

A. three
B. four
C. five
D. six

29. Which is the functional unit of the kidney?

A. renin
B. renal valve
C. pacer
D. nephron

30. What is the last step in protein synthesis?

A. Endation
B. Transcription
C. Translation
D. Helixation

31. Mitosis is the process by which eukaryotic cells

A. develop function.
B. die.
C. multiply.
D. develop structure.

32. Which statement is FALSE?

A. Ribose is the sugar found in RNA.
B. DNA is double stranded.
C. RNA is mostly double stranded.
D. Deoxyribose is the sugar found in DNA.

33. During meiosis the number of chromosomes

A. remains the same.
B. decreases by 50 percent.
C. increases by 50 percent.
D. none of the above

34. A cell will shrivel in a

A. hypertonic medium.
B. hypotonic medium.
C. isotonic medium.
D. ionic medium.

35. The stage in cell division marked by chromosome separation is

A. anaphase.
B. interphase.
C. prophase.
D. telophase.

36. Organisms that produce their own food are

A. autotrophic.
B. heterotrophic.
C. monotrophic.
D. chronotropic.

37. Fungi are

A. autotrophic.
B. heterotrophic.
C. monotrophic.
D. chronotropic.

38. Characteristics used to separate organisms into the five kingdoms include

A. cell type.
B. number of cells in each organism.
C. mechanism for acquiring energy.
D. All the above

39. The simplest kingdom of life is

A. Protista.
B. Monera.
C. Fungi.
D. Plantae.

40. What is the smallest unit of life?

A. DNA

B. Organ

C. Cell

D. Chromosome

41. Which of the following cells excavate bone cavities?

A. Osteoclasts

B. Osteoblasts

C. Osteomasts

D. Osteocytes

42. Which of the following hormones is involved in calcium homeostasis?

A. Parathyroid hormone

B. Calcitonin

C. Insulin

D. A and B

43. Which of the following cells form bone matrix?

A. Osteoclasts

B. Osteocytes

C. Osteoblasts

D. Osteomasts

44. The bones of the skeleton articulate with each other at

A. the appendicular skeleton.

B. the joints.

C. the axial skeleton.

D. cartilage.

45. Ball and socket, plane, gliding, hinge, and condylar are all types of

A. bones.

B. muscles.

C. cartilage.

D. joints.

46. Which of the following is (are) included in the function(s) of the circulatory system?

   A. Supplies nutrients and oxygen to the tissues
   B. Removes waste material
   C. Initiates clotting
   D. All of the above

47. Hormones are distributed throughout the body by means of the

   A. blood.
   B. gallbladder.
   C. pancreas.
   D. stomach.

48. The classification of organisms is based on which of the following characteristics?

   A. Ancestry
   B. Structure
   C. Development
   D. All of the above

49. Blood is delivered to the heart from the lungs by the

   A. renal veins.
   B. pulmonary veins.
   C. mitral arteries.
   D. pulmonary arteries.

50. Which statement is FALSE?

   A. Red blood cells transport oxygen.
   B. Backflow of blood in the circulatory system is prevented by valves.
   C. The liver returns blood via the hepatic veins to the inferior vena cava.
   D. Plasma constitutes less than 23 percent of the blood volume.

51. What is another name for red blood cells?

A. Erythrocytes
B. Leukocytes
C. Lymphocytes
D. Basophils

52. Which statement is NOT characteristic of red blood cells?

A. Hemoglobin is present in red blood cells.
B. Mature red blood cells lack a nucleus.
C. The normal life span of red blood cells is about 30 days.
D. Red blood cells carry oxygen from the lungs to the tissues.

53. Which are NOT leukocytes?

A. Neutrophils
B. Eosinophils
C. Basophils
D. Thrombophils

54. The primary function of platelets involves

A. blood formation.
B. blood clotting.
C. metabolism.
D. defense against infections.

55. What is (are) the primary function(s) of white blood cells?

A. Phagocytosis
B. Proteolysis
C. Antibody formation
D. All of the above

56. Albumin is

A. an electrolyte.
B. a trace element.
C. a plasma protein.
D. a mineral.

57. What is the functional unit of the nervous system?

A. Neuron
B. Nerve
C. Synapse
D. None of the above

58. Which of the following statements is (are) TRUE concerning the respiratory system?

A. Respiration refers to the gaseous exchanges that occur between the body and the environment.
B. During inspiration the thoracic cavity expands.
C. During inspiration air rushes into the respiratory tract because of the creation of negative pressure.
D. All of the above

59. The affinity of hemoglobin for oxygen is affected by

A. pH level.
B. Carbon dioxide.
C. Neither A nor B.
D. A and B.

60. Which of the following statements is (are) TRUE concerning the urinary system?

A. The urinary system functions to help maintain homeostasis of the body by excreting waste and regulating the content of the blood.
B. The urinary system consists of two kidneys, two ureters, a urinary bladder, and a urethra.
C. The urinary system regulates the acid-base balance of the body.
D. All of the above

61. Which of the following is (are) NOT normally reabsorbed in the kidney?

A. Glucose
B. Creatinine
C. Sodium
D. A and C

62. Which statement concerning the liver is FALSE?

  A. The liver is one of the smallest organs of the body.

  B. The liver synthesizes and stores glycogen.

  C. The liver detoxifies toxic substances in the blood.

  D. The liver synthesizes albumin.

63. Which statement concerning the skin is FALSE?

  A. The function of the skin is to protect the body against damage.

  B. The skin acts as a barrier to infectious organisms.

  C. The skin aids in regulating the temperature of the body.

  D. The skin plays a role in the production of hydrochloric acid.

64. What is the name of the thin, mucus-secreting epithelial membrane that lines the interior surface of the eyelid?

  A. Tarsal plate

  B. Lacrimal gland

  C. Conjunctiva

  D. Sclera

65. Where does digestion start?

  A. Mouth

  B. Esophagus

  C. Stomach

  D. Intestine

66. The term *oral cavity* refers to the

  A. stomach.

  B. intestine.

  C. mouth.

  D. liver.

67. The fat-soluble vitamins include all of the following EXCEPT

  A. vitamin D.

  B. vitamin K.

  C. vitamin A.

  D. vitamin B_1.

68. Which statement is FALSE concerning the digestive system?

A. The small intestine has three major regions—the duodenum, jejunum, and ileum.
B. Most nutrients are absorbed by the large intestine.
C. The pancreas synthesizes and secretes a number of digestive enzymes.
D. Water is resorbed from the residue of the food mass as it passes through the large intestine.

69. All of the following are digestive enzymes EXCEPT

A. amylase.
B. gastrin.
C. lipase.
D. trypsin.

70. The water-soluble vitamins include all of the following EXCEPT

A. thiamine.
B. niacin.
C. folic acid.
D. vitamin E.

71. What is the primary function of the gallbladder?

A. To store gastrin
B. To store bile
C. To synthesize insulin
D. To store amylase

72. The spleen is involved with

A. blood cell formation.
B. blood cell storage.
C. blood filtration.
D. All of the above

73. Which of the following enhance(s) the intestinal absorption of fatty acids?

   A. Bile salts
   B. Amylase
   C. Hydrochloric acid
   D. Pepsin

74. If the blood pH of a subject is measured immediately before and after hyperventilation, which of the following results is expected?

   A. There is no difference between the pH measurements.
   B. The pH will be lower after hyperventilating.
   C. The pH will be higher after hyperventilating.
   D. The pH will be higher before hyperventilating but will rapidly fall.

75. Which is NOT a function of the medulla oblongata?

   A. Arteriole wall contraction
   B. Respirations
   C. Heartbeat
   D. Verbal communication

76. Which of the following is (are) included among the function(s) of the thyroid gland?

   A. Controlling the rate of metabolism
   B. Controlling the growth of the organism
   C. Influencing nervous system activity
   D. All of the above

77. The testes is involved in the

   A. production of sperm.
   B. production of testosterone.
   C. production of prolactin.
   D. A and B

78. Which statement is TRUE concerning the parathyroid glands and/or the hormone they produce?

   A. There are usually four parathyroid glands, which are embedded in the thyroid gland.
   B. The parathyroid glands produce parathyroid hormone.
   C. Parathyroid hormone regulates calcium levels.
   D. All of the above

79. Major functions of the ovaries include

   A. production of estrogen.
   B. production of progesterone.
   C. A and B
   D. Neither A nor B.

Figure 4 is needed to answer question 80.

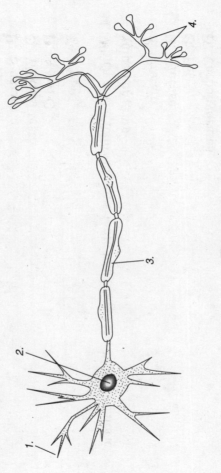

Figure 4.

80. Figure 4 illustrates a typical neuron. Which number on the figure indicates where impulses from other neurons are picked up?

   A. 1
   B. 2
   C. 3
   D. 4

81. Which of the following is NOT a neurotransmitter?

A. Albuterol
B. Serotonin
C. Acetylcholine
D. Norepinephrine

82. Which of the following is (are) responsible for the removal and destruction of erythrocytes?

A. Liver
B. Gallbladder
C. Kidneys
D. Pancreas

83. In humans, which of the following is (are) NOT vestigial in nature?

A. Appendix
B. Stomach
C. Wisdom teeth
D. A and C

84. Which of the following nutrients has (have) the highest caloric value per gram?

A. Protein
B. Glucose
C. Fat
D. Carbohydrates

85. In humans, which blood type is the universal recipient?

A. O
B. A
C. B
D. AB

86. Which of the following is (are) essential to blood clotting?

   A. Heparin
   B. Warfarin
   C. Thrombones
   D. Thromboplastin

87. Normal red blood cells have an average life span of

   A. 1 month.
   B. 4 months.
   C. 6 months.
   D. 9 months.

88. In humans, which blood type is the universal donor?

   A. A
   B. B
   C. AB
   D. O

89. The Rh factor in blood is a

   A. protein.
   B. carbohydrate.
   C. blood cell.
   D. nuclear acid.

90. How many chromosomes are normally found in a human cell?

   A. 23
   B. 46
   C. 92
   D. None of the above

91. If Y represents yellow (dominant color) and y represents green (recessive color), which of the following crosses would be expected to result in 75 percent yellow offspring?

   A. Yy × yy
   B. YY × yy
   C. Yy × Yy
   D. Yy × YY

92. If Y represents yellow (dominant color) and y represents green (recessive color), which of the following crosses would be expected to result in 50 percent green offspring?

    A. Yy × yy
    B. YY × yy
    C. Yy × Yy
    D. Yy × YY

93. Blue (B) is the dominant color for the Figbird, whereas white (w) is the alternative recessive color. When a homozygous blue bird is crossed with a homozygous white bird, what percentage of the offspring is expected to be white?

    A. 0
    B. 25
    C. 50
    D. 100

94. Blue (B) is the dominant color for the Figbird, whereas white (w) is the alternative recessive color. When a homozygous blue bird is crossed with a homozygous white bird, what percentage of the offspring is expected to be blue heterozygous?

    A. 0
    B. 25
    C. 50
    D. 100

95. Which of the following provide(s) daylight color vision and is (are) responsible for visual acuity?

    A. Rods
    B. Cones
    C. Optic disc
    D. Retina

96. The offspring of matings between two pure strains are called

    A. mutants.
    B. alleles.
    C. hybrids.
    D. genes.

97. A person who is heterozygous at the gene locus of a disorder, but shows no signs of the disorder, is called _____ of the disorder.

    A. an infector
    B. a carrier
    C. infectious
    D. a holder

98. Cystic fibrosis develops in individuals who inherit two copies of a recessive gene (c). If a man with cystic fibrosis marries a woman who does not have the disease but is a carrier of it, what percentage of their offspring is expected to have the disease?

    A. 0
    B. 25
    C. 50
    D. 75

99. Sickle-cell anemia develops in individuals who inherit two copies of a recessive gene(s). If a man with sickle-cell anemia marries a woman who does not have the disease but is a carrier of it, what percentage of their offspring is expected to have the disease or to be a carrier of it?

    A. 25
    B. 50
    C. 75
    D. 100

100. If green eyes are dominant and blue eyes are recessive, what percentage of the offspring can be expected to have blue eyes if one parent has green eyes and one parent has blue eyes?

    A. 0
    B. 25
    C. 50
    D. Cannot be determined from the information given

BIOLOGY ANSWER KEY

1. **D**	21. **C**	41. **A**	61. **B**	81. **A**
2. **C**	22. **B**	42. **D**	62. **A**	82. **A**
3. **C**	23. **C**	43. **C**	63. **D**	83. **B**
4. **A**	24. **D**	44. **B**	64. **C**	84. **C**
5. **B**	25. **B**	45. **D**	65. **A**	85. **D**
6. **C**	26. **D**	46. **D**	66. **C**	86. **D**
7. **D**	27. **B**	47. **A**	67. **D**	87. **B**
8. **D**	28. **C**	48. **D**	68. **B**	88. **D**
9. **A**	29. **D**	49. **B**	69. **B**	89. **A**
10. **C**	30. **C**	50. **D**	70. **D**	90. **B**
11. **D**	31. **C**	51. **A**	71. **B**	91. **C**
12. **B**	32. **C**	52. **C**	72. **D**	92. **A**
13. **A**	33. **B**	53. **D**	73. **A**	93. **A**
14. **A**	34. **A**	54. **B**	74. **C**	94. **D**
15. **B**	35. **A**	55. **D**	75. **D**	95. **B**
16. **D**	36. **A**	56. **C**	76. **D**	96. **C**
17. **C**	37. **B**	57. **A**	77. **D**	97. **B**
18. **D**	38. **D**	58. **D**	78. **D**	98. **C**
19. **A**	39. **B**	59. **D**	79. **C**	99. **D**
20. **B**	40. **C**	60. **D**	80. **A**	100. **D**

BIOLOGY EXPLANATORY ANSWERS

1. <u>Answer is **D**</u>. An animal cell has a plasma membrane (B) and a nucleus (C). Animal cells also have a nucleolus, endoplasmic reticulum, mitochondria, and ribosomes. Unlike a plant cell, an animal cell does not have a cell wall (A).

2. <u>Answer is **C**</u>. There are two different kinds of cells, prokaryotic (procaryotic) and eukaryotic (eucaryotic). Remember prokaryotic means *before the nucleus*, thus hinting that these cells were the first life forms. They existed roughly 3.5 billion years ago and are limited in size and complexity. The Monera Kingdom, which is mostly bacteria, is made of prokaryotic cells.

3. <u>Answer is **C**</u>. The Protista, Fungi, Plantae, and Animalia Kingdoms are made of eukaryotic cells. Remember, eukaryotic means *true nucleus*, thus suggesting that these cells constitute all organisms other than the bacteria and cyanobacteria (A). They have diameters of approximately 10–100 μm (B). Additionally, eukaryotic cells also differ from prokaryotic cells by having enclosed structures such as a nucleus and other organelles.

4. <u>Answer is **A**</u>. Mitochondria are organelles of the cell cytoplasm. Each consists of two sets of membranes, a smooth continuous outer coat and an inner membrane arranged in folds that form cristae. Mitochondria are sites for cellular respiration (A) and are the principal energy source of the cell. They are not directly involved in elimination (B), protection (C), or movement (D). Cilia and flagella provide cellular locomotion or movement.

5. <u>Answer is **B**</u>. Chromosomes (B) contain genetic instructions within the cell. The nuclear envelope (A) sets the nucleus apart from the rest of the cell and is made of two membranes that regulate the passage of molecules between the nucleus and the cytoplasm. The nucleoplasm (C) is the protoplasm of the cell nucleus. The nucleolus (D) is in the cell nucleus and produces ribonucleoprotein.

6. <u>Answer is **C**</u>. Both flagella (C) and cilia (B) provide cell locomotion. However, human sperm cells move by means of flagella.

7. Answer is **D**. Chloroplasts are found in plants and unicellular algae. They contain chlorophyll molecules and other pigments capable of capturing energy from sunlight. Remember, mitochondria (A) are the site for cellular respiration in the cell, and the cell wall (C) is found outside of the cell membrane of plants, fungi, bacteria, and plantlike protist cells. Choice (B) is irrelevant.

8. Answer is **D**. The nucleolus, a small, rounded mass in the cell nucleus, is where ribonucleoprotein is produced. See explanatory answer for question 5.

9. Answer is **A**. The nuclear envelope forms a boundary between the nucleus and cytoplasm. See explanatory answer for question 5.

10. Answer is **C**. Nucleoplasm, meaning protoplasm of the nucleus, is the fluid medium of the nucleus.

Figure 1 (Questions 11–14)

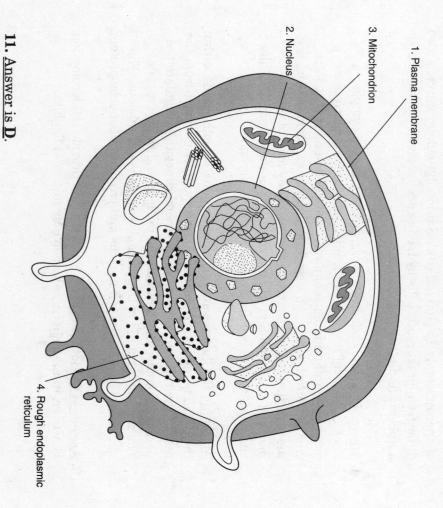

1. Plasma membrane

2. Nucleus

3. Mitochondrion

4. Rough endoplasmic reticulum

11. Answer is **D**.

12. Answer is **B**.

13. Answer is __A__.

14. Answer is __A__.

Figure 2 (Questions 15–18)

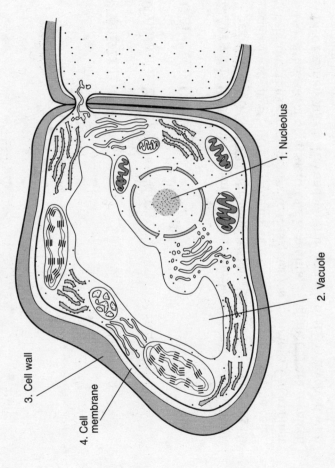

1. Nucleolus

2. Vacuole

3. Cell wall

4. Cell membrane

15. Answer is __B__.

16. Answer is __D__.

17. Answer is __C__.

18. Answer is __D__.

Figure 3 (Questions 19–21)

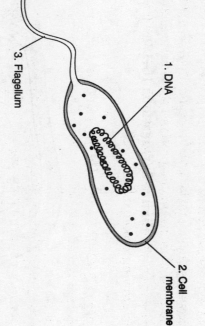

1. DNA

2. Cell membrane

3. Flagellum

19. Answer is **A**.

20. Answer is **B**.

21. Answer is **C**.

22. Answer is **B**. If you remember that mitochondria (B) are the cells' primary source of ATP (adenosine triphosphate) and ATP is associated with most energy-requiring reactions carried out by the cells, selecting the correct answer to this question is simple. Chloroplast (A) is the site of photosynthesis in plants. Flagella (C) are involved with cell movement. The endoplasmic reticulum (D) is involved with protein biosynthesis.

23. Answer is **C**. The nucleus of the cell is responsible for synthesizing RNA and DNA (C). Flagella and cilia are responsible for locomotion or mobility (D), and mitochondria are the primary source of cellular energy.

24. Answer is **D**. No explanation needed.

25. Answer is **B**. Plant, fungus, and some protist cells have cell walls.

26. Answer is **D**. An enzyme is a protein that acts as a catalyst (a catalyst regulates the rate of a reaction). The rate of enzyme activity is temperature and pH dependent.

27. Answer is **B**. Messenger RNA (mRNA) carries the code for the amino acid sequences of proteins from the genes of DNA out of the nucleus and into the cytoplasm. Each transfer RNA (A) carries an amino acid to a ribosome during protein synthesis, recognizes a codon of messenger RNA, and positions its amino acid for incorporation into the growing protein chain.

28. Answer is **C**. The sugar found in DNA is deoxyribose, and it is a 5-carbon sugar.

29. Answer is **D**. The nephron is the functional unit of the kidney. There are approximately one million nephrons per kidney.

30. Answer is **C**. Transcription (B) is the earlier step in protein synthesis. During transcription, RNA polymerase synthesizes a strand of RNA from the DNA template of the genes in the nucleus. The last step in protein synthesis is translation (C), whereby the sequence of messenger RNA nucleotides is converted into the sequence of amino acids of a protein. Choices A and D are irrelevant.

31. Answer is **C**. No explanation needed.

32. Answer is **C**. While DNA consists of a double strand, RNA is mostly single stranded (certain viruses are exceptions).

33. Answer is **B**. Meiosis is a process of cell division comprising two nuclear divisions in succession. It results in four gametocytes, each containing half the number of chromosomes (B) as the parent cell.

34. Answer is **A**. In a hypertonic medium (A), water will leave the cell. This will cause the cell to shrivel until the concentrations of water inside and outside the cell are equal. In a hypotonic medium (B), water will enter the cell, causing it to swell. In an isotonic medium (C), the concentrations of water and particles inside and outside the cell are equal; therefore, water does not leave or enter the cell. Choice D is irrelevant.

35. Answer is **A**. The stages of cellular division include prophase, metaphase, anaphase, and telophase. During prophase (C) the chromosomes condense, the nuclear membrane deteriorates, and the spindle microtubules attach to the chromosomes. During metaphase the chromosomes move to the center of the cell. During anaphase (A) each kinetochore divides, and the chromosomes separate. During telophase (D) the nuclear membrane reforms around each new daughter cell's nucleus.

36. <u>Answer is **A**</u>. The big distinction here is between the terms autotroph and heterotroph. Autotrophic organisms are capable of producing their own food. In contrast, heterotrophic organisms obtain their energy from organic compounds.

37. <u>Answer is **B**</u>. Since fungi obtain their energy from organic compounds, they are heterotrophic in nature. (See table in explanatory answer 38).

38. <u>Answer is **D**</u>. Characteristics used to separate organisms into the five kingdoms include cell type, number of cells in each organism, and the mechanism in which energy is acquired.

Kingdom	Cell Type	Cell Number	Energy Source
Monera	Prokaryotic	One, occasionally chains	Autotrophic Heterotrophic
Protista	Eukaryotic	One, occasionally chains	Autotrophic Heterotrophic
Fungi	Eukaryotic	Multicellular, occasionally unicellular	Heterotrophic
Plantae	Eukaryotic	Multicellular	Autotrophic
Animalia	Eukaryotic	Multicellular	Heterotrophic

39. <u>Answer is **B**</u>. Monerans are single-celled prokaryotes, and they are the simplest form of life. See table in explanatory answer 38.

40. <u>Answer is **C**</u>. No explanation needed.

41. <u>Answer is **A**</u>. In the bone remolding cycle, osteoclasts (A) are cells that remove bone, and osetoblasts (B) are cells that form bone. Choices C and D are irrelevant.

42. <u>Answer is **D**</u>. Both parathyroid hormone (A) and calcitonin (B) are involved in calcium homeostasis. Parathyroid hormone, secreted by the parathyroid glands, causes (1) bones to release calcium into the bloodstream, (2) the kidneys to conserve calcium lost through the urine, and (3) intestinal absorption of calcium. Calcitonin promotes a decrease in blood calcium, thereby antagonizing the effects of parathyroid hormone. Insulin (C) promotes glucose utilization and glycogen storage.

43. Answer is **C**. See explanatory answer for question 41.

44. Answer is **B**. Joints (B) are the place of union between two or more bones whereas cartilage (D) is a type of connective tissue with a solid elastic matrix. Choices A and C are irrelevant.

45. Answer is **D**. No explanation needed.

46. Answer is **D**. Blood in the circulatory system supplies nutrients and oxygen to tissues, removes waste material, and initiates clotting. Oxygen is supplied to the tissues primarily by the lungs and red blood cells. Erythrocytes (red blood cells) carry oxygen to the tissues' cells. In the lungs, oxygen from the inhaled air attaches to hemoglobin molecules within the erythrocytes and is transported to the cells for aerobic respiration. The lungs also eliminate carbon dioxide produced by cell respiration. Metabolic waste is filtered through the capillaries of the kidneys and excreted in urine. Platelets (thrombocytes) in the blood play a major role in blood clotting.

47. Answer is **A**. Hormones are secreted in the blood from a specific gland and are distributed by the blood to a specific target site. Blood (A), not choices B, C, or D, plays a role in the general distribution of hormones.

48. Answer is **D**. No explanation needed.

49. Answer is **B**. To answer this question correctly, it is important to remember two principles: (1) arteries carry blood away from the heart, while veins carry blood to the heart; and (2) the pulmonary circulation consists of blood vessels that transport blood to the lungs and then to the heart. Therefore, the correct choice is pulmonary veins (B), not pulmonary arteries (D). Choices A and C are irrelevant.

50. Answer is **D**. All of the statements are true (A, B, and C) except D. Approximately 55 percent, not 23 percent, of the blood is plasma.

51. Answer is **A**. No explanation needed.

52. Answer is **C**. Statements A, B, and D are correct. The only false statement is C. The life span of normal red blood cells is approximately 120 days, not 30 days.

53. Answer is **D**. White blood cells are called leukocytes. Neutrophils (A), eosinophils (B), basophils (C), lymphocytes, and monocytes are types of white blood cells.

54. Answer is **B**. No explanation needed.

55. Answer is **D**. No explanation needed.

56. Answer is **C**. Protein in the blood is composed of albumin and globulin, with albumin being the most abundant serum protein. The total quantity of albumin is two to three times the level of globulin. Choices A, B, and D are irrelevant.

57. Answer is **A**. No explanation needed.

58. Answer is **D**. No explanation needed.

59. Answer is **D**. Since hemoglobin in red blood cells transports oxygen and carbon dioxide to provide oxygen to the body's tissues, it should come as no surprise that factors affecting the affinity of hemoglobin for oxygen include the body's pH (acid-base level) and level of carbon dioxide present.

60. Answer is **D**. No explanation needed.

61. Answer is **B**. Glucose (A) and sodium (C) are reabsorbed in the kidney. However, creatinine is not absorbed by the kidneys, thereby making it a good indicator of renal function.

62. Answer is **A**. The liver is one of the largest, not the smallest (A), organs of the body. The other choices B, C, and D are true. The primary responsibilities of the liver include synthesizing and storing glycogen, detoxifying toxic substances in the blood, and synthesizing albumin.

63. Answer is **D**. The skin protects the body against damage (A), acts as a barrier (B), and aids in regulating the temperature of the body (C). The skin does not play a role in the production of hydrochloric acid (D).

64. Answer is **C**. The tarsal plates (A) are made of dense fibrous connective tissue and are important in maintaining the shape of the eyelids. The lacrimal gland (B) secretes lacrimal fluid through the ducts into the conjunctival sac of the upper eye. The answer is (C), the conjunctiva is the thin, mucus-secreting epithelial membrane that lines the interior surface of the eyelid.

65. Answer is **A**. Digestion begins far before food reaches the esophagus, stomach, or intestine. It begins in the mouth. Saliva in the mouth contains enzymes that digest fat and starch.

66. Answer is **C**. No explanation needed.

67. Answer is **D**. Fat-soluble vitamins include vitamins A, D, E, and K. B_1 is a water-soluble vitamin, not a fat-soluble vitamin.

68. Answer is **B**. All of the statements are true except B. Most nutrients are absorbed by the small intestines rather than the large intestines.

69. Answer is **B**. Amylase (A), lipase (C), and trypsin (D) are digestive enzymes. Amylase cleaves starch and glycogen, lipase cleaves fat, and trypsin hydrolyzes peptides and amides. Gastrin (B) is a hormone that stimulates the production of HCl (hydrochloric acid).

70. Answer is **D**. Vitamin E is a fat-soluble vitamin. Fat-soluble vitamins include vitamins A, D, E, and K. Thiamine (B_1), riboflavin (B_2), and folic acid (B_9) are water-soluble vitamins.

71. Answer is **B**. The gallbladder serves as a reservoir for bile (B). Bile aids in the emulsification of fats. The beta cells of the pancreas produce insulin (C), not the gallbladder. Choices A and D are irrelevant.

72. Answer is **D**. No explanation needed.

73. Answer is **A**. Bile salts enhance the intestinal absorption of fatty acids. The other three choices are involved in the digestion of food.

74. Answer is **C**. If an individual hyperventilates, a change in blood pH is likely to occur, thus ruling out choice A. To reason the correct solution, one must know that hyperventilation (rapid breathing) results in a loss of CO_2—thereby increasing blood pH. Therefore, choices B and D are incorrect.

75. Answer is **D**. The medulla oblongata controls autonomic respirations and functions of the cardiac centers (e.g., heartbeat) and the vasomotor center (e.g., arteriole wall constriction). Verbal communication is a function of the frontal lobe of the brain, not the medulla oblongata.

76. Answer is **D**. No explanation needed.

77. Answer is **D**. Testes, the male reproductive glands, are involved with the production of sperm (A) and testosterone (B). Prolactin, a hormone secreted from the hypothalamus, stimulates the secretion of milk.

78. Answer is **D**. No explanation needed.

79. Answer is **C**. No explanation needed.

80. Answer is **A**. Impulses from other neurons are picked up by dendrites (A).

81. Answer is **A**. A neurotransmitter is a specific chemical agent in the body released by presynaptic cells, upon excitation, that crosses the synapse to stimulate or inhibit the postsynaptic cells. Serotonin (B), acetylcholine (C), and norepinephrine (D) are neurotransmitters. On the other hand, albuterol (D) is not. Albuterol is a medication used to bronchodilate.

82. Answer is **A**. No explanation needed.

83. Answer is **B**. Although the stomach (B) is not vestigial (remnants of organs that do not serve a true function, but are believed to have served a function in the past), the appendix (A) and the wisdom teeth (C) are vestigial in nature.

84. Answer is **C**. No explanation needed.

85. Answer is **D**. Blood type AB (choice D) is the universal recipient, and blood type O (choice A) is the universal donor.

86. Answer is **D**. Thrombocytes, the blood-clotting cells, contain thromboplastin (D). Thromboplastin is essential to blood clotting. Choices A, B, and C are irrelevant.

87. Answer is **B**. Since the life span of normal red blood cells is approximately 120 days (4 months), the correct choice is B.

88. Answer is **D**. No explanation needed.

89. Answer is **A**. No explanation needed.

90. Answer is **B**. No explanation needed.

91. Answer is **C**. The best way to solve this problem is to find the cross that will most likely result in 75 percent yellow offspring given that yellow is dominant over green. After making your selection from the four possible choices, you should perform the cross by using a Punnett square. For example, let's cross choice C (Yy and Yy):

	Y	y
Y	YY	Yy
y	Yy	yy

YY = homozygous yellow;
Yy = heterozygous yellow;
yy = green

This cross will result in 75 percent yellow offspring.

To check the other choices, set up each of them in a Punnett square. Choice A will result in 50 percent yellow and 50 percent green. Choice B will result in 100 percent yellow offspring. Choice D will result in 100 percent yellow.

92. Answer is **A**. Similar to question 91, Choice A will result in:

	y	y
Y	Yy	Yy
y	yy	yy

Yy = yellow; yy = green

This cross will result in 50 percent green offspring.

93. Answer is **A**. A homozygous, having the same pair, blue bird is represented by BB, and a homozygous white bird is represented by ww. Cross the two in the following Punnett square:

	w	w
B	Bw	Bw
B	Bw	Bw

Bw = blue

A cross between a homozygous blue bird (BB) and a homozygous white bird (ww) will result in 0 percent white birds.

94. <u>Answer is **D**</u>. Follow the same procedure as in question 93:

	w	w
B	Bw	Bw
B	Bw	Bw

Bw = blue

A cross between a homozygous blue bird and a homozygous white bird will result in 100 percent blue heterozygous (Bw) birds.

95. <u>Answer is **B**</u>. Cones (B) provide daylight color vision and are responsible for visual acuity. Rods (A) respond to dim light for black-and-white vision. The optic disc (C) is a small region of the retina where the fibers of the ganglion neurons exit from the eyeball. The retina (D) is the inner layer of eyeball, and it contains the rods and cones.

96. <u>Answer is **C**</u>. No explanation needed.

97. <u>Answer is **B**</u>. No explanation needed.

98. <u>Answer is **C**</u>. Set up the cross between the individual carrying the disease (represented by Cc) and the individual with the disease (represented by cc = two recessive genes):

	C	c
c	Cc	cc
c	Cc	cc

Cc = do not have disease but are carriers;

cc = have the disease

Therefore, 50 percent will have the disease.

99. <u>Answer is **D**</u>. Similar to question 98, set up the cross between the individual carrying the disease (Ss) and the individual with the disease (ss):

	s	s
S	Ss	Ss
s	ss	ss

Ss = carrier of disease;
ss = have the disease

Therefore, 100 percent will either be a carrier or have the disease.

100. <u>Answer is **D**</u>. The percentage cannot be determined from the information given. You need to know if the parent is heterozygous green or homozygous green.

Inorganic and Organic Chemistry Review and Practice

TIPS FOR THE CHEMISTRY SECTION

The Chemistry section of the PCAT consists of approximately 60 questions. Both inorganic and organic chemistry questions are asked. "Watch" the time, and answer every question.

INORGANIC CHEMISTRY REVIEW OUTLINE

I. **Matter and the Periodic Table**
    A. Three states of matter
       1. Solid
       2. Liquid
       3. Gas
    B. Chemical and physical properties
    C. Elements, compounds, and mixtures
    D. Metals and nonmetals
    E. Electrolytes and nonelectrolytes
    F. Sizes of atoms
    G. Electronegativity
    H. Phase changes

II.   Simple mathematics

A. Density

B. Percent composition

C. Average atomic weight

D. Conversions (e.g., English and metric systems; see Appendix)

III.   Atomic structure

A. Atomic particles

   1. Protons

   2. Neutrons

   3. Electrons

B. Atomic number

C. Atomic mass (atomic weight)

D. Molecular weight

E. Formula weight

F. Isotopes

G. Allotropes

H. Moles and Avogadro's number

IV.   Oxidation and reduction

A. Oxidation number

B. Formal charge

C. Oxidizing agents

D. Reducing agents

V.   Balancing equations

A. Simple equations

B. Redox equations

VI.   Solutions

A. Concentration

   1. Molarity

   2. Molality

   3. Percent composition

   4. Mole fraction

B. Dilution of solutions

C. Colligative properties

   1. Depression of vapor pressure

   2. Elevation of boiling point

   3. Depression of freezing point

   4. Osmosis

D. Solubility rules

VII. Gas laws
   A. Boyle's law
   B. Charles' law
   C. Ideal gas law
   D. Dalton's law of partial pressure
   E. Real gases
   F. Effusion and diffusion

VIII. Bonding
   A. Ionic
   B. Covalent
   C. Polar covalent
   D. Intermolecular forces
      1. Hydrogen bonding
      2. Van der Waals forces

IX. Stoichiometry and equations
   A. Molar relationships
   B. Volume relationships
   C. Limiting reagent
   D. Percent yield

X. Nomenclature and writing formulas

XI. Molecular geometry
   A. Hybridization
   B. Bond angles
   C. Dipole moment

XII. Resonance

XIII. Electromagnetic spectrum
   A. Quantum theory and quantum numbers
   B. Electron configuration
   C. Lewis dot structures

XIV. Calorimetry
   A. Specific heat
   B. Heat capacity

XV. Acids and bases
   A. Definitions—Arrhenius, Brönsted-Lowry (conjugate
      pairs), Lewis
   B. Strengths of acids and bases

C. pH
D. Neutralization
E. Buffers
F. Acidic, basic, and amphoteric oxides

XVI. Kinetics

A. First-order reactions
B. Second-order reactions
C. Half-life
D. Determination of reaction orders
E. Graphs

XVII. Equilibrium

A. Equilibrium constants
   1. Acid
   2. Base
   3. Solubility product
   4. Complex ion formation
B. Le Châtelier's principle

XVIII. Electrochemistry

A. Electrolytic and galvanic cells
B. Oxidation and reduction
C. Anode and cathode

XIX. Radioactivity

A. Nuclear particles
B. Balancing equations
C. Fission
D. Fusion

ORGANIC CHEMISTRY REVIEW OUTLINE

I. **Formulas for families**
   A. RCOOH, carboxylic acid, etc.
   B. General (e.g., C_nH_n)
   C. Empirical, molecular, and structural formulas

II. **Physical properties of various organic families**

III. **Nomenclature**

IV. **Isomerism**
   A. Geometric
   B. Optical
      1. Enantiomer
      2. Diastereomer
      3. Stereocenter
      4. Racemic mixture

V. **Examples of simple reactions**
   A. Oxidation
   B. Addition
   C. Dehydration
   D. Reduction
   E. Esterification
   F. Elimination
   G. Nucleophilic substitution
   H. Free-radical substitution

VI. **Structures of biomolecules**
   A. Lipids
   B. Carbohydrates
   C. Proteins

VII. **Resonance—benzene**

CHEMISTRY ANSWER SHEET

1 (A) (B) (C) (D)
2 (A) (B) (C) (D)
3 (A) (B) (C) (D)
4 (A) (B) (C) (D)
5 (A) (B) (C) (D)
6 (A) (B) (C) (D)
7 (A) (B) (C) (D)
8 (A) (B) (C) (D)
9 (A) (B) (C) (D)
10 (A) (B) (C) (D)
11 (A) (B) (C) (D)
12 (A) (B) (C) (D)
13 (A) (B) (C) (D)
14 (A) (B) (C) (D)
15 (A) (B) (C) (D)
16 (A) (B) (C) (D)
17 (A) (B) (C) (D)
18 (A) (B) (C) (D)
19 (A) (B) (C) (D)
20 (A) (B) (C) (D)

21 (A) (B) (C) (D)
22 (A) (B) (C) (D)
23 (A) (B) (C) (D)
24 (A) (B) (C) (D)
25 (A) (B) (C) (D)
26 (A) (B) (C) (D)
27 (A) (B) (C) (D)
28 (A) (B) (C) (D)
29 (A) (B) (C) (D)
30 (A) (B) (C) (D)
31 (A) (B) (C) (D)
32 (A) (B) (C) (D)
33 (A) (B) (C) (D)
34 (A) (B) (C) (D)
35 (A) (B) (C) (D)
36 (A) (B) (C) (D)
37 (A) (B) (C) (D)
38 (A) (B) (C) (D)
39 (A) (B) (C) (D)
40 (A) (B) (C) (D)

41 (A) (B) (C) (D)
42 (A) (B) (C) (D)
43 (A) (B) (C) (D)
44 (A) (B) (C) (D)
45 (A) (B) (C) (D)
46 (A) (B) (C) (D)
47 (A) (B) (C) (D)
48 (A) (B) (C) (D)
49 (A) (B) (C) (D)
50 (A) (B) (C) (D)
51 (A) (B) (C) (D)
52 (A) (B) (C) (D)
53 (A) (B) (C) (D)
54 (A) (B) (C) (D)
55 (A) (B) (C) (D)
56 (A) (B) (C) (D)
57 (A) (B) (C) (D)
58 (A) (B) (C) (D)
59 (A) (B) (C) (D)
60 (A) (B) (C) (D)

61 (A) (B) (C) (D)
62 (A) (B) (C) (D)
63 (A) (B) (C) (D)
64 (A) (B) (C) (D)
65 (A) (B) (C) (D)
66 (A) (B) (C) (D)
67 (A) (B) (C) (D)
68 (A) (B) (C) (D)
69 (A) (B) (C) (D)
70 (A) (B) (C) (D)
71 (A) (B) (C) (D)
72 (A) (B) (C) (D)
73 (A) (B) (C) (D)
74 (A) (B) (C) (D)
75 (A) (B) (C) (D)
76 (A) (B) (C) (D)
77 (A) (B) (C) (D)
78 (A) (B) (C) (D)
79 (A) (B) (C) (D)
80 (A) (B) (C) (D)

81 (A) (B) (C) (D)
82 (A) (B) (C) (D)
83 (A) (B) (C) (D)
84 (A) (B) (C) (D)
85 (A) (B) (C) (D)
86 (A) (B) (C) (D)
87 (A) (B) (C) (D)
88 (A) (B) (C) (D)
89 (A) (B) (C) (D)
90 (A) (B) (C) (D)
91 (A) (B) (C) (D)
92 (A) (B) (C) (D)
93 (A) (B) (C) (D)
94 (A) (B) (C) (D)
95 (A) (B) (C) (D)
96 (A) (B) (C) (D)
97 (A) (B) (C) (D)
98 (A) (B) (C) (D)
99 (A) (B) (C) (D)
100 (A) (B) (C) (D)

CHEMISTRY PRACTICE QUESTIONS

100 Questions

<u>Directions</u>: Select the best answer to each of the following questions.

1. Which of the following statements describes a chemical property?

   A. Liquid water is converted to water vapor by application of heat.
   B. Salt, NaCl, dissolves in water.
   C. A stone displaces its volume in a liquid.
   D. Milk sours more readily at room temperature than in the refrigerator.

2. Which of the following substances is a pure element?

   A. Salt
   B. Water
   C. Gold
   D. Brass

3. A sample of metal, weighing 5.5 grams, is placed in a graduated cylinder containing 15.5 milliliters of water. The volume of water increases to 20 milliliters. What is the density, in grams per milliliter, of the metal?

   A. 1.22
   B. 0.35
   C. 0.28
   D. 1.06

4. How many minutes are there in 1 week?

   A. 1.01×10^4
   B. 1.75×10^4
   C. 2.06×10^4
   D. 2.80×10^4

5. Given the following equation:

$$°C = \frac{5°C}{9°F} \ (°F - 32 \ °F)$$

convert $-10°F$ to $°C$.

A. -12
B. -26
C. -23
D. -37

6. How many neutrons are contained in the following atom of the element scandium: $^{45}_{21}Sc$?

A. 21
B. 66
C. 45
D. 24

7. Calculate the average atomic mass, in atomic mass units (amu), of the fictional element pharmaceia, Ph, given the following data:

Element	Atomic Mass of Isotope of Ph	Relative Abundance of Isotope of Ph
Ph	30 amu	20.0%
Ph	32 amu	80.0%

A. 30.5
B. 31.0
C. 31.6
D. 31.9

8. The mass of 1 mole of copper, (Cu), atoms equals 63.55 grams. What is the weight, in grams, of one atom of Cu?

[Avogadro's number = 6×10^{23}]

A. 1.06×10^{-24}
B. 9.47×10^{-23}
C. 9.47×10^{-21}
D. 1.06×10^{-22}

9. Calculate the formula weight, in atomic mass units (amu), of the salt ammonium sulfate, $(NH_4)_2SO_4$. ($S = 32$ amu, $O = 16$ amu, $N = 14$ amu, $H = 1$ amu)

A. 72
B. 132
C. 128
D. 114

10. What is the percentage of hydrogen, H, present in ammonium sulfate, $(NH_4)_2SO_4$? ($S = 32$ amu, $O = 16$ amu, $N = 14$ amu, $H = 1$ amu)

A. 11
B. 6
C. 3
D. 4

11. What is the correct formula for hypochlorous acid?

A. $HClO_3$
B. HCl
C. $HClO$
D. $HClO_2$

12. When the following equation is balanced with the smallest set of whole numbers, what is the coefficient of H_2SO_4?

___ Na_2CO_3 + ___ H_2SO_4 ⟶ ___ $NaHSO_4$ + ___ H_2O + ___ CO_2

A. 1
B. 2
C. 3
D. 5

13. What is the oxidation number of sulfur, S, in H_2SO_3?

A. 2
B. 4
C. 5
D. 6

14. What is the reducing agent in the following equation?

$$Zn + CuSO_4 \longrightarrow ZnSO_4 + Cu$$

A. Zn
B. $CuSO_4$
C. $ZnSO_4$
D. Cu

15. When the following equation is balanced with the smallest set of numbers, what is the coefficient of Fe^{3+}?

$$\_Fe^{2+} + \_MnO_4^{-1} + \_H^+ \longrightarrow \_Fe^{3+} + \_Mn^{2+} + \_H_2O$$

A. 1
B. 4
C. 5
D. 8

16. In the following reaction, how many moles of O_2 are necessary to react with 5 moles of NH_3? ($O = 16$ amu, $N = 14$ amu, $H = 1$ amu)

$$4NH_3 + 5O_2 \longrightarrow 4NO + 6H_2O$$

A. 4.0
B. 5.0
C. 5.5
D. 6.3

17. How many liters of oxygen gas, O_2, will react completely with 3.5 liters of carbon disulfide gas, CS_2, in the following reaction?

$$CS_2 + 2O_2 \longrightarrow CO_2 + 2SO_2$$

A. 14.0
B. 3.5
C. 7.0
D. 1.8

18. In the following reaction, how many grams of NO are produced from 17.0 g of NH_3? ($O = 16$ amu, $N = 14$ amu, $H = 1$ amu)

$$4NH_3 + 5O_2 \longrightarrow 4NO + 6H_2O$$

A. 5.7
B. 30
C. 17
D. 170

19. In the following reaction, how many liters of NO are produced from 1.70 g of NH_3 at standard temperature and pressure conditions? ($O = 16$ amu, $N = 14$ amu, $H = 1$ amu)

$$4 NH_3 + 5 O_2 \longrightarrow 4 NO + 6 H_2O$$

- **A.** 2.24
- **B.** 1.70
- **C.** 8.96
- **D.** 0.026

20. In the following reaction, how many molecules of NO are produced from 0.17 g of NH_3? ($O = 16$ amu, $N = 14$ amu, $H = 1$ amu)

$$4 NH_3 + 5 O_2 \longrightarrow 4 NO + 6 H_2O$$

- **A.** 6.0×10^{21}
- **B.** 1.4×10^{22}
- **C.** 4.0×10^{23}
- **D.** 2.9×10^{23}

21. A 100-milliliter sample of oxygen, O_2, is collected over water at 25°C and 750 mmHg pressure. The pressure of water vapor at 25°C is 23.76 mmHg. Which of the following equations is correct to calculate the number of grams of oxygen collected? ($R = 0.082$ L-atm/K-mole)

A. $750 \, mm (100 \, ml) = \dfrac{x}{16 \, g/mole} \left(\dfrac{0.082 \, \text{L-atm}}{\text{K-mole}} \right) (25°C)$

B. $\dfrac{726.24 \, mm (100 \, ml)}{760 \, mm/atm} = \dfrac{x}{16 \, g/mole} \left(\dfrac{0.082 \, \text{L-atm}}{\text{K-mole}} \right) (25°C)$

C. $\dfrac{750 \, mm (100 \, ml)}{760 \, mm/atm} = \dfrac{x}{32 \, g/mole} \left(\dfrac{0.082 \, \text{L-atm}}{\text{K-mole}} \right) (298K)$

D. $\dfrac{726.24 \, mm (0.100 \, liter)}{760 \, mm/atm} = \dfrac{x}{32 \, g/mole} \left(\dfrac{0.082 \, \text{L-atm}}{\text{K-mole}} \right) (298K)$

E. $726.24 \, mm (100 \, ml) = \dfrac{x}{16 \, g/mole} \left(\dfrac{0.082 \, \text{L-atm}}{\text{K-mole}} \right) (25°C)$

22. What is the molarity (M) of a solution prepared by dissolving 1.8 grams of sugar, $C_6H_{12}O_6$, in 1000 milliliters of solution? (O = 16 amu, C = 12 amu, H = 1 amu)

   A. 0.01

   B. 1.80

   C. 0.0018

   D. 0.10

23. How many grams of oxygen gas are present in a bulb of volume 2.0 liters, at 7°C and 1 atmosphere? (R = 0.082 liter-atm/mole-K, O = 16 amu)

   A. 1.30

   B. 112

   C. 2.60

   D. 55.8

24. How many milliliters of 5.0 M, sodium hydroxide, NaOH, solution must be used to prepare 200 milliliters of 2.5 M solution?

   A. 440

   B. 36

   C. 500

   D. 100

25. How many moles of sulfuric acid, H_2SO_4, are needed to neutralize 1.5 moles of sodium hydroxide, NaOH, according to the following equation?

$H_2SO_4 + 2NaOH \longrightarrow Na_2SO_4 + 2H_2O$

   A. 3.0

   B. 0.75

   C. 2.0

   D. 0.50

26. How many milliliters of 2.0 M lithium hydroxide, LiOH, solution are necessary to neutralize 10 milliliters of 3.0 M sulfuric acid, H_2SO_4, according to the following equation?

$$2\,LiOH + H_2SO_4 \longrightarrow Li_2SO_4 + 2H_2O$$

A. 60
B. 30
C. 15
D. 12

27. A bubble of gas (1.2 mL) is at the bottom of a lake where the temperature and pressure are 7°C and 2.8 atmosphere, respectively. The temperature and pressure at the surface of the lake are 27°C and 1.0 atmosphere. What is the volume, in milliliters, of a gas bubble at the surface of the lake?

A. 1.6
B. 3.6
C. 0.5
D. 13.0

28. Ammonia, NH_3, and oxygen, O_2, are gases at standard temperature and pressure. They are combined to produce nitrous oxide gas, NO, and water vapor. How many liters of NO can be produced at 27°C and 0.80 atmospheres from 1.7 g of NH_3? (O = 16 amu,

$$N = 14\ \text{amu},\ H = 1\ \text{amu}\left(R = 0.082\ \frac{\text{L-atm}}{\text{K-mole}}\right)$$

$$4NH_3 + 5O_2 \longrightarrow 4NO + 6H_2O$$

A. 4.4
B. 3.1
C. 5.8
D. 2.7

29. Two gases—oxygen, O_2, and hydrogen, H_2—effuse (escape from one part of a container to another part by passing through a small hole). What is the rate of effusion of hydrogen as compared to that of oxygen at the same temperature and pressure? (O = 16 amu, H = 1 amu)

A. 16.0
B. 0.25
C. 4.00
D. 0.06

30. Gases obey the ideal gas laws most closely under what conditions of temperature and pressure?

A. High temperature and high pressure
B. High temperature and low pressure
C. Low temperature and high pressure
D. Low temperature and low pressure

31. The specific heat of copper, Cu, is 0.385 joule per gram-°C. What is the heat capacity, in joules per °C, of 10.0 grams of copper?

A. 0.03
B. 15.4
C. 3.85
D. 38.9

32. The wavelength of a light wave is 150 nanometers. What is its frequency, in cycles per second? (The speed of light is 3.00×10^8 m/s.)

A. 2.0×10^{-3}
B. 2.0×10^{15}
C. 5.0×10^{16}
D. 5.0×10^{-3}

Use the small portion of the periodic table below in order to answer questions 33–47.

H							He
Li	Be	B	C	N	O	F	Ne
Na	Mg	Al	Si	P	S	Cl	Ar

33. Which of the following substances would NOT be expected to conduct electricity?

A. Al
B. Li
C. Cl
D. Na

34. Which of the following is a possible set of quantum numbers for the last electron added to an atom of aluminum, Al?

	n	l	m_l	m_s
A.	3	2	–1	$+\frac{1}{2}$
B.	3	1	2	$-\frac{1}{2}$
C.	3	3	–1	$+\frac{1}{2}$
D.	3	2	3	$+\frac{1}{2}$

35. The electron configuration for the sulfide ion, S^{2-}, is

A. $1s^2 2s^2 2p^6 3s^2 3p^6$.
B. $1s^2 2s^2 2p^6 3s^2 3p^4$.
C. $1s^2 2s^2 2p^6 3s^2 3p^2$.
D. $1s^2 2s^2 2p^6 3s^2 3p^6 4s^2$.

36. In which of the following are the sizes of the atoms listed in the correct order?

A. Li < B < F
B. Cl < Si < Na
C. Na < Li < Be
D. Cl < F < O

37. What is the maximum number of electrons possible in the p orbitals of an atom?

A. 6
B. 10
C. 5
D. 3

38. The elements are arranged in the periodic table according to increasing

   A. atomic mass.
   B. number of neutrons.
   C. number of protons.
   D. number of protons plus neutrons.

39. How many electrons are represented around the phosphorus ion, P^{3-}, in a Lewis dot symbol?

   A. 15
   B. 8
   C. 5
   D. 3

40. What is the formal charge on the carbon atom in the carbonate ion, CO_3^{2-}, when the Lewis structure has two single bonds and one double bond drawn to the central carbon atom?

   A. 0
   B. +1
   C. –1
   D. +4

41. The compound with the greatest amount of ionic bonding character is

   A. CO_2
   B. LiO
   C. CH_4
   D. NH_3

42. What is the molecular geometry of the silicon hydride, SiH_4, molecule?

   A. Linear
   B. Bent
   C. Tetrahedral
   D. Trigonal pyramid

43. What is the approximate value of the bond angle for the H-S-H bond in hydrogen sulfide, H_2S?

A. 105°
B. 120°
C. 180°
D. 90°

44. What is the hybridization state of the aluminum, Al, atom in $AlCl_3$?

A. sp
B. sp^2
C. sp^3
D. sp^3d^2

45. Which of the following elements has the greatest electronegativity value?

A. Al
B. Cs
C. F
D. Li

46. Which of the following bonds is a strongly polar covalent bond?

A. C-C
B. Li-Cl
C. H-F
D. B-C

47. Which of the following molecules has a dipole moment of zero?

A. CO_2
B. H_2O
C. HF
D. NH_3

48. Which of the following oxides is a basic oxide?

A. CO_2
B. K_2O
C. SO_2
D. P_2O_5

49. How many resonance structures are possible for the carbonate ion, CO_3^{2-}, when the Lewis structure has one double bond and two single bonds drawn to the central carbon atom?

A. 1
B. 2
C. 3
D. 4

50. Which of the following compounds has fewer than eight outer shell electrons around the underlined atom?

A. $\underline{H}_2O$
B. $\underline{C}H_4$
C. $\underline{P}F_5$
D. $\underline{Be}F_2$

51. Which of the following compounds has more than eight outer shell electrons around the underlined atom?

A. $\underline{H}_2O$
B. $\underline{C}H_4$
C. $\underline{P}F_5$
D. $\underline{Be}F_2$

52. Which of the following solutes dissolved in water will elevate the boiling temperature of the water to the greatest extent?

A. 1 mole of sugar, $C_6H_{12}O_6$
B. 1 mole of sodium chloride, $NaCl$
C. 1 mole of calcium carbonate, $CaCO_3$
D. 1 mole of sodium sulfate, Na_2SO_4

53. What is the freezing point, in degrees Celsius, of 100 grams of H_2O containing 1.8 grams of sugar, $C_6H_{12}O_6$?

(K_f for $H_2O = 1.86°C$ / m; O = 16 amu, C = 12 amu, H = 1 amu)

A. +0.372
B. −0.00186
C. −0.186
D. +0.00186

54. The initial concentration of a reactant in a first-order reaction having a rate constant of 3.5×10^{-2} per second is 0.50 M. What is the molarity of the reactant after 5 minutes?

A. 0.42
B. 0.60
C. 1.8×10^4
D. 1.4×10^{-5}

55. What is the half life, in seconds, for a first-order reaction having a rate constant of 6.93×10^2 per second?

A. $1.0 \times 10^{+1}$
B. 1.0×10^{-3}
C. 1.0×10^{-1}
D. $1.0 \times 10^{+5}$

56. In a second-order reaction, a straight line is obtained by plotting which of the following expressions of concentration, A, versus time, t?

A. ln A vs. t
B. $1/A$ vs. t
C. A vs. t
D. ln $1/A$ vs. t

57. The rate law for the following reaction:

$$A + B \longrightarrow C + D$$

is given below:

Rate = $k [A][B]^2$

The overall order of this reaction is

A. zero order.

B. first order.

C. second order.

D. third order.

58. What is the equilibrium constant for the following reaction when $[H_2] = 0.50$ M, $[I_2] = 0.60$ M and $[HI] = 0.80$ M?

$$H_2 + I_2 \longleftrightarrow 2HI$$

A. 2.1

B. 2.7

C. 0.38

D. 0.47

59. Which of the following changes will NOT cause the reaction equilibrium shown below to shift toward the products on the right?

$$Heat + N_2O_4(g) \longleftrightarrow 2NO_2(g)$$

A. A decrease in temperature

B. Addition of more N_2O_4

C. Removal of some NO_2

D. An increase in temperature

60. Which of the following changes will cause the reaction equilibrium shown below to shift toward the products on the right?

$$Heat + N_2O_4(g) \longleftrightarrow 2 NO_2(g)$$

A. A decrease in pressure

B. Addition of a catalyst

C. A decrease in temperature

D. An increase in pressure

61. A Brönsted-Lowry acid, by definition, is a substance that

- **A.** accepts a share in an electron pair.
- **B.** forms a hydrogen ion when dissolved in water.
- **C.** donates a proton.
- **D.** donates a share in an electron pair.

62. Which of the following is NOT a Brönsted-Lowry acid?

- **A.** HCl
- **B.** Ag^+
- **C.** H_2O
- **D.** HCO_3^{2-}

63. In which of the following are the compounds listed correctly in the order of their strength as acids, (with the strongest acid first and the weakest acid last)?

- **A.** $CH_4 > NH_3 > H_2O > HF$
- **B.** $HF > H_2O > NH_3 > CH_4$
- **C.** $NH_3 > H_2O > HF > CH_4$
- **D.** $HF > NH_3 > CH_4 > H_2O$

64. In which of the following are the acids listed correctly in the order of their acidity, with the weakest acid first and the strongest acid last?

- **A.** $HClO < HClO_3 < HClO_2 < HClO_4$
- **B.** $HClO < HClO_2 < HClO_3 < HClO_4$
- **C.** $HClO_4 < HClO_3 < HClO_2 < HClO$
- **D.** $HClO_4 < HClO < HClO_2 < HClO_3$

65. What is the pH of a solution having a hydroxide ion concentration, $[OH^-]$, equal to 0.01 M?

- **A.** 2
- **B.** 10
- **C.** 12
- **D.** 14

66. Which of the following reactions will produce an acidic solution?

    A. Strong acid with strong base

    B. Weak acid with strong base

    C. Strong acid with weak base

    D. Weak acid with weak base

67. Which of the following oxides is an amphoteric oxide?

    A. Li_2O

    B. Al_2O_3

    C. N_2O_5

    D. I_2O_7

68. Which of the following is **not** a Lewis acid?

    A. $HCO_3{}^{-1}$

    B. $AlCl_3$

    C. BI_3

    D. Li^+

69. What is the conjugate base of $NH_4{}^+$ in the following reaction?

$$NH_3 + H_2O \longleftrightarrow NH_4{}^+ + OH^{-1}$$

    A. NH_3

    B. H_2O

    C. OH^{-1}

    D. None of the above

70. What is the hydroxide ion concentration, $[OH^{-1}]$, in 2.50 M $Mg(OH)_2$?

    A. 2.50 M

    B. 1.25 M

    C. 5.00 M

    D. 7.25 M

71. When the solution of a complex ion appears red, what is the color of the wavelength of the light absorbed?

A. Yellow
B. Violet
C. Green
D. Blue

72. What is the pH of a 1.0 M solution of acetic acid, HAc? K_A for acetic acid = 1.8×10^{-5}

A. 2.37
B. 1.40
C. 4.74
D. 4.57

73. If the value of K_A for acetic acid, HAc, is 1.8×10^{-5}, what is the value of K_B for the acetate ion, Ac^-?

A. 5.6×10^{-10}
B. 5.6×10^{-8}
C. 1.8×10^{-8}
D. 1.8×10^{-9}

74. Which of the following weak acids is the strongest acid? (The ionization constants are given.)

	K_A
A. Benzoic acid	6.5×10^{-5}
B. Nitrous acid	4.5×10^{-4}
C. Formic acid	1.7×10^{-4}
D. Acetic acid	1.8×10^{-5}

75. How many minutes are there in 1 day?

A. 1440
B. 1660
C. 2440
D. 2660

76. Which of the following compounds is insoluble in water?

    A. NaOH
    B. NH_4Cl
    C. $LiNO_3$
    D. $CaCO_3$

77. The solubility product constant, K_{sp}, for silver chloride, AgCl, is 1.6×10^{-10}. What is the solubility, in moles per liter, of AgCl in water?

    A. 1.3×10^{-10}
    B. 1.6×10^{-5}
    C. 1.6×10^{-10}
    D. 1.3×10^{-5}

78. Which of the following slightly soluble salts is the most soluble? (The solubility product constants are given)

	K_{sp}
A. Copper (II) sulfide	6.0×10^{-37}
B. Nickel (II) sulfide	1.4×10^{-24}
C. Silver chloride	1.6×10^{-10}
D. Lead (II) chromate	2.0×10^{-14}

79. Which of the following complex ions is the most stable? (The formation constants, K_f, are given)

	K_f
A. $Ag(NH_3)_2^{+1}$	1.5×10^7
B. $Zn(NH_3)_4^{2+}$	2.0×10^9
C. HgI_4^{2-}	2.0×10^{30}
D. $Cd(CN)_4^{2-}$	7.1×10^{16}

80. Which of the following salts—copper bromide, CuBr; copper iodide, CuI; copper hydroxide, $Cu(OH)_2$; copper sulfide, CuS—will be much more soluble in acidic solution than in neutral water?

    A. CuBr, CuI, $Cu(OH)_2$, CuS
    B. CuBr, CuI, $Cu(OH)_2$
    C. $Cu(OH)_2$, CuS
    D. CuS

81. In which of the following solutions will aluminum hydroxide, $Al(OH)_3$, be the LEAST soluble?

A. H_2O

B. 0.5 M $Al(NO_3)_3$

C. 1.6 M NaOH

D. 0.3 M HCl

Use the following table of standard reduction potentials to answer questions 82–84.

		emf°
Li^+ (aq) + e^- $\longrightarrow$ Li (s)		-3.05
Ca^{2+} (aq) + $2e^-$ $\longrightarrow$ Ca (s)		-2.87
Zn^{2+} (aq) + $2e^-$ $\longrightarrow$ Zn (s)		-0.76
Sn^{+2} (aq) + $2e^-$ $\longrightarrow$ Sn (s)		-0.14
$2 H^+$ (aq) + $2e^-$ $\longrightarrow$ H_2 (g)		0.00
Cu^{2+} (aq) + $2e^-$ $\longrightarrow$ Cu (s)		$+0.34$
Fe^{3+} (aq) + e^- $\longrightarrow$ Fe^{2+}		$+0.77$
Br_2 (ℓ) + $2e^-$ $\longrightarrow$ $2 Br^{-1}$		$+1.07$

82. Which of the following reactions would have to be carried out in an electrolytic cell rather than a voltaic cell?

A. $Zn(s) + Cu^{2+} \longrightarrow Zn^{2+} + Cu$ (s)

B. $Sn(s) + 2 H^+ \longrightarrow Sn^{2+} + H_2$ (g)

C. $2 Fe^{3+} + 2 Br^- \longrightarrow 2 Fe^{2+} + Br_2$ (g)

D. $2 Li(s) + Ca^{2+} \longrightarrow Ca(s) + 2 Li^+$

83. In the following overall reaction:

$$Zn (s) + Cu^{+2} \longrightarrow Zn^{2+} + Cu (s)$$

which partial reaction shows the reagent that is oxidized?

A. Zn^{2+} (aq) + $2e^-$ $\longrightarrow$ Zn (s)

B. Cu^{2+} (aq) + $2e^-$ $\longrightarrow$ Cu (s)

C. Zn (s) $\longrightarrow$ Zn^{2+} (aq) + $2e^-$

D. Cu (s) $\longrightarrow$ Cu^{2+} (aq) + $2e^-$

84. Which of the following species is the strongest reducing agent?

A. Li^+
B. Br_2
C. Br^{-1}
D. Li

85. Which of the following statements describes the reaction which occurs at the cathode in an electrochemical cell?

A. The cathode is the electrode at which electrons are lost and oxidation occurs.
B. The cathode is the electrode at which electrons are lost and reduction occurs.
C. The cathode is the electrode at which electrons are gained and oxidation occurs.
D. The cathode is the electrode at which electrons are gained and reduction occurs.

86. The general formula RCOOH is the formula for

A. an aldehyde.
B. a ketone.
C. an ester.
D. a carboxylic acid.

87. What is the general formula for a cycloalkane?

A. C_nH_{2n+2}
B. C_nH_{2n}
C. C_nH_n
D. C_nH_{2n-2}

88. Which of the following formulas represents an unsaturated compound?

A. C_2H_6
B. C_3H_6
C. C_2H_6O
D. CH_3Cl

89. How many different structural isomers can be formed by the compound having the molecular formula C_4H_9Cl?

- **A.** 1
- **B.** 2
- **C.** 3
- **D.** 4

90. How many different compounds can be formed by the monochlorination of C_2H_5Cl?

- **A.** 2
- **B.** 3
- **C.** 4
- **D.** 5

91. What is the name of the following compound?

$$CH_3 - CH_2 - CH_2 - CH - CH - CH - CH_3$$
$$\qquad\qquad\qquad\qquad Br \quad CH_3 \quad CH_2 - CH_3$$

- **A.** 5-Bromo-3,4-dimethyloctane
- **B.** 4-Bromo-2-ethyl-3-methylheptane
- **C.** 4-Bromo-6-ethyl-5-methylheptane
- **D.** 4-Bromo-5,6-dimethyloctane

92. A stereocenter is one to which are attached

- **A.** four groups that are the same.
- **B.** three groups that are the same, one group that is different.
- **C.** four groups that are different.
- **D.** two groups that are the same, and another two groups which are the same yet different from the first two groups.

93. The two formulas shown below represent

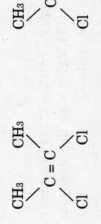

- **A.** geometric isomers.
- **B.** a racemic mixture.
- **C.** enantiomers.
- **D.** diastereomers.

94. The carbon atom in methane, CH_4, has the hybridization

A. sp.
B. sp^2.
C. sp^3.
D. sp^3d^2.

95. The carbon atom in ethylene, $H_2C = CH_2$, has the hybridization

A. sp.
B. sp^2.
C. sp^3.
D. sp^3d^2.

96. Oxidation of the secondary alcohol 2-propanol:

$$CH_3 - CH - CH_3$$
$$|$$
$$OH$$

yields

A. ethanol.
B. propanone.
C. propanal.
D. dimethyl ether.

97. Which of the following compounds is the most water soluble?

A. Ethyl ether, $CH_3CH_2OCH_2CH_3$
B. Ethyl chloride, CH_3CH_2Cl
C. Ethane, CH_3CH_3
D. Benzene, C_6H_6

98. After reaction workup, the reaction of the Grignard reagent, methyl magnesium bromide, CH_3MgBr, with the aldehyde, acetaldehyde, CH_3CHO, produces as a product

A. methyl ethyl ether.
B. 2-propanol.
C. 1-propanol.
D. dimethyl ketone.

99. Dehydration of an alcohol produces

   A. a ketone.
   B. an alkene.
   C. an aldehyde.
   D. an alkyl halide.

100. A mixture of equal amounts of a pair of enantiomers is called a

   A. pair of diastereomers.
   B. conformational mixture.
   C. meso compound.
   D. racemic mixture.

CHEMISTRY ANSWER KEY

1. **D**	21. **D**	41. **B**	61. **C**	81. **C**
2. **C**	22. **A**	42. **C**	62. **B**	82. **C**
3. **A**	23. **C**	43. **A**	63. **B**	83. **C**
4. **A**	24. **D**	44. **B**	64. **B**	84. **D**
5. **C**	25. **B**	45. **C**	65. **C**	85. **D**
6. **D**	26. **B**	46. **C**	66. **C**	86. **D**
7. **C**	27. **B**	47. **A**	67. **B**	87. **B**
8. **D**	28. **B**	48. **B**	68. **A**	88. **B**
9. **B**	29. **C**	49. **C**	69. **A**	89. **D**
10. **B**	30. **B**	50. **D**	70. **C**	90. **A**
11. **C**	31. **C**	51. **C**	71. **C**	91. **A**
12. **B**	32. **B**	52. **D**	72. **A**	92. **C**
13. **B**	33. **C**	53. **C**	73. **A**	93. **A**
14. **A**	34. **A**	54. **D**	74. **B**	94. **C**
15. **C**	35. **A**	55. **B**	75. **A**	95. **B**
16. **D**	36. **B**	56. **B**	76. **D**	96. **B**
17. **C**	37. **A**	57. **D**	77. **D**	97. **A**
18. **B**	38. **C**	58. **A**	78. **C**	98. **B**
19. **A**	39. **B**	59. **A**	79. **C**	99. **B**
20. **A**	40. **A**	60. **A**	80. **C**	100. **D**

CHEMISTRY EXPLANATORY ANSWERS

1. Answer is **D**. Physical changes are illustrated by answers A, B, and C. Most physical changes are reversible. For example, water vapor can be converted back to liquid water by cooling, salt can be separated from water by evaporating the water, and the volume of the liquid returns to its original volume when the stone is removed. Answer *D*, however, represents a chemical change. Once milk sours, the original chemicals present in the milk are converted to new compounds and the change is not reversible. Some chemical changes are reversible, but most are not.

2. Answer is **C**. Salt, NaCl, and water, H_2O are compounds. Brass is a mixture of zinc, Zn, and tin, Sn. Only gold, Au, is a pure element.

3. Answer is **A**. Density is defined as mass divided by volume. The density of the sample is the mass, 5.5 g, divided by the volume, which is the difference between the final volume and the initial volume of the water, 20.0 mL – 15.5 mL, displaced by the metal. The correct answer is 1.22 g / mL.

4. Answer is **A**. The easiest way to solve this problem is to use the factor label method of solution. Write down all the equalities that are needed.

$$60 \text{ min} = 1 \text{ hr} \quad 24 \text{ hr} = 1 \text{ da} \quad 7 \text{ da} = 1 \text{ wk}$$

Convert each of these equalities into a fraction, for example, 60 min / 1 hr or 1 hr / 60 min. Then multiply appropriate fractions so that the only label remaining is min / wk.

$$\frac{60 \text{ min}}{1 \text{ hr}} \times \frac{24 \text{ hr}}{1 \text{ da}} \times \frac{7 \text{ da}}{1 \text{ wk}} = 10,080 = 1.01 \times 10^4 \frac{\text{min}}{\text{wk}}$$

5. Answer is **C**. To convert a temperature from the Fahrenheit to the Celsius scale, use the following equation:

$$°C = \frac{5°C}{9°F} \ (°F - 32°F)$$

$$°C = \frac{5°C}{9°F} \ (-10°F - 32°F)$$

$$°C = -23°C$$

6. Answer is D. In the symbol $_{21}^{45}Sc$, 45 is the mass number, or atomic weight (number of protons plus number of neutrons), 21 is the atomic number (number of protons) of scandium, Sc. Subtracting 21 from 45 gives the number of neutrons, 24.

7. Answer is C. The average atomic weight or mass of an atom is a weighted average calculated in the following manner:

$$30\ (0.20) = \quad 6.00$$
$$32\ (0.80) = + \ \underline{25.60}$$
$$31.60$$

8. Answer is D. Again, use the factor-label method to calculate the weight of one atom of Cu.

Avogadro's number $\cong 6 \times 10^{23}$ atoms = 1 mole

$$63.55\text{ g Cu} = 1\text{ mole}$$

$$\frac{63.55\text{ g}}{1\text{ mole}} \times \frac{1\text{ mole}}{6 \times 10^{23}\text{ atoms}} = 10.59 \times 10^{-23} = 1.06 \times 10^{-22}\text{ g}$$

9. Answer is B. A formula weight (or molecular weight) is calculated by adding the number of atoms of each element multiplied by its atomic mass, or weight, a total weight in atomic mass units, for $(NH_4)_2SO_4$.

$$
\begin{array}{ll}
2N & = 2(14) = 28 \\
8H & = 8(1) \ \ = 8 \\
1S & = 1(32) = 32 \\
4O & = 4(16) = \underline{64} \\
& \quad \ \ 132\text{ amu}
\end{array}
$$

10. Answer is B. Percentage equals part divided by whole times 100.

$$\frac{\text{Part}}{\text{Whole}} \times 100 = \%$$

$$\frac{8\text{ H}}{(NH_4)_2\ SO} \times 100 = \frac{8}{132} \times 100 = 6.06\%$$

11. Answer is C. The formula for hypochlorous acid is HClO. The formula for chlorous acid is $HClO_2$; $HClO_3$ is chloric acid, and $HClO_4$ is perchloric acid. HCl is hydrogen chloride or when dissolved in water, HCl (aq), hydrochloric acid.

12. Answer is B. The coefficient of H_2SO_4 is 2 as shown in the balanced equation below:

$$Na_2CO_3 + 2H_2SO_4 \longrightarrow 2\ NaHSO_4 + H_2O + CO_2$$

13. Answer is **B**. The oxidation number of hydrogen, H, in a compound is +1, except when that element is present as a hydride [eg. LiH (–1)], and the oxidation number of oxygen, O, in a compound is –2, except when that element is present as a peroxide, [eg. Na_2O_2 (–1)].

$$\begin{array}{cc} +2 & -6 \\ 2(+1) & 3(-2) \\ \multicolumn{2}{c}{H_2SO_3} \end{array}$$

Since sulfurous acid, H_2SO_3, is a neutral compound, the sum of the oxidation numbers for hydrogen, sulfur, and oxygen must equal zero; +2 (for H) plus +4 (for S) combine with –6 (for O) to equal zero.

14. Answer is **A**. Oxidation is the loss of electrons; the substance oxidized is the reducing agent. Reduction is the gain of electrons; the substance reduced is the oxidizing agent. In the given equation, Zn loses electrons while Cu^{2+} gains electrons. Thus, Zn^0 (which is oxidized to Zn^{2+}) is the reducing agent; Cu^{2+} (which is reduced to Cu^0) is the oxidizing agent.

$$Zn + CuSO_4 \longrightarrow ZnSO_4 + Cu$$
$$Zn^0 \longrightarrow Zn^{2+} + 2\,e^-$$
$$Cu^{2+} + 2\,e^- \longrightarrow Cu$$

15. Answer is **C**. To balance a redox equation, separate the equation into two parts.

$$Fe^{2+} + H^+ + MnO_4^- \longrightarrow Fe^{3+} + Mn^{2+} + H_2O$$
$$Fe^{2+} \longrightarrow Fe^{3+} \qquad MnO_4^- \longrightarrow Mn^{2+}$$

Begin with the equation involving oxygen. Add 4 molecules of water to the right side of the equation to balance the 4 atoms of oxygen present in the permanganate ion.

$$MnO_4^- \longrightarrow Mn^{2+} + 4H_2O$$

Since H^+ is present in the equation, the reaction is carried out in acid solution. Add 8 hydrogen ions to the left side of the equation to balance the 8 hydrogen atoms present in the 4 molecules of water.

$$8H^+ + MnO_4^- \longrightarrow Mn^{2+} + 4H_2O$$

The sum of the charges on both sides of the equation must be the same. On the left side, 8 positive charges and 1 negative charge equal +7, while on the right side the sum is +2. To balance the charges on the two sides, add 5 electrons to the left side.

$$5e^- + 8H^+ + MnO_4^- \longrightarrow Mn^{2+} + 4H_2O$$

Now the atoms and charges are balanced.

Next, since 5 electrons are gained by the permanganate ion, 5 electrons must be lost by the ferrous ion, Fe^{2+}. However, each ferrous ion loses only 1 electron.

$$Fe^{2+} \longrightarrow Fe^{3+} + e^-$$

Therefore, multiply the equation by 5.

$$5Fe^{2+} \longrightarrow 5Fe^{3+} + 5e^-$$

Now the atoms and charges are balanced.

Add the two equations together; the 5 electrons on each side will cancel to yield, as the final equation:

$$5Fe^{2+} + 8H^+ + MnO_4^- \longrightarrow Mn^{2+} + 4H_2O + 5Fe^{3+}$$

Finally, check to be sure that the numbers of atoms and the total charges on both sides of the equation are balanced. The coefficient of Fe^{3+} in the balanced equation is 5.

16. <u>Answer is D</u>. The coefficients of the reactants and products in a balanced equation represent *volume* for gases, as well as *molecules* and *moles*. These are the only direct relationships involving coefficients that exist in a balanced equation. Use the factor-label method to calculate the number of moles of oxygen formed when the reaction begins with 4 moles of ammonia.

$$4NH_3(g) + 5O_2(g) \longrightarrow 4NO(g) + 6H_2O(g)$$

Two fractions are possible from the relationship that 4 moles NH_3 require 5 moles O_2:

$$\frac{4 \text{ moles } NH_3}{5 \text{ moles } O_2} \qquad \frac{5 \text{ moles } O_2}{4 \text{ moles } NH_3}$$

Having 5 moles of NH_3, multiply by the appropriate fraction so that only moles of O_2 remain.

$$5 \text{ moles } NH_3 \times \frac{5 \text{ moles } O_2}{4 \text{ moles } NH_3} = 6.3 \text{ moles } O_2$$

17. <u>Answer is C</u>. Refer to the explanation for question 16.

18. <u>Answer is B</u>. Given 17.0 gm NH_3 and asked for the number of grams of NO produced, follow the scheme shown below using the factor label method since the coefficients in front of the formulas do represent moles but do not represent grams.

$$4NH_3(g) + 5O_2(g) \longrightarrow 4NO(g) + 6H_2O(g)$$

molecular weights NH_3 = 17 g / mole, NO = 30 g / mole

$$\text{g } NH_3 \longrightarrow \underline{\text{moles } NH_3} \longrightarrow \underline{\text{moles NO}} \longrightarrow \text{g NO}$$

$\underline{\text{g } NH_3}$

17.0 g

$\underline{\text{moles } NH_3}$

$\dfrac{17.0 \text{ g}}{17 \text{ g / mole}}$ = 1.0 mole NH_3

$\underline{\text{moles NO}}$

1.0 mole $NH_3 \times \dfrac{4 \text{ moles NO}}{4 \text{ moles } NH_3}$ = 1.0 mole NO

$\underline{\text{g NO}}$

1.0 mole NO $\times \dfrac{30 \text{ g NO}}{\text{mole NO}}$ = 30 g NO

Although the mathematics in this problem is simple, the same procedure can be used to solve any problem like this having different numbers.

19. <u>Answer is **A**</u>. Follow the same method as shown in the explanation to problem 18, except convert from moles NO to liters NO. Remember, 1 mole of any gas at standard temperature and pressure, STP, 0°C and 1 atm, occupies 22.4 liters.

$$\text{g } NH_3 \longrightarrow \underline{\text{moles } NH_3} \longrightarrow \underline{\text{moles NO}} \longrightarrow \underline{\text{liters NO}}$$

$\underline{\text{g } NH_3}$

17.0 g NH_3

$\underline{\text{moles } NH_3}$

$\dfrac{1.70 \text{ g}}{17 \text{ g / mole}}$ = 0.10 mole NH_3

$\underline{\text{moles NO}}$

0.10 mole $NH_3 \times \dfrac{4 \text{ moles NO}}{4 \text{ moles } NH_3}$ = 0.10 mole NO

$\underline{\text{liters NO}}$

0.10 mole NO $\times \dfrac{22.4 \text{ liters NO}}{1 \text{ mole NO}}$ = 2.24 liters NO

20. **Answer is A.** Follow the same method as shown in the explanations to problems 18 and 19, except convert from moles NO to molecules NO. Remember, 1 mole of any substance contains 6×10^{23} particles.

g NH_3 —> moles NH_3 —> moles NO —> molecules NO

g NH_3

0.17 g NH_3

moles NH_3

$\dfrac{0.17 \text{ g } NH_3}{17 \text{ g / mole}}$ = 0.01 mole NH_3

moles NO

0.01 mole $NH_3 \times \dfrac{4 \text{ moles NO}}{4 \text{ moles } NH_3}$ = 0.01 mole NO

molecules NO

0.01 mole NO $\times \dfrac{6 \times 10^{23} \text{ molecules NO}}{1 \text{ mole NO}}$ = 6×10^{21} molecules NO

21. **Answer is D.** The equation used to solve the problem is

PV = nRT

The symbol P is pressure in atmospheres, V is volume in liters, n is number of moles, which equals grams/molar mass, R is the gas constant, and T is temperature in Kelvin. Because the oxygen is collected over water, both water and oxygen contribute to the pressure of the gas. The contribution of water, 23.76 mm, must be subtracted from the total pressure, 750 mm, in order to determine the pressure contributed by the oxygen, 726.24 mm. Pressure must be converted to atmospheres, volume converted to liters, and temperature converted to Kelvin. In addition oxygen is a diatomic gas and, consequently, its molar mass is 32 amu.

22. **Answer is A.** Molarity is defined as moles of solute divided by liters of solution.

$M = \dfrac{\text{moles of solute}}{\text{liters of solution}} = \dfrac{\text{g/mol. wt.}}{\text{liters of solution}}$

Sugar, $C_6H_{12}O_6$, has a molecular weight of 180 g/mole. Substitute 1.8 g, 180 g/mole, and 1.0 L into the above equation to obtain the molarity of the solution.

$$M = \frac{1.8 \text{ g } / 180 \text{ g/mole}}{1.0 \text{ L}} = 0.01 \frac{\text{moles}}{\text{liter}} = 0.01 \text{ M}$$

23. Answer is **C**. The ideal gas law, $PV = nRT$, is used to solve this problem. Pressure is used in atmospheres, volume in liters, and temperature in Kelvin. Moles of gas is represented by n. The molar mass of oxygen is 32 grams/mole since oxygen is a diatomic molecule, O_2. Substituting the given data into the above formula gives:

$$1 \text{ atm } (2.0 \text{ liters}) = \frac{x}{32 \text{ grams/mole}} \left(0.082 \frac{\text{l-atm}}{\text{K-mole}}\right)(273 + 7) \text{ K}$$

$$x = 2.60 \text{ g}$$

24. Answer is **D**. In a dilution problem, # moles of solute before dilution = # moles of solute after dilution. Therefore

Molarity × volume   = Molarity × volume
(before dilution)   (after dilution)

$$\frac{2.5 \text{ moles} \times 0.2 \text{ L}}{\text{L}} = \frac{5.0 \text{ moles} \times \text{volume}}{\text{L}}$$

$$0.100 \text{ L} = \text{volume}$$

To prepare the 2.5 M solution of NaOH, dilute 100 mL of the 5.0M solution to 200 mL.

25. Answer is **B**. Refer to the explanation for question 16.

26. Answer is **B**. Neutralization is the reaction of acid plus base to produce salt plus water.

$$2LiOH + H_2SO_4 \longrightarrow Li_2SO_4 + 2H_2O$$

The balanced equation shows that twice as many moles of LiOH are needed to completely react with H_2SO_4. Given the volume and molarity of the sulfuric acid, 10 mL of 3 M H_2SO_4, calculate the number of moles of sulfuric acid.

$$M = \frac{\text{\# moles}}{\text{\# liters}} \qquad 3M = \frac{\text{\#moles}}{0.01 \text{ L}} \qquad \text{\# moles } H_2SO_4 = 0.03$$

Multiply the moles of acid by 2 (factor-label method from balanced equation) to determine the number of moles of lithium hydroxide.

$$0.03 \text{ mole } H_2SO_4 \times \frac{2 \text{ moles LiOH}}{1 \text{ mole } H_2SO_4} = 0.06 \text{ mole LiOH}$$

Finally, determine the volume of lithium hydroxide necessary to contain that number of moles of 2 M lithium hydroxide.

$$M = \frac{\#\text{moles}}{\#\text{liters}} \qquad 2M = \frac{0.06 \text{ mole}}{\#\text{liters}} \qquad \#\text{liters LiOH} = 0.03 \text{ (30 mL)}$$

27. <u>Answer is **B**</u>. The bubble at the bottom of the lake has a volume of 1.2 mL at (7 + 273)K and 2.8 atm pressure. To determine the volume of the bubble at the surface of the lake at (27 + 273)K and 1.0 atm pressure, use the equation shown below.

$$\frac{P_1V_1}{T_1} = \frac{P_2V_2}{T_2} = \frac{2.8 \text{ atm } (1.2 \text{ mL})}{280 \text{ K}} = \frac{1 \text{ atm } V_2}{300 \text{ K}} \quad V_2 = 3.6 \text{ mL}$$

Since pressure and volume are present on both sides of the equation, any pressure or volume term (mL, liters, etc.) can be used as long as it is the same on both sides of the equation. The pressure units cancel, and the volume term is part of the answer.

28. <u>Answer is **B**</u>. This problem involves calculating the number of liters of NO produced at STP, 0°C and 1.0 atm, and converting that volume to the new volume at 27°C and 0.80 atm.

$$4NH_3(g) + 5 O_2(g) \longrightarrow 4NO(g) + 6 H_2O(g)$$

g NH$_3$ --> moles NH$_3$ --> moles NO --> liters NO at STP

$$1.7 \qquad \frac{1.7}{17} = 0.10 \qquad \frac{0.10(4)}{4} = 0.10 \qquad 0.10(22.4) = 2.2L$$

After finding the volume at STP, convert this volume to the volume at 0.80 atm and (27 + 273)K,

$$\frac{P_1V_1}{T_1} = \frac{P_2V_2}{T_2} = \frac{1 \text{ atm } (2.2 \text{ L})}{(0+273) \text{ K}} = \frac{0.80 \text{ atm } V_2}{(27+273) \text{ K}}$$

$$V_2 = 3.1 \text{ L at } 27°C \text{ and } 0.80 \text{ atm}$$

An alternative solution involves use of the ideal gas law equation.

$$PV = nRT$$

$$(0.80 \text{ atm})V = \frac{1.7 \text{ g}}{17 \text{ g / mole}} \left(0.082 \frac{\text{L-atm}}{\text{k-mole}}\right)(27 + 273) \text{ K}$$

$$V = 3.1 \text{ liters at } 27°C \text{ and } 0.8 \text{ atm}$$

29. <u>Answer is **C**</u>. The rate of effusion or diffusion (mixing of gases) of a gas is inversely proportional to the square root of its molecular weight. The rates of effusion can be compared by using the following equation:

$$\frac{\text{Rate 1}}{\text{Rate 2}} = \sqrt{\frac{\text{molecular weight 2}}{\text{molecular weight 1}}}$$

Let the rate of hydrogen be rate 1, and the rate of oxygen be rate 2. The molecular weight 1 is the molecular weight of hydrogen gas and molecular weight 2 is the molecular weight of oxygen gas.

$$\frac{\text{Rate 1}}{\text{Rate 2}} = \sqrt{\frac{32}{2}} = \sqrt{16} = 4$$

Therefore the rate of effusion of hydrogen is 4 times faster than that of oxygen. Lighter gases move faster than heavier ones.

30. <u>Answer is **B**</u>. Gases behave most nearly as ideal gases when the temperature is high and the pressure is low. At low temperature and high pressure, gases tend to be converted to liquids.

31. <u>Answer is **C**</u>. The heat capacity, C, of a substance equals the specific heat, s, times the mass of the material, m.

$$C = ms$$

$$C = 10.0 \text{ g} \left(0.385 \frac{\text{J}}{\text{g}^\circ\text{C}}\right) = 3.85 \text{ J/}^\circ\text{C}$$

32. <u>Answer is **B**</u>. The wavelength times the frequency of light equals the speed of light, c. The wavelength is given in nanometers. Since the speed of light, c, is given in meters per second, convert the wavelength to meters: 1 m = 10^9 nm.

$$\text{Wavelength} \times \text{Frequency} = c = 3.00 \times 10^8 \text{m/s}$$

$$150 \text{ nm} \frac{(1\text{m})}{10^9 \text{ nm}} \times \text{Frequency} = 3.00 \times 10^8 \text{ meters/second}$$

$$\text{Frequency} = 2.0 \times 10^{15} \text{cycles/second}$$

33. <u>Answer is **C**</u>. Metals conduct electricity, while nonmetals do not. In the periodic table metals are located on the left, nonmetals, on the right. A diagonal line extending from boron, B, to astatine, At, approximately divides the metals from the nonmetals. An element along this diagonal is amphoteric; that is, it can behave either as a metal or as a nonmetal, depending on the conditions.

The correct answer is chlorine, Cl, because this element is a nonmetal, and therefore cannot conduct electricity, whereas the other elements listed—aluminum, Al, lithium, Li, and sodium, Na—are metals.

34. Answer is A. Every electron in an atom has four quantum numbers. The first number is n, an integer that represents the number of the orbit. This number increases as the distance of the orbit increases from the nucleus.

The second quantum number, ℓ, represents the type of orbital and can be any integer up to $n-1$. The value of $\ell = 0$ represents an s orbital; $\ell = 1$, a p orbital; $\ell = 2$, a d orbital; and $\ell = 3$, an f orbital.

The third quantum number, m_ℓ, can assume any integer value from $-\ell$ to $+\ell$. For example, if $\ell = 2$, m_ℓ can be $-2, -1, 0 +1, +2$, a total of five values. The value m_ℓ indicates the number of s, p, d, and f orbitals. When $\ell = 0$, there is one value for m_ℓ, 0, and one s orbital. When $\ell = 1$, there are three m_ℓ values, $-1, 0, +1$, and three p orbitals. When $\ell = 2$, there are five m_ℓ values, $-2, -1, 0$, $+1, +2$, and five d orbitals. When $\ell = 3$, there are seven m_ℓ values, $-3, -2, -1, 0, +1, +2, +3$, and seven f orbitals.

The fourth quantum number, m_s, represents the spin of the electron and can be either of two values, $+1/2$ or $-1/2$.

For the last electron added to an atom of aluminum, m_s,

n = the number of the orbit, 1, 2, 3, 4...

$\ell = n - 1$

$m_\ell = -\ell.....0....+\ell$

$m_s = \pm^{1}/_{2}$

35. Answer is A. The correct electron configuration for the sulfide ion, S^{2-}, is $1s^2 2s^2 2p^6 3s^2 3p^6$. The letters s, p, d, and f indicate the type of orbital. The number in front of the symbols, as in 1s, indicates the number of the orbit, in this case 1. The superscript, as in $1s^2$, indicates the number of electrons present in the orbital, in this case 2. The electron configuration for the sulfur atom, S, which is $1s^2 2s^2 2p^6 3s^2 3p^4$, shows the 16 electrons present in the atom. The sulfur ion, S^{2-}, has two more electrons in the p orbital:

$1s^2 2s^2 2p^6 3s^2 3p^6$.

36. Answer is B. The size of atoms decreases as one progresses from left to right across a row in the periodic table. For example, in the row beginning with Li and ending with F, Li is the largest atom and F is the smallest. Answer B is correct; Na is larger than Si, which is larger than Cl.

The size of atoms increases as one progresses from top to bottom down a family. For example, Li is the smallest and Cs the largest in the alkali metal family.

37. <u>Answer is **A**</u>. In the first shell around the nucleus of the atom, there is one *s* orbital. In the second shell there are one *s* orbital and three *p* orbitals. In the third shell there are one *s* orbital, three *p* orbitals and five *d* orbitals. In the fourth shell there are one *s* orbital, three *p* orbitals, five *d* orbitals, and ten *f* orbitals. Each orbital is capable of containing a maximum of two electrons. Therefore there are six electrons possible in the three *p* orbitals.

38. <u>Answer is **C**</u>. The elements in the periodic table are arranged according to increasing atomic number, that is, number of protons.

39. <u>Answer is **B**</u>. In a Lewis dot symbol, 8 electrons are shown around the phosphorus ion, P^{3-}. In a Lewis dot symbol, only the electrons in the outermost shell are indicated. Thus, for the phosphorus atom, which has 2 electrons in the first shell, 8 in the second, and 5 in the third, only five electrons are shown.

The ion P^{3-} has 3 additional electrons, and so 8 electrons $(5 + 3)$ would be shown in a Lewis dot symbol.

40. <u>Answer is **A**</u>. The formal charge on a bonded atom equals the number of valence electrons in the nonbonded atom minus the number of nonbonded electrons in the bonded atom minus one-half the number of bonding electrons in the bonded atom.

The number of valence electrons in the non-bonded atom (Lewis dot formula)

$$\cdot \overset{\cdot}{\underset{\cdot}{C}} \cdot \; = 4$$

The number of nonbonded electrons in the bonded atom (Lewis dot structure)

$$= \overset{|}{\underset{|}{C}} - \quad = 0$$

One-half the number of bonding electrons in the bonded atom

$$= \overset{|}{\underset{|}{C}} - \quad -\frac{1}{2}(8) = 4$$

The formal charge on a bonded atom

$$4 - 0 - 4 = 0$$

41. <u>Answer is **B**</u>. The farther two elements are from each other in the periodic table, one being a metal and the other a nonmetal, the more ionic the bond between them. Consequently, of the compounds listed, LiO has the most ionic bond.

For the other compounds, CO_2, CH_4, and NH_3, the bonding is covalent because the atoms are close to each other and the compounds are nonmetals. Although hydrogen, H, may be located a distance from carbon, C, and from nitrogen, N, this element is an anomaly and has unique properties.

42. <u>Answer is **C**</u>. The molecular geometry of SiH_4, like that of CH_4, is tetrahedral. Carbon is above silicon in the periodic table; consequently, if the same number of bonds is formed by the 4 hydrogen atoms to the central atom, Si or C, the geometry of the molecule is the same.

If there are 2 bonding electron pairs around the central atom, as in BeF_2, the molecule is linear. If there are 3 bonding electron pairs around the central atom, as in BF_3, the molecule is trigonal planar. With 4 bonding electron pairs, as in SiH_4 or CH_4, the molecule is tetrahedral. In the molecule NH_3, there are 4 electron pairs but 1 is a nonbonding pair (only 3 hydrogen atoms), and the molecule is described as being a trigonal pyramid. In H_2O there are 4 electron pairs but only 2 pairs participate in bonding to the 2 hydrogen atoms, and the molecule is bent.

43. **Answer is A.** The molecule H_2S has the same geometry as does H_2O, which is bent. Sulfur, S, is under oxygen, O, in the periodic table and has the same number of atoms bonded to it, two hydrogens in each case. A bent molecule has a bond angle of about $105°$, a trigonal pyramid an angle of $107°$, a tetrahedron an angle of $109°$, a trigonal planar molecule an angle of $120°$, and a linear molecule an angle of $180°$.

44. **Answer is B.** The molecule $AlCl_3$, a trigonal planar molecule, has sp^2 hybridization. The linear molecule BeF_2 is sp hybridized. The tetrahedral CH_4, as well as the trigonal pyramid, NH_3, and the bent molecule, H_2O, are all sp^3 hybridized.

45. **Answer is C.** Electronegativity is the ability of an atom to draw electrons in a covalent bond to itself, as in the C – F bond. The electron pair covalently shared between carbon, C, and fluorine, F, are drawn more toward F because F is more electronegative than C. Electronegativity increases in the same row as one progresses from left to right, for example Li —> F, and decreases in a family as one progresses from top to bottom, for example Li —> Cs, cesium. The most electronegative element in the periodic table is F at the top right, and the least electronegative is Cs at the bottom left.

46. **Answer is C.** An example of a polar covalent bond is the H – F bond (Answer C). The two electrons forming the bond are shared between the two atoms but not equally. Fluorine is more electronegative than hydrogen and therefore the electrons are drawn more strongly toward fluorine than toward hydrogen.

The C – C bond is a nonpolar covalent bond since the electrons between the carbon atoms are shared equally. The B – C bond is very slightly polar since the boron and the carbon have very slightly different electronegativities. The Li – Cl bond is ionic, as explained in the answer to question 41.

47. **Answer is A.** The dipole moment is a measure of the polarity of a molecule, that is, one part of the molecule is partially positive and one part partially negative. The greater the dipole moment, the more polar a molecule is. Carbon dioxide, CO_2, has a dipole moment of zero because the molecule is linear with carbon in the middle and one oxygen atom on either side of the carbon. Although each individual C – O bond is polar, the two bonds balance each other to produce a nonpolar molecule.

H_2O, HF, and NH_3 are all polar molecules. The water molecule is bent with the electrons being drawn toward the oxygen. The hydrogen fluoride molecule is linear, but the H – F bond is polar with the electrons drawn toward the fluorine. The ammonia molecule is trigonal pyramidal with the electrons drawn toward the nitrogen.

48. **Answer is B.** A basic oxide is a substance that, when it reacts with water, produces a base; another name for a basic oxide is a basic anhydride. Potassium oxide, K_2O, reacts with water to produce potassium hydroxide, KOH, according to the following equation:

$$K_2O + H_2O \longrightarrow 2KOH$$

The other oxides, CO_2, SO_2, and P_2O_5, are all acid oxides or acid anhydrides.

$$CO_2 + H_2O \longrightarrow H_2CO_3$$
$$SO_2 + H_2O \longrightarrow H_2SO_3$$
$$P_2O_5 + 3H_2O \longrightarrow 2H_3PO_4$$

49. **Answer is C.** Three structures may be drawn for the carbonate ion, CO_3^{-2}.

The double bond between the carbon atom and one of the oxygen atoms may be in any one of three possible positions.

50. **Answer is D.** The compound BeF_2 has 4 electrons, 2 electron pairs, around the central Be atom. The compound $AlCl_3$ has 6 electrons, 3 electron pairs, around the central Al atom. The compounds H_2O and CH_4 both have 8 electrons, 4 electron pairs, around the central O and C atoms. The compound PF_5 has 10 electrons, 5 electron pairs, around the central P atom because of the availability of empty d orbitals for the third shell elements.

51. Answer is C. Refer to the explanation for question 50.

52. Answer is D. Colligative properties are properties of solutions that depend on the number, not the nature, of the solute particles dissolved in a solvent. The four colligative properties are depression of vapor pressure, elevation of boiling point, depression of freezing point, and osmosis. The more particles of solute dissolved in the solvent, the greater the depression of the vapor pressure, the elevation of the boiling point, the depression of the freezing point, and the osmotic pressure.

One mole of Na_2SO_4 produces the most particles, 3 moles: 2 moles of Na^+ and 1 mole of SO_4^{2-}. One mole of $C_6H_{12}O_6$ produces only 1 mole of particles because sugar does not ionize but remains as molecules. One mole of $CaCO_3$ produces two moles of particles: 1 mole of Ca^{2+} and 1 mole of CO_3^{2-}. One mole of NaCl produces 2 moles of particles, 1 mole of Na^+ and 1 mole of Cl^-.

53. Answer is C. The depression of the freezing temperature of water, a colligative property, can be calculated in the following manner. First find the molality of the solution, 1.8 g $C_6H_{12}O_6$ in 100 g water.

$$\text{Molality} = \frac{\text{\# moles solute}}{\text{\# kg solvent}} = \frac{\text{\# g / mol. wt.}}{\text{\# kg solvent}} = \frac{1.8\,g/180g/mole}{0.100\ kg}$$

$$= 0.100\ m$$

Next substitute the molality into the expression used to calculate the change in freezing temperature.

$$K_f\,m = T_f^{\,0} - T_f$$

In this equation, K_f is the molal freezing point depression constant for water, m is the molality of the solution, $T_f^{\,0}$ is the original freezing point of water before adding the solute, and T_f is the freezing point after adding the solute.

$$\frac{1.86°C\,(0.100\ m)}{m}$$

$$-0.186°C = T_f$$

$$= 0°C - T_f$$

54. Answer is D. For a first-order reaction, that is, a reaction in which the rate depends on the concentration of one reactant raised to the first power, the following equation connects original concentration, A_0, 0.5 M; final concentration, A; time t, 5 min.; and the rate constant, k, 3.5×10^{-2}/sec.

If sugar ionized into two particles, the molality would have been the value calculated times the two particles: $-0.186\ m \times 2 = -0.372\ m$.

$$\ln \frac{[A_0]}{[A]} = kt$$

$$\ln 0.5 - \ln [A] = \frac{3.5 \times 10^{-2}}{\text{sec}} \left(5\,\text{min} \times \frac{60\,\text{sec}}{1\,\text{min}} \right)$$

$$[A] = 1.4 \times 10^{-5} M$$

This answer may be estimated in the following manner and the most probable answer of those given may be selected.

$$\frac{0.035\,\text{decrease}}{\text{sec}} \left(60\,\frac{\text{sec}}{\text{min}} \right) (5\,\text{min}) = 10.5\,\text{decrease}$$

Since the answers given include 0.42, 0.60, 1.8×10^4, and 1.4×10^{-5}, the only reasonable answer of those listed, the only one showing a large decrease, is 1.4×10^{-5}.

55. <u>Answer is **B**</u>. In a first-order reaction, the half-life, that is, the length of time for one-half of the concentration to be reacted, is dependent only on the rate constant, not on the original concentration. If the rate constant, k, is 6.93×10^2 / sec, the length of time needed for one-half of the starting material to be reacted is

$$t_{1/2} = \frac{0.693}{k}$$

$$t_{1/2} = \frac{0.693}{6.93 \times 10^2 / \text{sec}} = 1.0 \times 10^{-3}\,\text{sec}$$

56. <u>Answer is **B**</u>. The equation for a second-order reaction is as follows:

$$\frac{1}{[A]} = kt + \frac{1}{[A_0]}$$

The graph of the equation is in the form of a straight line $y = mx + b$. If one plots $1/[A]$ on the y-axis and t on the x-axis for a second-order reaction, a straight line is obtained with a y-intercept of $1/[A_0]$, and a positive slope, $+k$.

For a first-order reaction, a rearrangement of the equation shown for question 54 gives

$$\ln[A] = -kt + \ln[A_0]$$

$$y = mx + b$$

A plot of $\ln [A]$ on the y-axis vs. t on the x-axis gives a straight line with a negative slope, $-k$, and with a y-intercept equal to $\ln [A_0]$.

57. Answer is D. The order of a reaction is determined by adding the powers to which each of the concentrations is raised in the rate equation.

$$\text{Rate} = k\,[A]\,[B]^2$$

The value of [A] is raised to the first power, and the value of [B] is raised to the second power. Therefore, the order is $1 + 2 = 3$, and the given reaction is a third-order reaction.

58. Answer is A. An equilibrium constant may be written for the following reaction. An equilibrium constant is equal to the product of the products divided by the product of the reactants, each raised to the power as indicated in the balanced equation.

$$H_2 + I_2 \longleftrightarrow 2HI \qquad K = \frac{[HI]^2}{[I_2][H_2]}$$

$$K = \frac{(0.80)^2}{(0.50)(0.60)} = 2.1$$

59. Answer is A. According to Le Châtelier's principle, any stress applied to a system in equilibrium will cause the equilibrium to shift so as to relieve the stress. For example, in the given system:

$$\text{Heat} + N_2O_4\,(g) \longleftrightarrow 2NO_2\,(g)$$

think of heat as one of the reactants. An increase in any reactant concentration on the left will cause the equilibrium to shift to the right, the products. An increase in the product concentration on the right will cause the equilibrium to shift left, to the reactants. A decrease in any reactant concentration will cause the equilibrium to shift to the left. A decrease in any product concentration will cause the equilibrium to shift to the right. Therefore a decrease in temperature or heat will cause the reaction to shift to the left, NOT to the right.

An increase in the concentration of N_2O_4, a decrease in the concentration of NO_2, and an increase in temperature will all cause the equilibrium to shift to the right.

60. Answer is A. This question involves Le Châtelier's principle as does question 59. The question here is which stress will shift the equilibrium to the right. When pressure is increased, the equilibrium shifts in the direction to produce the smaller gas volume. When pressure is decreased, the equilibrium shifts in the direction to produce the larger gas volume. For the given reaction:

$$\text{Heat} + N_2O_4\,(g) \longleftrightarrow 2NO_2\,(g)$$

a decrease in pressure favors a shift to the right of the present equilibrium, 2 volumes of gas in the product versus 1 volume of gas in the reactant.

Adding a catalyst changes the activation energy of a reaction and either speeds up or slows down the reaction; it has no effect on the equilibrium of the reaction.

61. <u>Answer is **C**</u>. There are three definitions of acid and base indicated in this question. An Arrhenius acid produces an H^+ when dissolved in water, for example $HCl \longrightarrow H^+ + Cl^-$. An Arrhenius base produces an OH^- when dissolved in water, for example, $NaOH \longrightarrow Na^+ + OH^-$.

A Brönsted-Lowry acid donates an H^+ ion, that is, a proton, to water to form the hydronium ion; for example,

$$HCl + H_2O \Longleftrightarrow H_3O^{+1} + Cl^{-1}.$$

A Brönsted-Lowry acid and an Arrhenius acid are really the same thing. However, a Brönsted-Lowry base, for example, OH^-, SO_4^{-2}, H_2O, NH_3, accepts an H^+ ion.

$$OH^- + H^+ \longrightarrow H_2O \qquad SO_4^{-2} + 2\,H^+ \longrightarrow H_2SO_4$$
$$H_2O + H^+ \longrightarrow H_3O^+ \qquad NH_3 + H^+ \longrightarrow NH_4^+$$

A Brönsted-Lowry base includes both negatively charged ions, OH^- and SO_4^{2-}, and molecules with nonbonded pairs of electrons, H_2O and NH_3. The Brönsted-Lowry base is a much broader concept than the Arrhenius base.

A Lewis base donates a share in an electron pair, for example, SO_4^{2-} and NH_3, while a Lewis acid accepts a share in an electron pair, for example BF_3 and Ag^+.

$$BF_3 + NH_3 \longrightarrow F_3BNH_3 \qquad Ag^{+1} + 2NH_3 \longrightarrow Ag(NH_3)_2^+$$

A Lewis base is essentially the same thing as a Brönsted-Lowry base, that is, a negatively charged ion or a molecule with nonbonded pairs of electrons. The Lewis acid is a much broader concept, however, than the Brönsted-Lowry acid. The Lewis acid can be a molecule with an empty orbital, that is, one with fewer than 8 electrons around the central atom, as in BF_3, or a positively charged ion, Ag^+.

62. <u>Answer is **B**</u>. Refer to the explanation for question 61.

63. Answer is **B**. The H - F bond is more polar than the C - H bond because fluorine is more electronegative than carbon. The more polar the bond, that is, the more the shared electrons are drawn to one atom rather than the other, the easier it is to break the bond. In the H - F bond, the shared electron pair is drawn more to the fluorine than to the hydrogen. Therefore, when the bond breaks, the fluorine gains, while the hydrogen loses, the electron pair:

HF ——> H$^+$ + F$^-$. For the compounds listed, the H - F is the most polar and the C - H bond is the least polar. Therefore, H - F is the most acidic and CH$_4$ is the least acidic.

64. Answer is **B**. Oxygen is a strongly electronegative element. The more oxygen atoms present in a series of homologous acids, the more electrons are drawn away from the hydrogen atoms, the weaker the O - H bond is, and the more acidic the compound is. Therefore, HClO < HClO$_2$ < HClO$_3$ < HClO$_4$.

65. Answer is **C**. The acidity of a solution can be measured by determining the pH or the pOH.

$$pH = -\log [H^+] \qquad pOH = -\log [OH^-]$$

The pH and pOH values are related by the following equations:

$$pH + pOH = 14 \text{ and } [H^+] [OH^-] = 10^{-14}$$

Calculating the pH when the [OH$^-$] = 0.01 M gives

$$pOH = -\log [OH^-] = -\log (10^{-2}) = -(-2) = 2$$
$$pH + 2 = 14$$
$$pH = 12$$

66. Answer is **C**. When a strong acid and a strong base react, a salt and water are produced.

$$HCl + NaOH \longrightarrow NaCl + H_2O$$

Sodium chloride, NaCl, being the salt formed from a strong acid and a strong base, does not react further with water, and the solution is neutral. The sodium ion, the conjugate acid of the strong base sodium hydroxide, is a weak acid and does not react further with water to produce other than a neutral solution. The chloride ion, the conjugate base of the strong acid hydrochloric acid, is a weak base and does not react further with water to produce other than a neutral solution.

When a weak acid and a strong base react, a salt and water are produced.

$$HAc + NaOH \longrightarrow NaAc + H_2O$$

Sodium acetate, NaAc, being the salt formed from a weak acid and a strong base, does react further with water. The acetate ion, Ac^{-1}, is a strong base, being the conjugate base of a weak acid. The acetate ion does react with water to produce a slightly basic solution according to the following equation:

$$Ac^{-1} + H_2O \longrightarrow HAc + OH^{-1}$$

When a strong acid and a weak base react, a salt is produced.

$$HCl + NH_3 \longrightarrow NH_4Cl$$

Ammonium chloride, NH_4Cl, being the salt formed from a strong acid and a weak base, does react further with water. The ammonium ion, NH_4^{+1}, is a strong acid, being the conjugate acid of a weak base, NH_3. The ammonium ion does react with water to produce a slightly acidic solution according to the following equation:

$$NH_4^{+1} + H_2O \longrightarrow H_3O^{+1} + NH_3$$

When a weak acid and a weak base react, a salt is produced.

$$HAc + NH_3 \longrightarrow NH_4Ac$$

Since both the ammonium ion and the acetate ion are capable of reacting with water, the relative concentrations of the acid and base determine whether the solution will be acidic or basic.

In summary, the conjugate acid of a weak base is a strong acid. The conjugate base of a weak acid is a strong base. Both the strong conjugate acid and the strong conjugate base react with water to change the pH of the water from a neutral value of 7. The solution becomes either slightly acidic or slightly basic. The conjugate acid of a strong acid is a weak acid. The conjugate base of a strong acid is a weak base. Both the weak conjugate acid and the weak conjugate base do not react with water to change the pH of the water from a neutral value of 7.

67. <u>Answer is **B**</u>. An amphoteric oxide is a substance that can react with either an acid or a base and is formed from an amphoteric element, that is, one that can react as either a metal or a nonmetal. Aluminum trioxide, Al_2O_3, fits the definition of an amphoteric oxide, as shown by the following reactions:

$$Al_2O_3 + 6HCl \longrightarrow 2AlCl_3 + 3H_2O$$
$$Al_2O_3 + 2NaOH + 3H_2O \longrightarrow 2NaAl(OH)_4$$

Of all the possible answers, Li is a metal, while N and I are nonmetals.

68. Answer is <u>A</u>. Refer to the explanation for question 61.

69. Answer is <u>A</u>. In the equilibrium reaction between ammonia, NH_3, and water, H_2O, ammonium ion, NH_4^{+1}, and hydroxide ion, OH^{-1}, are formed as products.

$$NH_3 + H_2O \longrightarrow NH_4^{+1} + OH^{-1}$$

Using the Brönsted-Lowry definitions of acid and base, NH_3 is the base accepting an H^{+1} ion from the acid H_2O to form the NH_4^{+1} ion. The NH_4^{+1} ion is the acid donating the H^{+1} ion to the base, OH^{-1} ion, to form H_2O.

$$\begin{array}{cccc} NH_3 & + \; H_2O & \longrightarrow & NH_4^{+1} & + \; OH^{-1} \\ \text{base} & \text{acid} & & \text{acid} & \text{base} \end{array}$$

The NH_4^{+1} and the NH_3 are a conjugate acid-base pair and the H_2O and the OH^{-1} are a conjugate acid-base pair.

70. Answer is <u>C</u>. Magnesium hydroxide, $Mg(OH)_2$, is a strong base. Strong bases ionize completely.

$$Mg(OH)_2 \longrightarrow Mg^{2+} + 2OH^{-}$$

From the balanced equation above, we see that, for every 1 mole of magnesium hydroxide, 2 moles of hydroxide ion are formed. If the concentration of magnesium hydroxide is 2.5 M, or 2.5 moles/L, then the concentration of the hydroxide ion, $[OH^{-}]$, is 2×2.5 M 5.0 M, that is, 5.0 moles/L.

Strong acids also ionize completely and their concentrations are calculated in the same manner as shown above for NaOH. A balanced equation for hydrochloric acid, HCl, is shown below.

$$HCl \longrightarrow H^{+} + Cl^{-}$$

71. Answer is <u>C</u>. Color occurs in an object because the object absorbs some of the light and transmits or reflects some of the light which originates from the sun.

Absorbed light	Color seen
<u>v</u>iolet	<u>y</u>ellow
<u>b</u>lue	<u>o</u>range
<u>g</u>reen	<u>r</u>ed
<u>y</u>ellow	<u>v</u>iolet
<u>o</u>range	<u>b</u>lue
<u>r</u>ed	<u>g</u>reen

ROYGBV   GBVROY

Reading both columns of colors from the bottom gives the acronym of the first letters of the colors, ROYGBV and GBVROY.

72. Answer is **A**. Acetic acid is a weak acid and ionizes only partially. An equilibrium expression may be written for the ionization of a weak acid.

$$HAc \longleftrightarrow H^{+1} + Ac^{-1} \qquad K_A = \frac{[H^{+1}][Ac^{-1}]}{[HAc]}$$

The concentration of hydrogen ion formed at equilibrium is unknown, x, and the concentration of acetate ion is the same, x, since the same number of hydrogen and acetate ions are formed in the balanced equation above. The concentration of acetic acid remaining at equilibrium is the initial concentration minus x, $1.0 - x$. These values are substituted into the equilibrium expression and set equal to the ionization constant for acetic acid.

$$K_A = 1.8 \times 10^{-5} = \frac{(x)(x)}{(1.0 - x)}$$

The value of x in $(1.0 - x)$ may be dropped since it is very small relative to the 1.0 M concentration because the value of K_A is small. Therefore the denominator becomes (1.0) and the equation is simplified.

$$K_A = 1.8 \times 10^{-5} = \frac{(x)(x)}{(1.0)} = x^2$$

In taking the square root of an exponential term, move the decimal so that the exponential term is an even number and divide by 2.

$$x^2 = 1.8 \times 10^{-5} = 18 \times 10^{-6}$$

The square root of 10^{-6} is 10^{-3}. Although you probably don't know the square root of 18, remember that the square root of 16 is 4 and the square root of 25 is 5. Therefore the square root of 18 is just a little larger than 4, say 4^+. The actual value is also shown below.

$$x = [H^{+1}] = 4^+ \times 10^{-3} = 4.24 \times 10^{-3} \quad \text{(Actual value with a calculator)}$$

Having the hydrogen ion concentration, it is possible to find the pH of the solution, either an estimated value, within one pH unit, or the actual value with the aid of a calculator.

$$pH = -\log [H^{+1}] = -\log [4^+ \times 10^{-3}] \qquad = -\log [4.24 \times 10^{-3}]$$

$$= -\log [4^+] -\log [10^{-3}] \qquad = -\log [4.24] -\log [10^{-3}]$$

$$= -(\text{a number between 0 \& 1}) - (-3) \qquad = -0.63 - (-3)$$

$$= 3 - (\text{a number between 0 \& 1}) \qquad = 3 - 0.63$$

$$= 2 \text{ to } 3 \qquad = 2.37$$

73. Answer is A. The constant K_B may be defined for the acetate ion, Ac^-, a base. The acetate ion reacts with water, which is the acid, and an equilibrium expression for a base can be written.

$$Ac^- + H_2O \longleftrightarrow HAc + OH^- \qquad K_B = \frac{[HAc][OH^-]}{[Ac^-]}$$

Since water is present in large excess in a dilute solution, its concentration does not change significantly and therefore its concentration is included in the constant K_B.

The relationship that exists between K_A and K_B is as follows:

$$(K_A)(K_B) = K_W = 1 \times 10^{-14}$$

where K_W is the ionization constant for water.

Substituting the given K_A value for acetic acid, 1.8×10^{-5}, into the above equation gives a value of 5.6×10^{-10} for K_B for the acetate ion.

74. Answer is B. The larger the value of the equilibrium constant, K_A, the greater the amount of products, the greater the amount of ionization of the acid (or base), or the stronger the acid (or base). Conversely, the smaller the equilibrium constant, the weaker the acid (or base). See the equation below for acetic acid, a weak acid. Therefore

$$HAc \longleftrightarrow H^+ + Ac^- \qquad K_A = \frac{[H^+][Ac^-]}{[HAc]}$$

Of the acids listed, nitrous acid, HNO_2 has the largest ionization constant and is the strongest acid. Conversely, the smaller the equilibrium constant, the weaker the acid (or base).

75. Answer is A. There are 1440 minutes in 1 day.

$$\frac{60 \text{ min}}{1 \text{ hr}} \times \frac{24 \text{ hr}}{1 \text{ day}} = 1440 \text{ min/day}$$

76. Answer is D. Calcium carbonate, $CaCO_3$, marble, is insoluble in water. The other compounds—$NaOH$, NH_4Cl, and $LiNO_3$—are all water soluble. The solubility rules include the following:

All salts formed with the alkali metals, for example, any member of the lithium family, are soluble.

All ammonium salts, NH_4^+, and all nitrate salts, NO_3^-, are soluble.

Many chlorides, Cl^-, bromides, Br^-, and iodides, I^-, are soluble.

Many sulfates, SO_4^{2-}, are soluble.

77. Answer is D. The solubility product constant, K_{sp}, is defined in the same fashion as the equilibrium constant for acids, K_A. The K_{sp} for silver chloride, $AgCl$, is shown below:

$$AgCl(s) \longleftrightarrow Ag^{+1}(aq) + Cl^{-1}(aq) \qquad K_{sp} = [Ag^{+1}][Cl^{-1}]$$

Since the *concentration* of a solid does not change, the concentration of the AgCl (s) is included in the equilibrium constant, K_{sp}.

Let $x = [Ag^{+1}] = [Cl^{-1}]$ and substitute into the equilibrium expression.

$$K_{sp} = [Ag^{+1}][Cl^{-1}] \qquad 1.6 \times 10^{-10} = (x)(x) = x^2$$

$$1.3 \times 10^{-5} = x$$

In taking the square root of an exponential term, move the decimal point (if necessary, although that is not necessary in this case) so that the exponential term is an even number and divide by 2. Take the square root of the number, in this case 1.6. Obviously the square root of 1.6 will be smaller than 1.6. It is possible to estimate the answer.

78. <u>Answer is **C**</u>. The solubility product constant, K_{sp}, is defined in question 77 above. As can be seen from the definition of K_{sp}, the larger the value of K_{sp}, the more silver and chloride ions are present in solution (on the right side of the equation) and hence the more soluble the salt. Of the salts listed, silver chloride is the most soluble.

79. <u>Answer is **C**</u>. The formation constant for the formation of a complex ion, K_f, may be defined for the silver ammonia complex, $Ag(NH_3)_2^{+1}$, as shown below.

$$Ag^{+1} + 2NH_3 \xleftrightarrow{\hspace{1cm}} Ag(NH_3)_2^{+1} \qquad K_f = \frac{[Ag(NH_3)_2]_2^{+1}}{[Ag^{+1}][NH_3]^2}$$

The concentration of each of the species in the equation is raised to the power shown in the balanced equation. As can be seen from the equation above, K_f will have a large value when the concentration of the complex ion, $[Ag(NH_3)_2^{+1}]$ is high. When much complex ion is formed the ion must be stable. Hence the largest value for the formation complex, 2.0×10^{30} for HgI_4^{-2}, gives the most stable ion.

80. <u>Answer is **C**</u>. Equations are shown for the ionization of the salts CuBr, CuI, Cu(OH)$_2$, and CuS.

1. $CuBr \xleftrightarrow{\hspace{1cm}} Cu^{+1} + Br^{-1}$

2. $CuI \xleftrightarrow{\hspace{1cm}} Cu^{+1} + I^{-1}$

3. $Cu(OH)_2 \xleftrightarrow{\hspace{1cm}} Cu^{+2} + 2OH^{-1}$

4. $CuS \xleftrightarrow{\hspace{1cm}} Cu^{+2} + S^{-2}$

Adding acid, H^{+1}, to either equation 1 or 2 will have no effect upon the equilibrium in those solutions since both hydrobromic acid, HBr, and hydroiodic acid, HI, which would form by the addition of the acid, H^{+1}, are strong acids and exist mostly as dissociated ions, not molecules.

$$Br^{-1}(aq) + H^{+1}(aq) \longleftrightarrow HBr(aq)$$

$$I^{-1}(aq) + H^{+1}(aq) \longleftrightarrow HI(aq)$$

However, adding acid, H^{+1}, to equations 3 or 4 will shift the equilibrium to the right since the resulting acids formed, H_2O and H_2S, are weak acids and exist mostly as the molecular species, not the ions.

$$OH^{-1}(aq) + H^{+1}(aq) \longleftrightarrow H_2O$$

$$S^{-2}(aq) + H^{+1}(aq) \longleftrightarrow H_2S$$

According to LeChatelier's Principle, if the hydroxide or sulfide ions, OH^{-1} or S^{-2}, are removed by reacting with H^{+1}, more of the solid salt will dissolve to replace the hydroxide and sulfide ions which were depleted.

81. Answer is **C**. Aluminum hydroxide, $Al(OH)_3$, dissolves in water to produce aluminum ions, Al^{+3}, and hydroxide ions, OH^{-1}.

$$Al(OH)_3(s) \longleftrightarrow Al^{+3}(aq) + 3OH^{-1}(aq)$$

An equilibrium exists in solution between undissolved aluminum hydroxide, $Al(OH)_3$ (s), and dissolved aluminum hydroxide, Al^{+3} (aq) + $3OH^{-1}$ (aq).

Dissolving aluminum hydroxide in either **B**, 0.5 M $Al(NO_3)_3$, or **C**, 1.6 M NaOH, will decrease its solubility relative to its solubility in water. Since aluminum nitrate, $Al(NO_3)_3$, is a soluble salt, the concentration of the aluminum ion, Al^{+3}, will be 0.5 M (0.5 moles/liter) in a solution of 0.5 M $Al(NO_3)_3$.

$$Al(NO_3)_3(s) \longrightarrow Al^{+3}(aq) + 3NO_3^{-1}(aq)$$

$$\frac{0.5\ moles}{liter} \qquad \frac{0.5\ moles}{liter} \qquad \frac{3(0.5\ moles)}{liter}$$

In the same way, the concentration of the hydroxide ion, OH^{-1}, in a solution of 1.6 M sodium hydroxide, NaOH (s), a soluble base, will be 1.6 M.

$$NaOH(s) \longrightarrow Na^{+1}(aq) + OH^{-1}(aq)$$

$$\frac{1.6\ moles}{liter} \qquad \frac{1.6\ moles}{liter} \qquad \frac{1.6\ moles}{liter}$$

Both the aluminum and hydroxide ions result in solution from dissolving solid aluminum hydroxide in water. According to LeChatelier's Principle, increasing the concentration of either ion on the right side of the equation will shift the equilibrium to the left and decrease the solubility of $Al(OH)_3$ (s). Therefore, the presence of aluminum ions in the aluminum nitrate solution and the presence of hydroxide ions in the sodium hydroxide solution decrease the solubility of aluminum hydroxide in either of these solutions. The concentration of hydroxide in the sodium hydroxide solution is 1.6 M which is larger than the concentration of the aluminum ion, 0.5 M, in the aluminum nitrate solution. The 1.6 M sodium hydroxide solution will decrease the solubility of aluminum hydroxide more than the 0.5 M aluminum nitrate solution will.

Adding solid aluminum hydroxide to the 0.3 M hydrochloric acid, HCl, will increase the solubility of the aluminum hydroxide relative to its solubility in water, since the hydroxide ion concentration would be reduced by reacting with the hydrogen ion, H^{+1}, of the hydrochloric acid, HCl, and the equilibrium would shift to the right. More aluminum hydroxide would dissolve.

82. Answer is **C**. A voltaic or galvanic cell may be constructed when a spontaneous oxidation-reduction, redox, reaction occurs. In an electrolytic cell, energy must be added to cause a reaction to take place, i.e. a nonspontaneous reaction is made to occur. When the standard electromotive force, emf^0, of a redox reaction is a positive value, the reaction is spontaneous. When the emf^0 is negative, energy must be added to cause the reaction to take place.

Using the following reactions from the standard reduction potential table as an example

$$Fe^{+3}(aq) + e^{-1} \longrightarrow Fe^{+2}(aq) \quad +0.77 \text{ volts}$$

$$Br_2(\ell) + 2e^{-1} \longrightarrow 2Br^{-1}(aq) \quad +1.07 \text{ volts}$$

and comparing them to one of the given equations

$$2Fe^{+3}(aq) + 2Br^{-1}(aq) \longrightarrow 2Fe^{+2}(aq) + Br_2(\ell)$$

one sees that it is possible to rearrange the two initial equations to obtain the final equation.

Keeping the first equation as it is and inverting the second equation gives

$$Fe^{+3}(aq) + e^{-1} \longrightarrow Fe^{+2}(aq) \quad +0.77 \text{ volts}$$

$$2Br^{-1}(aq) \longrightarrow Br_2(\ell) + 2e^{-1} \quad -1.07 \text{ volts}$$

Notice that the emf^0 is now negative for the inverted equation. Whenever a redox equation is reversed, the sign of the emf^0 changes.

In the first equation Fe^{+3} gains an electron and is reduced. In the second equation Br^{-1} loses two electrons and is oxidized. These two equations represent a redox couple. However the same number of electrons must be gained by Fe^{+3} as are lost by Br^{-1} for the reaction to occur. The first equation is therefore multiplied by 2.

$$2Fe^{+3}(aq) + 2e^{-1} \longrightarrow 2Fe^{+2}(aq) \quad +0.77 \text{ volts}$$

$$2Br^{-1}(aq) \longrightarrow Br_2(\ell) + 2e^{-1} \quad -1.07 \text{ volts}$$

Notice that multiplying the equation by a number does not in any way change the value of the emf^0. The two equations are now added to give the final equation. Equal numbers of electrons on each side of the reaction cancel.

$$2Fe^{+3}(aq) + 2Br^{-1}(aq) \longrightarrow 2Fe^{+2}(aq) + Br_2(\ell)$$

The emf^0 values are added to give a final cell value of -0.30 volts. Since this value is negative, the reaction does not occur spontaneously and would have to be carried out in an electrolysis rather than a voltaic or galvanic cell. Following the same procedure for each of the other equations given would give positive cell values, hence spontaneous reactions.

83. Answer is **C**. Oxidation is the loss of electrons; reduction is the gain of electrons. The oxidizing agent is the material reduced, and the reducing agent is the material oxidized.

In the given reaction between zinc and the ion Cu^{2+}:

$$Zn + Cu^{2+} \longrightarrow Zn^{2+} + Cu$$

Zn is oxidized because it has lost electrons to form Zn^{2+} as in answer C, and consequently is the reducing agent. The ion Cu^{2+} has gained electrons to form copper, Cu, and is the oxidizing agent.

84. Answer is **D**. Refer to the answer given to questions 14 and 83. The reducing agent is the species that loses electrons, Li or Br^{-1}. The equation with the more negative value for emf^0 indicates the species with the greater tendency to lose electrons, Li. The equation with the more positive value indicates the species with the greater tendency to gain the electrons, Br_2.

85. Answer is **D**. An electrochemical cell is made up of two electrodes connected in solution and by wires. One of the chemical species in solution loses electrons, the process of oxidation, to an electrode, the anode. Oxidation occurs at the anode. The electrons travel from the anode, through the wire, to the cathode where another species in solution gains the electrons, the process of reduction, supplied by the cathode. Reduction occurs at the cathode.

86. <u>Answer is **D**</u>. RCOOH is the general formula for a carboxylic acid.

$CH_3 - CH_3$ an alkane, specifically ethane

$CH_2 = CH_2$ an alkene, specifically ethene

$HC \equiv HC$ an alkyne, specifically ethyne

C_6H_6 benzene

CH_3CHO an aldehyde, specifically ethanal, acetaldehyde

CH_3COCH_3 a ketone, specifically propanone, acetone

CH_3CH_2Cl an alkyl halide, specifically chloroethane, ethyl chloride

CH_3COOH a carboxylic acid, specifically ethanoic acid, acetic acid

CH_3COOCH_3 an ester, specifically methyl ethanoate, methyl acetate

CH_3CH_2OH an alcohol, specifically ethanol, ethyl alcohol

CH_3CONH_2 an amide, specifically ethanamide, acetamide

$CH_3CH_2NH_2$ an amine, specifically aminoethane, ethyl amine

CH_3OCH_3 an ether, specifically dimethyl ether

87. <u>Answer is **B**</u>. The following general formulas represent the following general types of compounds:

C_nH_{2n+2} an alkane

C_nH_{2n} an alkene or a cycloalkane

C_nH_{2n-2} an alkyne or a cycloalkene (Answer D)

C_nH_n benzene when n = 6

88. <u>Answer is **B**</u>. The formula, C_3H_6, is one for either an alkene or a cycloalkane, both of which are unsaturated. The formula C_2H_6 represents an alkane; the formula C_2H_6O represents fully saturated compound and could be dimethyl ether or ethyl alcohol; the formula CH_3Cl represents an alkyl halide, methyl chloride.

89. <u>Answer is **D**</u>. Four different structural isomers can be formed by C_4H_9Cl.

$CH_3 - CH_2 - CH_2 - CH_2 - Cl$ 1-chlorobutane

$CH_3 - CH_2 - CHCl - CH_3$ 2-chlorobutane

$(CH_3)_2 - CH - CH_2Cl$ 1-chloro-2-methylpropane

$(CH_3)_3 - C - Cl$ 2-chloro-2-methylpropane

90. <u>Answer is **A**</u>. Two different structural formulas are possible for the monochlorination of C_2H_5Cl.

CH_3CHCl_2 1,1-dichloroethane

CH_2ClCH_2Cl 1,2-dichloroethane

91. <u>Answer is **A**</u>. Pick the longest straight chain for the base name of the alkane, in this case octane. Next name each of the substituents, two methyl groups and one bromo group. Give each substituent the lowest possible number and arrange the substituents in alphabetical order. The name is 5-bromo-3,4-dimethyloctane.

The base names are listed below for the straight-chain alkanes with the general formula C_nH_{2n+2}. The names of compounds in other families can be derived from these names by using the proper suffix.

1 Carbon	methane
2 Carbons	ethane
3 Carbons	propane
4 Carbons	butane
5 Carbons	pentane
6 Carbons	hexane
7 Carbons	heptane
8 Carbons	octane
9 Carbons	nonane
10 Carbons	decane

92. <u>Answer is **C**</u>. A stereocenter is an atom to which four different groups are attached. The different groups may be atoms such as the chlorine atom, Cl, or the bromine atom, Br, or they may be groups of atoms such as the methyl group, CH_3, or the ethyl group, CH_3CH_2. The underlined C in the following molecule, 2-bromo-2-chlorobutane, is a stereocenter.

$$CH_3$$
$$|$$
$$Cl - C - CH_2 - CH_3$$
$$|$$
$$Br$$

93. <u>Answer is **A**</u>. The two molecules pictured in question 93 have carbon-carbon double bonds. It is not possible to freely rotate around a carbon-carbon double bond as it is around a carbon-carbon single bond. Therefore, when a carbon-carbon double bond is present in a compound, two different compounds, geometric isomers, exist. In the example shown in question 93, the two chlorine atoms are on the same side of the double bond in one compound and on opposite sides of the double bond in the other compound. One could just as easily compare the positions of the two methyl groups relative to the carbon-carbon double bond and arrive at the same conclusion. Racemic mixture — Refer to the explanation for question 100.

Enantiomers are a form of stereoisomers, i.e. compounds which have the same groups within the molecules but differ from each other because of the arrangement of groups in the molecules. Enantiomers are two compounds having the same four different groups bonded to the stereocenter in each compound, but, because of the different positions in which these groups are placed relative to each other, i.e. because of different configurations, they are nonsuperimposable mirror images. Enantiomers are identical in almost all their physical and chemical properties. The enantiomers of 1-chloro-1-iodoethane are shown below.

$$
\begin{array}{cc}
CH_3 & CH_3 \\
| & | \\
H - C - Cl & Cl - C - H \\
| & | \\
I & I
\end{array}
$$

Diastereomers are also a form of stereoisomers. Diastereomers are two compounds, each having at least two different stereocenters. The diastereomers have the arrangement of the four different groups at one of the stereocenters identical in both molecules but the arrangement of another four different groups at the other stereocenter different in both compounds. In other words, diastereomers with two stereocenters have the same configuration at one of the stereocenter but opposite configurations at the other stereocenter. Diastereomers are nonsuperimposable and have different physical and chemical properties. One pair of diastereoisomers of 2-bromo-3-chlorobutane are shown below.

$$
\begin{array}{cc}
CH_3 & CH_3 \\
| & | \\
H - C - Cl & H - C - Cl \\
| & | \\
H - C - Br & Br - C - H \\
| & | \\
CH_3 & CH_3
\end{array}
$$

94. Answer is **C**. Refer to the explanation for question 44.

95. Answer is **B**. The carbon atom in ethylene has four pairs of electrons around it.

$$
\begin{array}{c}
H \\
| \\
H - C =
\end{array}
$$

Based upon the explanation given to questions 42, 43, and 44, one might expect the hybridization to be sp^3. However, when a multiple bond such as the carbon-carbon double bond in ethylene is present, the multiple bond is considered as one pair of electrons for the purpose of determining hybridization. The carbon atom is considered to have three pairs of electrons around it and consequently has sp² hybridization.

96. Answer is **B**. Oxidation may be defined as the loss of hydrogen. Oxidation of the secondary alcohol results in the loss the two underlined hydrogen atoms, one bonded to the carbon atom and one bonded to the oxygen atom. A double bond forms between the two atoms which lost the hydrogen atoms. The product is a ketone.

$$CH_3 - \underset{\underset{OH}{|}}{CH} - CH_3 \longrightarrow CH_3 - \underset{\underset{O}{\|}}{C} - CH_3$$

2-propanol   Propanone or acetone

97. Answer is **A**. Water-soluble compounds are substances whose structures are most like the structure of water. An ether, alkyl chloride, alkane, and benzene are given as possible answers. Ethyl ether or diethyl ether contains an oxygen atom, as does water. The hydrogen atoms in water are capable of hydrogen bonding to the oxygen atom in the ether, just as they can hydrogen bond to other water molecules.

Of the compounds listed, ether is not only the most soluble in water; it is the only one that is slightly soluble. The other functional groups are totally water insoluble.

98. Answer is **B**. A Grignard Reagent reacts with an aldehyde to produce, upon subsequent workup with water, a secondary alcohol. The reaction consists of addition across the carbon-oxygen double bond, with the alkyl group from the Grignard Reagent adding to the carbon atom and hydrogen adding to the oxygen atom. The methyl of the Grignard Reagent adds to the carbon atom of the double bond and the hydrogen adds to the oxygen to produce 2-propanol.

$$CH_3 - \underset{\underset{H}{\|}}{\overset{\overset{O}{}}{C}} - H \xrightarrow[H_2O]{CH_3MgBr} CH_3 - \underset{\underset{CH_3}{|}}{\overset{\overset{OH}{|}}{C}} - H$$

acetaldehyde   2 = propanol
or ethanal

99. Answer is B. The term dehydration means loss of water. When the elements of water are lost from an alcohol, the OH of the alcohol and the hydrogen atom on a carbon atom adjacent to the carbon atom bonded to the OH group are lost. The underlined atoms shown in the formula below are the ones most likely to be lost. An alkene is produced.

$$CH_3 - CH - \underset{\underline{OH}}{\underset{|}{\underset{|}{C}}} \overset{\overset{CH_3}{|}}{-} \underline{H} \qquad CH_3 - CH = C(CH_3)_2$$
$$\qquad\qquad\quad\; CH_3$$

3-methyl-2-butanol   2-methyl-2-butene

100. Answer is D. Each member of a pair of enantiomers rotates plane polarized light to an equal extent but in opposite directions. If one enantiomer rotates plane polarized light +42°, the other enantiomer of the pair rotates the light −42°. When the two enantiomers are mixed together in equal amounts, the mixture does not rotate plane polarized light and is called a racemic mixture (Answer D). A conformational mixture is a mixture of conformers, i.e. compounds that differ from each other only in orientation of groups but that can be converted into each other by rotation around a carbon-carbon single bond. A meso compound is one in which the molecule can be visualized as two parts which are nonsuperimposable mirror images of each other, i.e. a pair of enantiomers in one molecule. Refer to the answer given to question 93 for an explanation of diastereomers.

7
Quantitative Ability Review and Practice

TIPS FOR THE QUANTITATIVE ABILITY SECTION

The Quantitative Ability section of the PCAT consists of approximately 65 math problems. Some require only that you complete the algebraic operation(s) needed to solve an equation. Others are word problems that require you to decide what operations should be performed and what data from the information provided are useful. These word problems assess your problem-solving ability, and this ability will serve as a foundation for the skills you need to acquire during your pharmacy education.

This section is the one that most students say they are unable to finish. Therefore, it is important that you pace yourself and answer all questions. Remember, in order to complete as many questions as possible, work first on all the questions to which you know the answer, then go back and work on the more difficult questions.

Currently, as of 2002, the use of calculators during the PCAT is prohibited. Therefore, it is important to brush up on your math skills!

QUANTITATIVE ABILITY REVIEW OUTLINE

I.   **Whole numbers and their operations**
   A. Addition of negative and positive integers
   B. Subtraction of negative and positive integers
   C. Multiplication of negative and positive integers
   D. Division of negative and positive integers
   E. Absolute value
   F. Factorial
   G. Order of operations

II. **Fractions**
   A. Adding fractions
   B. Subtracting fractions
   C. Multiplying fractions
   D. Dividing fractions
   E. Comparing fractions: Which is larger or smaller?

III. **Decimals**
   A. Adding decimals
   B. Subtracting decimals
   C. Multiplying decimals
   D. Dividing decimals

IV. **Percentages**
   A. Calculating percents
   B. Adding percentages
   C. Subtracting percentages
   D. Multiplying percentages
   E. Dividing percentages
   F. Percent increase and decrease (percent change)
   G. Simple and compound interest

V. **Converting percents, fractions, and decimals**
   A. Converting fractions to percents
   B. Converting percents to fractions
   C. Converting fractions to decimals
   D. Converting decimals to fractions
   E. Converting percents to decimals
   F. Converting decimals to percents

VI. **Ratios and proportions**

VII. **Powers and exponents**

VIII. **Logarithms**
   A. Base 10 and natural logarithm
   B. Solving equations with logarithms or exponents
   C. Laws of logarithms
      1. Addition
      2. Subtraction
      3. Multiplication
      4. Division

IX. **Roots and radicals**
   A. Square root
   B. Cube root
   C. Addition of radicals
   D. Subtraction of radicals
   E. Multiplying radicals

X. **Statistics**
   A. Mean
   B. Median
   C. Mode
   D. Probability

XI. **Basic algebra**
   A. Linear equations
   B. Fractional equations
   C. Quadratic equations

XII. **Basic geometry**
   A. Calculating area
   B. Calculating perimeter
   C. Angles

XIII. **Operations concerning the conversion of basic units of measure (see Appendix)**

XIV. **Word-problem solving—analytical reasoning**

XV. **Interpretation of graphs and figures**

QUANTITATIVE ABILITY ANSWER SHEET

1 Ⓐ Ⓑ Ⓒ Ⓓ
2 Ⓐ Ⓑ Ⓒ Ⓓ
3 Ⓐ Ⓑ Ⓒ Ⓓ
4 Ⓐ Ⓑ Ⓒ Ⓓ
5 Ⓐ Ⓑ Ⓒ Ⓓ
6 Ⓐ Ⓑ Ⓒ Ⓓ
7 Ⓐ Ⓑ Ⓒ Ⓓ
8 Ⓐ Ⓑ Ⓒ Ⓓ
9 Ⓐ Ⓑ Ⓒ Ⓓ
10 Ⓐ Ⓑ Ⓒ Ⓓ
11 Ⓐ Ⓑ Ⓒ Ⓓ
12 Ⓐ Ⓑ Ⓒ Ⓓ
13 Ⓐ Ⓑ Ⓒ Ⓓ
14 Ⓐ Ⓑ Ⓒ Ⓓ
15 Ⓐ Ⓑ Ⓒ Ⓓ
16 Ⓐ Ⓑ Ⓒ Ⓓ
17 Ⓐ Ⓑ Ⓒ Ⓓ
18 Ⓐ Ⓑ Ⓒ Ⓓ
19 Ⓐ Ⓑ Ⓒ Ⓓ
20 Ⓐ Ⓑ Ⓒ Ⓓ

21 Ⓐ Ⓑ Ⓒ Ⓓ
22 Ⓐ Ⓑ Ⓒ Ⓓ
23 Ⓐ Ⓑ Ⓒ Ⓓ
24 Ⓐ Ⓑ Ⓒ Ⓓ
25 Ⓐ Ⓑ Ⓒ Ⓓ
26 Ⓐ Ⓑ Ⓒ Ⓓ
27 Ⓐ Ⓑ Ⓒ Ⓓ
28 Ⓐ Ⓑ Ⓒ Ⓓ
29 Ⓐ Ⓑ Ⓒ Ⓓ
30 Ⓐ Ⓑ Ⓒ Ⓓ
31 Ⓐ Ⓑ Ⓒ Ⓓ
32 Ⓐ Ⓑ Ⓒ Ⓓ
33 Ⓐ Ⓑ Ⓒ Ⓓ
34 Ⓐ Ⓑ Ⓒ Ⓓ
35 Ⓐ Ⓑ Ⓒ Ⓓ
36 Ⓐ Ⓑ Ⓒ Ⓓ
37 Ⓐ Ⓑ Ⓒ Ⓓ
38 Ⓐ Ⓑ Ⓒ Ⓓ
39 Ⓐ Ⓑ Ⓒ Ⓓ
40 Ⓐ Ⓑ Ⓒ Ⓓ

41 Ⓐ Ⓑ Ⓒ Ⓓ
42 Ⓐ Ⓑ Ⓒ Ⓓ
43 Ⓐ Ⓑ Ⓒ Ⓓ
44 Ⓐ Ⓑ Ⓒ Ⓓ
45 Ⓐ Ⓑ Ⓒ Ⓓ
46 Ⓐ Ⓑ Ⓒ Ⓓ
47 Ⓐ Ⓑ Ⓒ Ⓓ
48 Ⓐ Ⓑ Ⓒ Ⓓ
49 Ⓐ Ⓑ Ⓒ Ⓓ
50 Ⓐ Ⓑ Ⓒ Ⓓ
51 Ⓐ Ⓑ Ⓒ Ⓓ
52 Ⓐ Ⓑ Ⓒ Ⓓ
53 Ⓐ Ⓑ Ⓒ Ⓓ
54 Ⓐ Ⓑ Ⓒ Ⓓ
55 Ⓐ Ⓑ Ⓒ Ⓓ
56 Ⓐ Ⓑ Ⓒ Ⓓ
57 Ⓐ Ⓑ Ⓒ Ⓓ
58 Ⓐ Ⓑ Ⓒ Ⓓ
59 Ⓐ Ⓑ Ⓒ Ⓓ
60 Ⓐ Ⓑ Ⓒ Ⓓ

61 Ⓐ Ⓑ Ⓒ Ⓓ
62 Ⓐ Ⓑ Ⓒ Ⓓ
63 Ⓐ Ⓑ Ⓒ Ⓓ
64 Ⓐ Ⓑ Ⓒ Ⓓ
65 Ⓐ Ⓑ Ⓒ Ⓓ
66 Ⓐ Ⓑ Ⓒ Ⓓ
67 Ⓐ Ⓑ Ⓒ Ⓓ
68 Ⓐ Ⓑ Ⓒ Ⓓ
69 Ⓐ Ⓑ Ⓒ Ⓓ
70 Ⓐ Ⓑ Ⓒ Ⓓ
71 Ⓐ Ⓑ Ⓒ Ⓓ
72 Ⓐ Ⓑ Ⓒ Ⓓ
73 Ⓐ Ⓑ Ⓒ Ⓓ
74 Ⓐ Ⓑ Ⓒ Ⓓ
75 Ⓐ Ⓑ Ⓒ Ⓓ
76 Ⓐ Ⓑ Ⓒ Ⓓ
77 Ⓐ Ⓑ Ⓒ Ⓓ
78 Ⓐ Ⓑ Ⓒ Ⓓ
79 Ⓐ Ⓑ Ⓒ Ⓓ
80 Ⓐ Ⓑ Ⓒ Ⓓ

81 Ⓐ Ⓑ Ⓒ Ⓓ
82 Ⓐ Ⓑ Ⓒ Ⓓ
83 Ⓐ Ⓑ Ⓒ Ⓓ
84 Ⓐ Ⓑ Ⓒ Ⓓ
85 Ⓐ Ⓑ Ⓒ Ⓓ
86 Ⓐ Ⓑ Ⓒ Ⓓ
87 Ⓐ Ⓑ Ⓒ Ⓓ
88 Ⓐ Ⓑ Ⓒ Ⓓ
89 Ⓐ Ⓑ Ⓒ Ⓓ
90 Ⓐ Ⓑ Ⓒ Ⓓ
91 Ⓐ Ⓑ Ⓒ Ⓓ
92 Ⓐ Ⓑ Ⓒ Ⓓ
93 Ⓐ Ⓑ Ⓒ Ⓓ
94 Ⓐ Ⓑ Ⓒ Ⓓ
95 Ⓐ Ⓑ Ⓒ Ⓓ
96 Ⓐ Ⓑ Ⓒ Ⓓ
97 Ⓐ Ⓑ Ⓒ Ⓓ
98 Ⓐ Ⓑ Ⓒ Ⓓ
99 Ⓐ Ⓑ Ⓒ Ⓓ
100 Ⓐ Ⓑ Ⓒ Ⓓ

QUANTITATIVE ABILITY PRACTICE QUESTIONS

100 Questions

<u>Directions:</u> Select the best answer to each of the following questions.

1. $\dfrac{2}{5} + \dfrac{3}{4} =$

   A. $1\dfrac{3}{20}$

   B. $\dfrac{21}{20}$

   C. $1\dfrac{4}{20}$

   D. $1\dfrac{4}{5}$

2. A plane traveling 200 miles per hour is 50 miles from its landing site at 1:20 P.M. At what time will it land at the airport?

   A. 2:00 P.M.
   B. 1:30 P.M.
   C. 1:35 P.M.
   D. 1:45 P.M.

3. If $x^2 - 2x = 0$, $x =$

   A. 4, 0
   B. 3, 0
   C. 2, 0
   D. 1, 0

4. Which one of the following is a solution for $x^2 - 36 = 0$?

   A. 4
   B. 5
   C. 6
   D. 7

5. $100^0 =$

A. 100.
B. 10
C. 1
D. 0

6. $\frac{2}{5} =$

A. 20%
B. 40%
C. 50%
D. 60%

7. $1.2^2 =$

A. 14.4
B. 0.144
C. 144
D. 1.44

8. 20% of 50 =

A. 5
B. 10
C. 15
D. 20

9. 12% of 130 =

A. 10.6
B. 12.7
C. 15.6
D. 18.2

10. $\frac{3}{8} =$

A. 23.5%
B. 33.5%
C. 37.5%
D. 42.3%

11. $\dfrac{3}{5} =$

A. 30%

B. 40%

C. 50%

D. 60%

12. During a 6-hour flight, a plane flew at 400 miles per hour for the first 2 hours, 600 miles per hour for the next 3 hours and 160 miles per hour for the last hour. What was the average speed of the flight?

A. 340 mph

B. 400 mph

C. 200 mph

D. 460 mph

13. If a coin is tossed four times, what is the probability of obtaining tails on the last toss?

A. $\dfrac{1}{2}$

B. $\dfrac{3}{5}$

C. $\dfrac{2}{5}$

D. $\dfrac{5}{8}$

14. What is the median of this series of values: 5, 7, 3, 12, 10, and 1?

A. 3

B. 5

C. 6

D. 7

15. $\left(\dfrac{1}{x}\right)^6 + \left(\dfrac{2}{x^2}\right)^3 =$

A. $3x^4$

B. $\dfrac{9}{x^6}$

C. $6x$

D. $\dfrac{1}{2x^4}$

16. 0.01% of 100 =

A. 1
B. 0.1
C. 0.01
D. 0.001

17. $-4 - 3 \{2 + 1[3 - (2 + 3) + 2] + 2\} + 4 =$

A. -12
B. 0
C. 2
D. 8

18. 22% of 65 =

A. 14.3
B. 15.4
C. 17.3
D. 19.1

19. $5^3 + 2^5 =$

A. 100
B. 141
C. 157
D. 189

20. $2^3 \cdot 3^0 =$

A. 8
B. 12
C. 24
D. 30

21. $6^2 \cdot 10^2 =$

A. 3.6
B. 36
C. 360
D. 3,600

22. Bonnie invested $3,000 in Southern National Bank at 6% interest per year. She also has an account at Central City Bank that pays 12% interest per year. If she earns a total of $540 in interest in 1 year, what amount of money does she have in Central City Bank?

A. $3,600
B. $1,200
C. $3,000
D. $5,400

23. Parks leaves home for work and drives at 30 miles per hour. Twenty minutes later Susan, his wife, realizes he left his tool box at home. If Susan drives at 40 miles per hour, how far must she drive before she overtakes him?

A. 20 miles
B. 30 miles
C. 40 miles
D. 60 miles

24. $\log 1 =$

A. 0
B. 1
C. 10
D. 100

25. log 10 =

A. 0
B. 1
C. 10
D. 100

26. log 100 =

A. 0
B. 1
C. 2
D. 3

27. Tommy has $7.50 in nickels and dimes. If he has the same number of nickels and of dimes, how many of each does he have?

A. 35
B. 30
C. 65
D. 50

28. Find the perimeter of the figure below. ($\pi = 3.14$)

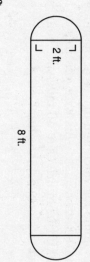

2 ft.

8 ft.

A. 22.28 ft.
B. 24.86 ft.
C. 40.54 ft.
D. 33.8 ft.

29. What is the area of the figure below?

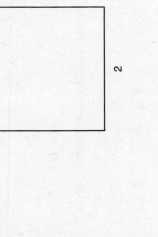

2

2

A. 2
B. 4
C. 8
D. 16

30. What is the slope of a line that contains points (2,3) and (4,6)?

A. 15
B. 10
C. 5
D. 1.5

31. Given log 2 = 0.3010, determine log 8.

A. 1.204
B. 0.602
C. 0.301
D. 0.903

32. If a scale has a 2.5% error in weighing, what is the range of possible weight for a tablet that weighs 160 milligrams on that scale?

A. 156 mg–164 mg
B. 152 mg–168 mg
C. 127 mg–154 mg
D. 125 mg–175 mg

33. 140 pounds are equivalent to how many kilograms?

A. 60.2
B. 63.6
C. 65.2
D. 67.7

34. 22 kilograms are equivalent to how many pounds?

A. 1.1
B. 39
C. 44.4
D. 48.4

35. 163 centimeters are equivalent to how many inches?

A. 60
B. 64
C. 68
D. 72

36. Given the following equation:

$$°C = \frac{5}{9} \ (°F - 32)$$

convert 10°F to °C.

A. –12.2
B. 12.2
C. 1.22
D. 0.122

37. $\dfrac{5}{30} + \dfrac{1}{8} =$

A. $\dfrac{6}{11}$
B. $\dfrac{7}{24}$
C. $\dfrac{3}{5}$
D. None of the above

38. $\dfrac{9}{81} \cdot 2 =$

A. $\dfrac{1}{9}$

B. $\dfrac{2}{9}$

C. $\dfrac{9}{162}$

D. None of the above

39. $\dfrac{8}{9} - \dfrac{1}{2} =$

A. $\dfrac{6}{18}$

B. $\dfrac{7}{18}$

C. $\dfrac{3}{18}$

D. None of the above

40. $\dfrac{5}{6} \cdot \dfrac{2}{11} =$

A. $\dfrac{11}{9}$

B. $\dfrac{31}{66}$

C. $\dfrac{5}{33}$

D. None of the above

41. 3! =

A. 3
B. 6
C. 9
D. 12

42. 2! =

A. 1
B. 2
C. 3
D. 4

43. Aminophylline injection is 80% theophylline content. The strength of aminophylline injection is 25 milligrams per milliliter. How many milliliters of aminophylline injection are needed to provide a dose of 320 milligrams theophylline?

A. 10.67
B. 12.8
C. 16
D. 20

44. A patient's creatinine clearance (CrCl) can be calculated by using the following formula:

$$CrCl = \frac{140 - age\ in\ years}{72 \cdot SCr} \cdot ideal\ body\ weight\ in\ kilograms$$

What is the CrCl for a 78-year-old patient who has a SCr of 2.8 and an ideal body weight of 150 pounds?

A. 21
B. 31
C. 41
D. 51

45. $\sqrt[3]{729}$ =

A. 7
B. 8
C. 9
D. None of the above

46. $\sqrt[3]{1331} =$

   A. 11
   B. 12
   C. 13
   D. 14

47. $\sqrt[3]{1} =$

   A. ½
   B. 1
   C. 2
   D. None of the above

48. $\sqrt[3]{0.125} =$

   A. 0.2
   B. 0.3
   C. 0.4
   D. 0.5

49. A mixture of gold and platinum is used to make crowns for teeth, usually in the ratio of 5 parts gold to 2 parts platinum by weight. If a crown made with these metals weighs 0.42 ounce, how many ounces of gold does the crown contain?

   A. 0.20
   B. 0.24
   C. 0.30
   D. 0.36

50. Larry's house is 12 miles from the park. Larry rode his bicycle from his house to the park at 12 miles per hour. He then walked the bicycle home from the park at 3 miles per hour. If he took the same route on both trips, what was his average speed?

   A. 4.8 mph
   B. 7.5 mph
   C. 1.6 mph
   D. 4.0 mph

51. $\sqrt{32} + \sqrt{50} =$

    A. $7\sqrt{2}$
    B. $8\sqrt{2}$
    C. $9\sqrt{2}$
    D. $10\sqrt{2}$

52. $0.04(10^3) =$

    A. 4
    B. 40
    C. 400
    D. 4,000

53. $0.7(10^4) =$

    A. 70
    B. 700
    C. 7,000
    D. 70,000

54. $x^2 + 2 = 27; x =$

    A. 4, –4
    B. 5, –5
    C. 6, –6
    D. None of the above

55. $x^2 + 5 = 149; x =$

    A. 11, –11
    B. 12, –12
    C. 13, –13
    D. None of the above

56. $x^3 + 23 = 50$; $x =$

A. 4
B. 5
C. 6
D. None of the above

57. Mr. Gammill can wash a car in 30 minutes, but his new helper takes twice as long to do the same job. If the two men work together, how many cars can they wash in 2 hours?

A. 4
B. 5
C. 6
D. 8

58. Jack is 3 years older than his younger brother Alan, who is twice as old as the youngest child, Marie. If the ages of the three add up to 28 years, how old is Alan?

A. 5 years
B. 8 years
C. 9 years
D. 10 years

59. Harvey noticed that his gas tank was only $\frac{1}{4}$ full. He completely filled the tank by putting 9 gallons into it. What is the capacity of the gas tank?

A. 10 gallons
B. 12 gallons
C. 14 gallons
D. 18 gallons

60. What is the perimeter of the figure below?

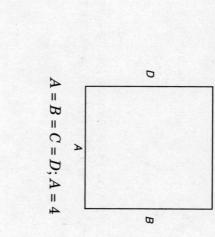

$A = B = C = D; A = 4$

A. 4
B. 16
C. 24
D. 32

61. $3x + 56 = 68; x =$

A. 2
B. 3
C. 4
D. 5

62. $\dfrac{50}{125} =$

A. 20%
B. 30%
C. 40%
D. 50%

63. $6x + 56 = 68; x =$

A. 2
B. 3
C. 4
D. 5

64. $5x - 15 = 45; x =$

A. 8
B. 10
C. 12
D. 14

65. $2x = \dfrac{1}{4}$

A. $\dfrac{1}{2}$

B. $\dfrac{1}{4}$

C. $\dfrac{1}{6}$

D. None of the above

66. Which line is perpendicular to the y-axis?

A. $y = 4$
B. $x = 3$
C. $x = 1 - y$
D. $y = 1 + x$

67. The sum of a number and 8 equals 4 less than the product of 4 and the number. Find the number.

A. 3
B. 2
C. 6
D. 4

68. The angles of a triangle are in the ratio of 1:2:3. How many degrees are in the largest angle?

A. 40°
B. 30°
C. 90°
D. 45°

69. What is the area of a square with a perimeter of 48 meters?

A. 2305 m^2
B. 96 m^2
C. 144 m^2
D. 24 m^2

70. What is the area of a square with a perimeter of 10 feet?

A. 2.5 ft.^{2}

B. 4.2 ft.^{2}

C. 5.1 ft.^{2}

D. 6.25 ft.^{2}

71. If 6 grams of powder X are needed to make 100 milliliters of product, how many grams of powder X are required to make 250 milliliters of product?

A. 10

B. 15

C. 20

D. 25

72. If a patient takes 2 teaspoonfuls of medicine three times daily, how many milliliters equal a 7 day supply? (1 tsp. = 5 mL).

A. 65

B. 70

C. 105

D. 210

73. If 500 milligrams of drug A equal 400 milligrams of drug B, what is the equivalent dose of drug B for a patient taking 250 mg of drug A?

A. 200 mg

B. 240 mg

C. 250 mg

D. 300 mg

74. Which of the following is equivalent to $-2 < \dfrac{x}{3} < 2$?

A. $-3 < x < 3$

B. $-4 < x < 4$

C. $-9 < x < 9$

D. $-6 < x < 6$

75. $\dfrac{\sqrt{36} \cdot \sqrt{16}}{\sqrt{9}} =$

A. $\dfrac{6 \cdot 4}{3} = 12$

B. $\dfrac{6 \cdot 4}{3} = 8$

C. $\dfrac{4 \cdot 4}{4} = 4$

D. $\dfrac{4 \cdot 3}{2} = 6$

76. 10% of 10 =

A. 10^2
B. 10^1
C. 10
D. 10^0

77. $2 - 3\{5 + 1[4 + (2 - 3) + 4] - 3\} + 6 =$

A. −19
B. 20
C. −13
D. 11

78. If 250 milligrams of drug K equal 200 milligrams of drug L, what is the equivalent dose of drug K for a patient taking 50 milligrams of drug L?

A. 52.5 mg
B. 58.5 mg
C. 62.5 mg
D. 68.5 mg

Use the graph below to answer questions 79 and 80.

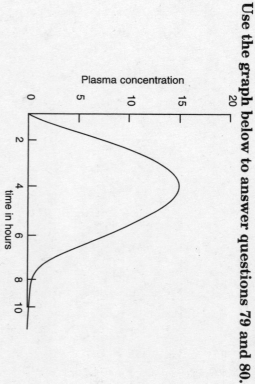

79. What is the maximum blood concentration of the drug in the graph?

A. 0 mg
B. 5 mg
C. 10 mg
D. 15 mg

80. How much time was required to achieve the maximum blood concentration?

A. 0 hr
B. 2 hr
C. 4 hr
D. 6 hr

81. 6!

A. 1250
B. 720
C. 400
D. 250

82. |−10| + 120 =

A. 110
B. 120
C. 125
D. 130

83. 1 liter − 573 milliliters =

    A. 1573 mL

    B. 527 mL

    C. 427 mL

    D. 0.5 L

84. How many ounces are there in 7 pounds?

    A. 56

    B. 112

    C. 140

    D. 160

85. A plane leaves the airport at 12 noon and flies for 2 hours at 450 miles per hour. A malfunction forces the plane to return to the airport, but at only one-third of the speed at which it left the airport. How long will the plane take to return?

    A. 3 hr.

    B. 5 hr.

    C. 6 hr.

    D. 8 hr.

86. Reading her bank statement, Beth realizes she has earned $400 in interest over the last year. If Beth started with $5,000 at the first of the year, what interest rate (per year) did she receive to earn $400?

    A. 4%

    B. 12%

    C. 8%

    D. 10%

87. Edward left for home driving at 40 miles per hour. Fifteen minutes later, he stopped for 15 minutes for gas. He resumed driving home at 30 miles an hour and reached home 20 minutes after he bought the gas. What distance did Edward drive to get home?

    A. 15 mi

    B. 20 mi

    C. 45 mi

    D. 30 mi

88. If a solution is 16% (16 g powder/100 mL), how many grams of powder are needed to make 25 milliliters of solution?

A. 2
B. 4
C. 6
D. 8

89. If a solution is 30% (30 g powder/100 mL), how many milligrams of powder are needed to make 20 milliliters of solution?

A. 3×10^3
B. 3×10^4
C. 6×10^3
D. 6×10^4

Use the figure below to answer questions 90 and 91.

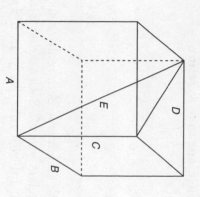

$(A = B = C; A = 3 \text{ inches})$

90. What is the total surface area of the cube?

A. 4 in.²
B. 16 in.²
C. 48 in.²
D. 54 in.²

91. What is the length of line D?

A. 9 in.
B. 3 in.
C. $3\sqrt{2}$ in.
D. $5\sqrt{2}$ in.

92. What is the median of the following numbers: 8, 35, 8, 9, 5, 10, 7, 3, 12?

   A. 5
   B. 8
   C. 35
   D. 12

93. $5! =$

   A. 25
   B. 50
   C. 60
   D. 120

94. $7! =$

   A. 49
   B. 98
   C. 5,040
   D. 9,604

95. $6x^3 = 162; x^3 =$

   A. 3
   B. 9
   C. 18
   D. 27

Use the figure below to answer questions 96 and 97.

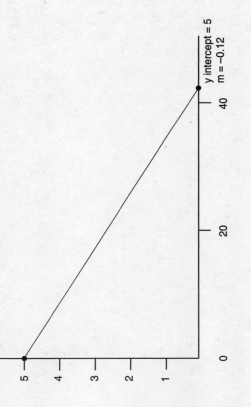

y intercept = 5
m = −0.12

96. What is the equation for the line shown in the figure?

A. $y = -0.12x + 5$
B. $5 = 0.12xy$
C. $y = 5x - 12$
D. $12 = 5xm$

97. If $y = 17$, what is value of x in the equation for the line?

A. -12
B. 100
C. 150
D. -100

98. $\sqrt{48} + \sqrt{12} =$

A. $7\sqrt{2}$
B. $6\sqrt{3}$
C. $9\sqrt{2}$
D. $5\sqrt{6}$

99. $\dfrac{1}{16} \div 4$

A. $\dfrac{1}{24}$
B. $\dfrac{1}{4}$
C. $\dfrac{3}{64}$
D. None of the above

100. $\dfrac{5}{9} \cdot \dfrac{1}{2} =$

A. $\dfrac{8}{9}$
B. $\dfrac{10}{9}$
C. $\dfrac{6}{11}$
D. $\dfrac{5}{18}$

QUANTITATIVE ABILITY ANSWER KEY

1. A	21. D	41. B	61. C	81. B
2. C	22. C	42. B	62. C	82. D
3. C	23. C	43. C	63. A	83. C
4. C	24. A	44. A	64. C	84. B
5. C	25. B	45. C	65. D	85. C
6. B	26. C	46. A	66. A	86. C
7. D	27. D	47. B	67. D	87. B
8. B	28. A	48. D	68. C	88. B
9. C	29. B	49. C	69. C	89. C
10. C	30. D	50. A	70. D	90. D
11. D	31. D	51. C	71. B	91. C
12. D	32. A	52. B	72. D	92. B
13. A	33. B	53. C	73. A	93. D
14. C	34. D	54. B	74. D	94. C
15. B	35. B	55. B	75. B	95. D
16. C	36. A	56. D	76. D	96. A
17. A	37. B	57. C	77. A	97. D
18. A	38. B	58. D	78. C	98. B
19. C	39. B	59. B	79. D	99. D
20. A	40. C	60. B	80. C	100. D

QUANTITATIVE ABILITY EXPLANATORY ANSWERS

1. <u>Answer is **A**</u>. Find the least common denominator of 5 and 4, 20. Rewrite the fractions using the least common denominator:

$$\frac{2 \cdot 4}{20} + \frac{3 \cdot 5}{20}.$$

$$\frac{8}{20} + \frac{15}{20} = \frac{23}{20} = 1\frac{3}{20}$$

2. <u>Answer is **C**</u>. At 200 mph the plane will fly 50 mi. in 15 min. (¼ hr.). Add 15 min. to 1:20 P.M. to arrive at the correct answer: 1:35 P.M.

3. <u>Answer is **C**</u>.

Factor the expression on the left-hand side:

Set each factor equal to 0:

Solve for x:

4. <u>Answer is **C**</u>. There are two methods for solving this problem.

(1) $(x + 6)(x - 6) = 0$ (2) $x^2 - 36 = 0$

$x + 6 = 0 \mid x - 6 = 0$ $x^2 = 36$

$x = -6 \mid x = 6$ $\sqrt{x^2} = \sqrt{36}$

$x = 6; \quad x = -6$

$x(x - 2) = 0$

$x = 0; x - 2 = 0$

$x = 0, x = 2$

5. <u>Answer is **C**</u>. Any number raised to zero power is 1: $100^0 = 1$.

6. <u>Answer is **B**</u>. $2 \div 5 = 0.40$. The decimal 0.40 can be converted to a percent by multiplying by 100, or by moving the decimal point to the right two spaces, to obtain 40%.

7. <u>Answer is **D**</u>. $1.2^2 = 1.2 \cdot 1.2 = 1.44$.

8. <u>Answer is **B**</u>. Convert 20% to a decimal. Divide by 100, or move the decimal point to the left two spaces: $20 \div 100 = 0.20$. Multiply: $0.20 \cdot 50 = 10$.

9. <u>Answer is **C**</u>. Convert 12% to a decimal. Divide by 100, or move the decimal point to the left two spaces: $12 \div 100 = 0.12$. Multiply: $0.12 \cdot 130 = 15.6$.

10. <u>Answer is **C**</u>. Convert $\dfrac{3}{8}$ to a decimal. $3 \div 8 = 0.375$. Convert 0.375 to a percent by multiplying by 100 or by moving the decimal to the right two spaces: $100 \cdot 0.375 = 37.5\%$.

11. <u>Answer is **D**</u>. Convert $\dfrac{3}{5}$ to a decimal: $3 \div 5 = 0.60$. Convert 0.60 to a percent by multiplying by 100, or by moving the decimal to the right two spaces: $100 \cdot 0.60 = 60\%$.

12. <u>Answer is **D**</u>. Calculate the total distance traveled:

$$[(400 \cdot 2) + (600 \cdot 3) + (160 \cdot 1)] = 2{,}760 \text{ mi}.$$

Then divide by the elapsed time, 6 hr., to obtain 460 mph.

13. <u>Answer is **A**</u>. Each time a coin is tossed, there are two possible outcomes, heads and tails. The probability of heads is $\dfrac{1}{2}$. The outcome of the fourth coin toss is independent of the outcomes of the three earlier tosses.

14. <u>Answer is **C**</u>. To find the median, arrange the numbers in increasing order: 1, 3, 5, 7, 10, 12. The median is the value in the middle of the list. The median (middle) value of an even-numbered set of numbers is the average of the two middle numbers in the set: (1, 3, <u>5</u>, <u>7</u>, 10, 12). The average of the middle two numbers is

$$\frac{5+7}{2} = \frac{12}{2} = 6.$$

15. <u>Answer is **B**</u>.

$$\left(\frac{1}{x}\right)^6 + \left(\frac{2}{x^2}\right)^3 = \frac{1^6}{x^6} + \frac{2^3}{(x^2)^3}$$

$$= \frac{1}{x^6} + \frac{8}{x^6}$$

$$= \frac{9}{x^6}$$

Rule: $\left(\dfrac{a}{b}\right)^n = \dfrac{a^n}{b^n}$

Rule: $(a^n)^m = a^{n \bullet m}$

16. <u>Answer is **C**</u>. Convert 0.01% to a decimal by dividing by 100, 0.0001. Multiply: $100 \cdot 0.0001 = 0.01$.

17. <u>Answer is **A**</u>. Begin with the innermost parentheses, and work outward.

$-4 - 3 \{2 + 1 [3 - (2 + 3) + 2] + 2\} + 4 =$

$-4 - 3 \{2 + 1 [3 - 5 + 2] + 2\} + 4 =$

$-4 - 3 \{2 + 1 \cdot 0 + 2\} + 4 =$

$-4 - 3 \cdot 4 + 4 =$

$-4 - 12 + 4 =$

-12

18. <u>Answer is **A**</u>. Convert 22% to a decimal: 0.22. Multiply:

$0.22 \cdot 65 = 14.3.$

19. <u>Answer is **C**</u>. $5^3 = (5 \cdot 5 \cdot 5) = 125;\ 2^5 = (2 \cdot 2 \cdot 2 \cdot 2 \cdot 2) = 32;$

$125 + 32 = 157.$

20. <u>Answer is **A**</u>. $2^3 = (2 \cdot 2 \cdot 2) = 8;\ 3^0 = 1;\ 8 \cdot 1 = 8.$

21. <u>Answer is **D**</u>. $6^2 = (6 \cdot 6) = 36;\ 10^2 = (10 \cdot 10) = 100;$

$36 \cdot 100 = 3,600.$

22. <u>Answer is **C**</u>. $3,000 \cdot 0.06 \ (6\%) = \$180$ interest in 1 year at Southern National Bank. Subtract $180 from $540 to obtain $360 in interest to be earned from Central City Bank. Let $D =$ dollars in Central City account; then

$$Dx \cdot 0.12 = \$360$$

$$D = \frac{360}{0.12} = \$3,000$$

23. <u>Answer is **C**</u>. In 20 min. $\left(\frac{1}{3}\ \text{hr.}\right)$, Parks has gone 10 mi. In another hour, he will have covered a total of 40 mi. (10 + 30). Therefore, Susan must drive 40 mi. (for 1 hr.) to catch him.

24. <u>Answer is **A**</u>. Read "log 1 =" as asking the question "To what power do I raise 10 to get 1?" Since $10^0 = 1$, the answer is 0.

25. <u>Answer is **B**</u>. You raise 10 to the power 1 to get 10, so the answer is 1.

26. <u>Answer is **C**</u>. You raise 10 to the power 2 to get 100, so the answer is 2.

27. Answer is **D**. Let x = the number of each kind of coin. $5x$ = value of the nickels, and $10x$ = value of the dimes.

$$5x + 10x = 750$$
$$15x = 750$$
$$x = 50$$

Fifty nickels = $2.50 and fifty dimes = $5.00 for a total of $7.50.

28. Answer is **A**. The length of the two straight sides is 16 ft. The circumference of a circle of diameter 2 is 2π = 6.28, so each end is $\dfrac{6.28}{2}$ = 3.14 ft. Therefore, the perimeter of the figure is

$16 + 2 \cdot 3.14 = 22.28$ ft.

29. Answer is **B**. The area of a square is calculated by multiplying the lengths of two sides: $(2 \cdot 2 = 4)$.

30. Answer is **D**. Use the slope formula and substitute the given values:

$$m = \frac{y_2 - y_1}{x_2 - x_1}$$

$$= \frac{6 - 3}{4 - 2}$$

$$= \frac{3}{2} \text{ or } 1.5.$$

31. Answer is **D**. $\log 8 = \log 2^3$, since $2^3 = 8$.

$\log 2^3 = 3 \log 2$, since $n \log a = \log a^n$.

$\therefore \log 8 = 3 \log 2 = 3 \cdot 0.3010 = 0.903$.

32. Answer is **A**. Convert 2.5% to a decimal: 0.025. Multiply: 0.025 × 160 mg = 4 mg. To calculate the range, subtract 4 from 160 and add 4 to 160: 156 mg − 164 mg.

33. Answer is **B**. $\dfrac{1\,\text{kg}}{2.2\,\text{lb.}} \cdot 140\,\text{lb.} = 63.6\,\text{kg.}$

34. Answer is **D**. $\dfrac{2.2\,\text{lb.}}{1\,\text{kg}} \cdot 22\,\text{kg} = 48.4\,\text{lb.}$

35. Answer is **B**. 1 in. = 2.54 cm; 163 cm ÷ 2.54 cm = 64 in.

36. <u>Answer is **A**</u>. $°C = \frac{5}{9}(10 - 32) = \frac{5}{9}(-22) = -12.2.$

37. <u>Answer is **B**</u>. Reduce $\frac{5}{30}$ to $\frac{1}{6}$. The least common denominator for $\frac{1}{6}$ and $\frac{1}{8}$ is 24. Rewrite the fractions using the least common denominator:

$$\frac{1 \cdot 4}{24} + \frac{1 \cdot 3}{24}.$$

$$\frac{4}{24} + \frac{3}{24} = \frac{7}{24}$$

38. <u>Answer is **B**</u>. Reduce $\frac{9}{81}$ to $\frac{1}{9}; \frac{1}{9} \cdot \frac{2}{1} = \frac{2}{9}.$

39. <u>Answer is **B**</u>. The least common denominator for $\frac{8}{9}$ and $\frac{1}{2}$ is 18. Rewrite the fractions, using the least common denominator:

$$\frac{8 \cdot 2}{18} - \frac{1 \cdot 9}{18}.$$

$$\frac{16}{18} - \frac{9}{18} = \frac{7}{18}$$

40. <u>Answer is **C**</u>. $\frac{5}{6} \cdot \frac{2}{11} = \frac{10}{66}.$ Reduce $\frac{10}{66}$ to $\frac{5}{33}.$

41. <u>Answer is **B**</u>. $3! = 3 \cdot 2 \cdot 1 = 6.$

42. <u>Answer is **B**</u>. $2! = 2 \cdot 1 = 2.$

43. <u>Answer is **C**</u>. Aminophylline is 80% theophylline; therefore, 25 mg (1 mL) of aminophylline will contain only 20 mg of theophylline. Divide 320 mg by 20 mg mL to obtain 16 mL.

44. Answer is **A**. Convert 150 lb. to kilograms: $150 \div 2.2 = 68.2$ kg. Substitute 68.2 kg for weight, 2.8 for SCr, and 78 for age in the given formula:

$$CrCl = \frac{(140 - 78)}{72 \cdot 2.8} \cdot 68.2 = 21$$

45. Answer is **C**. $\sqrt[3]{729} = 9$; $9^3 = 9 \cdot 9 \cdot 9 = 729$.

46. Answer is **A**. $\sqrt[3]{1331} = 11$; $11^3 = 11 \cdot 11 \cdot 11 = 1331$.

47. Answer is **B**. $\sqrt[3]{1} = 1$; $1^3 = 1 \cdot 1 \cdot 1 = 1$.

48. Answer is **D**. $\sqrt[3]{0.125} = 0.5$; $0.5^3 = 0.5 \cdot 0.5 \cdot 0.5 = 0.125$.

49. Answer is **C**. Add 5 parts and 2 parts to get 7 parts for the total amount of metal. Divide 0.42 by 7 to obtain a weight of 0.06 oz. per part. Multiply 0.06 oz. per part by 5 parts to obtain 0.30 oz. of gold.

50. Answer is **A**. If the house is 12 mi. from the park, at 12 mph Larry needed 1 hr. to make the trip. At only 3 mph, he needed 4 hr. to get back home. Thus, he traveled 24 mi. (2 · 12 mi.) in 5 hr. (1 + 4 hr.). Divide 24 by 5 to get an average speed of 4.8 mph.

51. Answer is **C**. $\sqrt{32} = \sqrt{16 \cdot 2} = 4\sqrt{2}$; $\sqrt{50} = \sqrt{25 \cdot 2} = 5\sqrt{2}$;

$$4\sqrt{2} + 5\sqrt{2} = 9\sqrt{2}.$$

52. Answer is **B**. $0.04(10^3) = 0.04(1,000) = 40.$

53. Answer is **C**. $0.7(10^4) = 0.7(10,000) = 7,000.$

54. Answer is **B**. Solve for x:

$$x^2 + 2 = 27$$
$$x^2 = 25$$
$$\sqrt{x^2} = \sqrt{25}$$
$$x = 5, -5$$

55. Answer is **B**. Solve for x:

$$x^2 + 5 = 149$$
$$x^2 = 144$$
$$\sqrt{x^2} = \sqrt{144}$$
$$x = 12, -12$$

56. <u>Answer is **D**</u>. Solve for x:

$$x^3 + 23 = 50$$
$$x^3 = 27$$
$$\sqrt[3]{x^3} = \sqrt[3]{27}$$
$$x = 3$$

57. <u>Answer is **C**</u>. Mr. Gammill can wash 2 cars per hour (60 min./hr. divided by 30 min./car). The helper can wash only 1 car per hour [30 min./car × 2]. Thus, the two men can wash 3 cars per hour if working together. In 2 hr. they can wash 6 cars.

58. <u>Answer is **D**</u>. Let x = age of Marie, the youngest. Alan is twice as old as Marie ($2x$). Jack is 3 years older than Alan ($2x + 3$). The sum of their ages is 28 yr. Set up the equation:

$$x + 2x + 2x + 3 = 28$$
$$x + 2x + 2x = 28 - 3$$
$$5x = 25$$
$$x = 5$$

Therefore, Marie (x) is 5 yr. old. Alan ($2x$) is 10 yr. old. Jack ($2x + 3$) is 13 yr. old for a total of 28 yr. The answer only asked for Alan's age: 10 yr.

59. <u>Answer is **B**</u>. Set up the following proportion: $\dfrac{3}{4}$ is to 9 gal. as 1 is to x gal. Then $x = 12$ gal.

60. <u>Answer is **B**</u>. The perimeter is the sum of the sides:
$$4 + 4 + 4 + 4 = 16.$$

61. <u>Answer is **C**</u>. Solve for x:

$$3x + 56 = 68$$
$$3x = 12$$
$$x = 4$$

62. <u>Answer is **C**</u>. $50 \div 125 = 0.4$. Convert to percent by multiplying by 100: $0.40 \cdot 100 = 40\%$.

63. <u>Answer is **A**</u>. Solve for x:

$$6x + 56 = 68$$
$$6x = 12$$
$$x = 2$$

64. <u>Answer is **C**</u>. Solve for x:

$$5x - 15 = 45$$
$$5x = 60$$
$$x = 12$$

65. <u>Answer is **D**</u>. Solve for x:

$$2x = \frac{1}{4}$$
$$x = \frac{1}{4} \div 2$$
$$x = \frac{1}{8}$$

66. <u>Answer is **A**</u>. If a line is perpendicular to the y-axis, it is a horizontal line. For any value of x, the y-value will be the same, c, so $y = c$. Only answer A is of this form.

67. <u>Answer is **D**</u>. This can be written as an equation, where x = number to be found: $x + 8 = 4x - 4$. Solve for x: $x = 4$.

68. <u>Answer is **C**</u>. The sum of the measures of the angles of a triangle is $180°$. Let x = measure of smallest angle. Then the other two angles can be represented as $2x$ and $3x$.

$$x + 2x + 3x = 180°$$
$$6x = 180°$$
$$x = 30°$$
$$\therefore 3x = 90°$$

69. <u>Answer is **C**</u>. A square has four equal sides. If the perimeter is 48 m, then each side is 12 m ($48 \div 4$). The area of a square is the product of two sides. Thus, the area is 144 m² ($12 \text{ m} \times 12 \text{ m}$).

70. <u>Answer is **D**</u>. If the perimeter of the square is 10 ft., then each side is 2.5 ft. ($10 \text{ ft.} \div 4$). The area of a square is the product of two sides. Thus, the area is 6.25 ft.² ($2.5 \text{ ft.} \cdot 2.5 \text{ ft.}$).

71. <u>Answer is **B**</u>. Set up a proportion:

$$\frac{6 \text{ g}}{100 \text{ mL}} = \frac{x \text{ g}}{250 \text{ mL}}$$

Cross multiply and divide:

$$6 \cdot 250 = 100x$$
$$1,500 = 100x$$
$$x = 15 \text{ g}$$

72. Answer is **D**. 2 tsp. per dose = 10 mL/dose. 10 mL/dose • 3 doses daily = 30 mL of medicine daily; 7-day supply = 7 • 30 mL = 210 mL.

73. Answer is **A**. Set up a proportion:

$$\frac{500 \text{ mg drug A}}{400 \text{ mg drug B}} = \frac{250 \text{ mg drug A}}{x \text{ mg drug B}}$$

Cross multiply and divide: 500x = 250 • 400

$$500x = 10,000$$
$$x = 200 \text{ mg}$$

74. Answer is **D**. Multiply each expression in the inequality by 3:

$$3(-2 < \frac{x}{3} < 2) = -6 < x \leq 6.$$

75. Answer is **B**. $\frac{\sqrt{36} \cdot \sqrt{16}}{\sqrt{9}} = \frac{6 \cdot 4}{3} = 8.$

76. Answer is **D**. Convert 10% to a decimal: 0.1. Multiply: 0.1 • 10 = 1 = 10^0 = 1.

77. Answer is **A**. Evaluate the innermost set of parentheses, then work outward.

$$2 - 3 \{5 + 1 [4 + (2 - 3) + 4] - 3\} + 6 =$$
$$2 - 3 \{5 + 1 [4 + (-1) + 4] - 3\} + 6 =$$
$$2 - 3 \{5 + 1(7) - 3\} + 6 =$$
$$2 - 3 \{9\} + 6 =$$
$$2 - 27 + 6 = -19$$

78. Answer is **C**. Set up a proportion:

$$\frac{250 \text{ mg drug K}}{200 \text{ mg drug L}} = \frac{x \text{ mg drug K}}{50 \text{ mg drug L}}$$

Cross multiply and divide: 200x = 250 • 50
$$200x = 12,500$$
$$x = 62.5 \text{ mg}$$

79. Answer is **D**. See figure.

80. Answer is **C**. See figure.

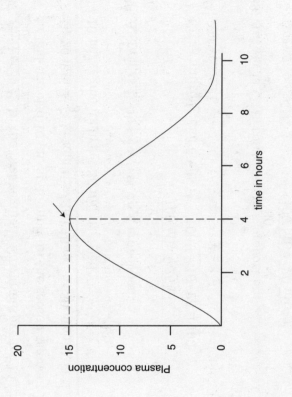

81. <u>Answer is **B**</u>. 6! = 6 factorial = 6 • 5 • 4 • 3 • 2 • 1 = 720.

82. <u>Answer is **D**</u>. When you see | |, drop the sign, so |–10| = 10;
10 + 120 = 130.

83. <u>Answer is **C**</u>. 1 L = 1,000 mL. Therefore, 1,000 mL – 573 mL =
427 mL.

84. <u>Answer is **B**</u>. $\dfrac{16 \text{ oz.}}{1 \text{ lb.}}$ • 7 lb. = 112 oz.

85. <u>Answer is **C**</u>. Distance flown from airport = 450 mph • 2 hrs =
900 mi. Speed of return trip = $\dfrac{1}{3}$ of 450 mph = 150 mph. To find the
time for the return trip, divide 900 mi. by 150 mph to obtain 6 hr.

86. <u>Answer is **C**</u>. Let x = interest rate.
  Then $x(5000) = 400$
  $x = 0.08$ or 8%

87. <u>Answer is **B**</u>. In the first segment Edward drove for 15 min. = $\frac{1}{4}$ hr and traveled 10 mi. at 40 mph. In the second segment he drove for 20 min = $\frac{1}{3}$ hr and traveled 10 mi. at 30 mph. Add the two 10 mi. segments to get 20 mi. traveled.

88. <u>Answer is **B**</u>. To solve, set up a proportion:

$$\frac{16 \text{ g}}{100 \text{ mL}} = \frac{x}{25 \text{ mL}}$$

Cross multiply and divide: $100x = 16 \cdot 25 = 400$

$$x = 4 \text{ g}$$

89. <u>Answer is **C**</u>. To solve, set up a proportion:

$$\frac{30 \text{ g}}{100 \text{ mL}} = \frac{x}{20 \text{ mL}}$$

Cross multiply and divide: $100x = 20 \cdot 30 = 600$

$$x = 6 \text{ g}$$

Convert 6 g into milligrams. Since 1 g = 1000 mg, multiply by 1,000: $6 \cdot 1,000 = 6,000$ mg $= 6 \cdot 10^3$

90. <u>Answer is **D**</u>. Each face of the cube has a surface area of 3 in. × 3 in. = 9 in². To calculate total surface area, multiply the surface area of each face by the number of faces. Since a cube has 6 faces: total surface area = 9 in.² · 6 = 54 in.².

91. <u>Answer is **C**</u>. Line D is the hypotenuse of an isosceles right triangle; each leg of this triangle has a length of 3, the given dimension of the six equal sides of the cube. To calculate hypotenuse D, use the Pythagorean theorem and substitute the given value of the legs:

$$(\text{Hypotenuse})^2 = (\text{leg 1})^2 + (\text{leg 2})^2$$

$$D^2 = 3^2 + 3^2$$

Solve for D: $\sqrt{D^2} = \sqrt{18}$

$$D = \sqrt{9 \cdot 2}$$

$$D = 3\sqrt{2}$$

92. <u>Answer is **B**</u>. In an ordered list, the median is the value that is in the middle of the list of data. To find the median arrange the given numbers in ascending order; 3, 5, 7, 8, 8, 9, 10, 12, 35. Since the list contains an odd number of values (9), the middle number, or median, is the fifth number in the list: 3, 5, 7, 8, <u>8</u>, 9, 10, 12, 25.

93. <u>Answer is **D**</u>. $5! = 5 \cdot 4 \cdot 3 \cdot 2 \cdot 1 = 120$.

94. <u>Answer is **C**</u>. $7! = 7 \cdot 6 \cdot 5 \cdot 4 \cdot 3 \cdot 2 \cdot 1 = 5{,}040$.

95. <u>Answer is **D**</u>. $6x^3 = 162$. Divide both sides by 6: $x^3 = 27$.

96. <u>Answer is **A**</u>. $y = mx + b$ is the slope-intercept equation for a line. Here, the slope, $m = -0.12$ and the y-intercept, $b = 5$, so the equation for the line shown is $y = -0, 12x + 5$.

97. <u>Answer is **D**</u>. First, write the equation of the line (see answer for question for 96). Then substitute 17 for y and solve for x.

$$17 = -0.12x + 5$$
$$12 = -0.12x$$
$$x = -100$$

98. <u>Answer is **B**</u>.

$\sqrt{48} = \sqrt{16 \cdot 3} = 4\sqrt{3}; \ \sqrt{12} = \sqrt{4 \cdot 3} = 2\sqrt{3}; \ 4\sqrt{3} + 2\sqrt{3} = 6\sqrt{3}$.

99. <u>Answer is **D**</u>. $\dfrac{1}{16} \div 4 = \dfrac{1}{16} \cdot \dfrac{1}{4} = \dfrac{1}{64}$.

100. <u>Answer is **D**</u>. $\dfrac{5}{9} \cdot \dfrac{1}{2} = \dfrac{5}{18}$.

8 Reading Comprehension Review and Practice

TIPS FOR THE READING COMPREHENSION SECTION

The Reading Comprehension section of the PCAT presents relatively short (usually 300–500 words) passages of science-oriented nonfiction. You are asked to read each passage carefully and then to answer questions related to it. For each passage, there are generally 4–8 questions, with a total of about 45 questions for this section. Keep in mind that the correct answer often is a direct statement taken from the reading passage.

Practice the reading passages and sample questions in this book. You may find one of the following strategies helpful. Try both, and see which works better for you.

Strategy 1. Read the passage first, and then answer the questions. Don't be concerned with how many times you need to refer to the passage to answer questions; just complete the section as quickly as possible, making sure you find the *correct* answer to every question. Underline the text in the passage that contains the answer to each question as you go.

Strategy 2. Read each question *before* you read the passage. Then, as you read the passage and come to a statement on which you know one of the questions was based, answer that question. Again, underline the section of the passage used to answer the question. Return to the passage and continue reading until you come to another statement that answers a question. Answer that question, and resume reading.

For each individual a slightly different process may be helpful in completing this section. Begin to formulate your own method by identifying which of the two strategies above works better for you as you answer the practice questions that follow. Make your decision based on (1) the time it takes you to answer the questions and (2) the number of correct answers you made. Remember to answer all the questions; if necessary, guess at a reasonable answer.

In addition to choosing strategy 1 or 2, try to determine where your general strengths and weaknesses as a reader lie. Do you tend to get a quick grasp of the overall sense of a passage but miss the details? Or do you, as a reader sometimes fail to see the forest for the trees? In other words, do you remember only the details and find yourself unable to state the basic meaning of the passage as a whole? In either case, take some time to improve your "weak" areas. Be patient with yourself as you practice. With adequate review, you should be able to work at your normal pace when you take the actual PCAT.

READING COMPREHENSION ANSWER SHEET

1 Ⓐ Ⓑ Ⓒ Ⓓ
2 Ⓐ Ⓑ Ⓒ Ⓓ
3 Ⓐ Ⓑ Ⓒ Ⓓ
4 Ⓐ Ⓑ Ⓒ Ⓓ
5 Ⓐ Ⓑ Ⓒ Ⓓ
6 Ⓐ Ⓑ Ⓒ Ⓓ
7 Ⓐ Ⓑ Ⓒ Ⓓ
8 Ⓐ Ⓑ Ⓒ Ⓓ
9 Ⓐ Ⓑ Ⓒ Ⓓ
10 Ⓐ Ⓑ Ⓒ Ⓓ

11 Ⓐ Ⓑ Ⓒ Ⓓ
12 Ⓐ Ⓑ Ⓒ Ⓓ
13 Ⓐ Ⓑ Ⓒ Ⓓ
14 Ⓐ Ⓑ Ⓒ Ⓓ
15 Ⓐ Ⓑ Ⓒ Ⓓ
16 Ⓐ Ⓑ Ⓒ Ⓓ
17 Ⓐ Ⓑ Ⓒ Ⓓ
18 Ⓐ Ⓑ Ⓒ Ⓓ
19 Ⓐ Ⓑ Ⓒ Ⓓ
20 Ⓐ Ⓑ Ⓒ Ⓓ

21 Ⓐ Ⓑ Ⓒ Ⓓ
22 Ⓐ Ⓑ Ⓒ Ⓓ
23 Ⓐ Ⓑ Ⓒ Ⓓ
24 Ⓐ Ⓑ Ⓒ Ⓓ
25 Ⓐ Ⓑ Ⓒ Ⓓ
26 Ⓐ Ⓑ Ⓒ Ⓓ
27 Ⓐ Ⓑ Ⓒ Ⓓ
28 Ⓐ Ⓑ Ⓒ Ⓓ
29 Ⓐ Ⓑ Ⓒ Ⓓ
30 Ⓐ Ⓑ Ⓒ Ⓓ

31 Ⓐ Ⓑ Ⓒ Ⓓ
32 Ⓐ Ⓑ Ⓒ Ⓓ
33 Ⓐ Ⓑ Ⓒ Ⓓ
34 Ⓐ Ⓑ Ⓒ Ⓓ
35 Ⓐ Ⓑ Ⓒ Ⓓ
36 Ⓐ Ⓑ Ⓒ Ⓓ
37 Ⓐ Ⓑ Ⓒ Ⓓ
38 Ⓐ Ⓑ Ⓒ Ⓓ
39 Ⓐ Ⓑ Ⓒ Ⓓ
40 Ⓐ Ⓑ Ⓒ Ⓓ

41 Ⓐ Ⓑ Ⓒ Ⓓ
42 Ⓐ Ⓑ Ⓒ Ⓓ
43 Ⓐ Ⓑ Ⓒ Ⓓ
44 Ⓐ Ⓑ Ⓒ Ⓓ
45 Ⓐ Ⓑ Ⓒ Ⓓ
46 Ⓐ Ⓑ Ⓒ Ⓓ
47 Ⓐ Ⓑ Ⓒ Ⓓ
48 Ⓐ Ⓑ Ⓒ Ⓓ
49 Ⓐ Ⓑ Ⓒ Ⓓ
50 Ⓐ Ⓑ Ⓒ Ⓓ

READING COMPREHENSION PRACTICE QUESTIONS

50 questions

<u>Directions</u>: Read each of the following passages, and choose the **best** answer to each question that follows.

Passage 1:

In the past two decades, people living in the northeastern, north-central, and western United States have unwittingly entered a dangerous enzootic cycle—a cycle of disease that typically is restricted to wildlife. Wild mammals and birds host a wide variety of disease agents, with effects ranging from mild symptoms to mortality, but in most cases the pathogen affects only one or a few host species and never causes disease in humans. However, as a result of a complicated sequence of events, people have become frequent accidental hosts for ticks and the disease agents they carry, including a corkscrew-shaped bacterium called *Borrelia burgdorferi*, the agent of Lyme disease. As of 1995, cases of Lyme disease had been reported in 48 of the 50 states and appear to be increasing, both in numbers of people affected and in geographic distribution.

Where does this disease come from, why has it emerged so rapidly, and what can people do to reduce their risk of exposure? It is possible to address these questions not from a medical point of view, but rather from an ecological one. All living organisms—from the *B. burgdorferi* bacterium and the ticks it infects to the mice and deer on which the ticks feed—form an ecological relationship with their habitats. Understanding the complex interactions between plant and animal species within those habitats may help people to predict the places where they are most likely to encounter disease-bearing ticks and become infected. Thus armed, individuals may ultimately be able to protect themselves from Lyme disease.

Currently, to prevent Lyme disease people wear protective clothing when they are in wooded areas and perform "tick checks" after leaving the woods. One underemphasized means to avoid exposure to Lyme disease, however, is avoiding the most heavily tick-infested habitats at the times of year when ticks are most abundant or dangerous. Recent research has suggested that such habitats can be predicted, often well in advance. Ultimately, it is the hope of ecologists studying this problem that we can use their expertise in pinpointing these habitats to warn the public away from areas that are likely to contain an abundance of disease-carrying ticks.

Excerpted from "The Ecology of Lyme-Disease Risk," by Richard S. Ostfeld, *The American Scientist*, Vol. 85, p. 338, reprinted by permission of *American Scientist*, magazine of Sigma Xi, The Scientific Research Society.

1. The agent of Lyme disease is

   A. an enzootic cycle.
   B. wild mammals and birds.
   C. people living in the northeastern, north-central, and western United States.
   D. a corkscrew-shaped bacterium called *Borrelia burgdorferi*.

2. The aim of understanding Lyme disease from an ecological as well as a medical point of view is

   A. to help preserve the mice and deer on which the ticks feed.
   B. to help people predict the places where they are most likely to encounter disease-bearing ticks and become infected.
   C. to develop a vaccine against the disease.
   D. to further our understanding of the relationship between ticks and their habitats.

3. To prevent Lyme disease people currently

   A. receive annual vaccinations.
   B. perform "tick checks" after leaving the woods.
   C. wear protective clothing in wooded areas.
   D. Both B and C

4. Which of the following statements is true?

   A. Since the ecological approach to Lyme disease was introduced in 1995, cases have been decreasing in the northeastern, north-central, and western United States.
   B. As of 1995, cases of Lyme disease had been reported in 48 of the 50 states and appear to be increasing, both in numbers of people affected and geographical distribution.
   C. While cases in the northeastern United States have decreased since 1995, because of alterations in the enzootic cycle, cases are still on the rise in other geographical areas.
   D. Cases of Lyme disease have remained relatively rare because of the inaccessibility of heavily tick-infested areas, but researchers still hope to keep as many people as possible away from areas where they might become infected.

5. One underemphasized means to avoid exposure to Lyme disease is

   A. wearing protective clothing.
   B. avoiding the most heavily tick-infested areas at certain times of the year.
   C. using insect repellent.
   D. remembering to get vaccinated before going into areas that are known to be heavily tick-infested.

Passage 2:

To the average physician, Lyme disease is suspected when a patient arrives at a clinic or hospital complaining of a strange bull's-eye rash, known as erythema migrans, or EM, together with one or more flulike symptoms, such as fever, chills, muscle aches, or lethargy. The physician will take a blood sample for laboratory confirmation, but will feel quite confident to make a diagnosis of Lyme disease after noting the telltale combination of symptoms, as well as the circumstances surrounding the infection. The patient will undoubtedly have been bitten by the black-legged tick *Ixodes scaplaris*, formerly called the deer tick, or a close relative, which transferred to him or her the *B. burgdorferi* bacterium. Most likely, the physician will prescribe an oral course of antibiotics and will duly report the case to the county or state health department, which will include it in the morbidity statistics for Lyme disease.

Accurate diagnosis and effective treatment of Lyme disease are not always so straightforward, particularly in regions of the country newly invaded by the epidemic. In these regions, health care professionals and the public need to be educated about the confusing and generalized symptoms, the generally poor, but growing, accuracy of lab tests, and the efficacy of various antibiotic treatments. If Lyme disease is left untreated for some time, *B. burgdorferi* may persist in the patient's tissues and can migrate to the central and peripheral nervous systems or to joints and cause more severe late-stage symptoms, which include arthritis and neurological disorders, such as dizziness, memory loss, and disorientation. Vaccines that protect against Lyme disease are now being field tested by pharmaceutical companies, but none has yet been approved by the Food and Drug Administration for public use. Even if an effective vaccine were certified and marketed, the primary means that individuals have of protecting themselves against the disease is avoiding the tick in the first place.

Excerpted from "The Ecology of Lyme-Disease Risk," by Richard S. Ostfeld, *The American Scientist*, Vol. 85, p. 338, reprinted by permission of *American Scientist*, magazine of Sigma Xi, The Scientific Research Society.

6. When a patient reports to a clinic or hospital with symptoms of Lyme disease, he or she has undoubtedly been bitten by

A. the black-legged tick *Ixodes scaplaris.*
B. a tick-bearing wild mammal.
C. *B. burgdorferi.*
D. none of the above; Lyme disease is generally believed to be spread by an airborne pathogen.

7. Symptoms of Lyme disease include fever, chills, muscle aches and

A. lethargy.
B. a bull's-eye rash.
C. vomiting.
D. Both A and B

8. Erythema migrans is best described as

A. a benign condition often mistaken for Lyme disease.
B. the microorganism believed to be an agent of Lyme disease.
C. the black-legged tick.
D. a strange, bull's-eye rash characteristic of Lyme disease.

9. In addition to noting the telltale combination of symptoms in a patient with Lyme disease, a physician is likely to

A. take a blood sample for laboratory confirmation.
B. prescribe an oral course of antibiotics.
C. report the case to the county or state health department.
D. All of the above

10. If Lyme disease is left untreated for some time,

A. health care professionals and the public will not be educated about its confusing and generalized symptoms.
B. the accuracy of diagnostic lab tests may be poor.
C. *B. burdorferi* may persist in the patient's tissues and cause more severe late-stage symptoms.
D. antibiotic treatments will no longer be effective.

Passage 3:

Rabies is a master dissembler. No other disease so completely manipulates its stricken host while barely leaving a trace of its presence. And rabies is preeminently adaptive: even if one host species is eliminated, the virus resurfaces in another. It bides its time, shadowing its victims, waiting for new hosts to emerge as people disrupt habitats and force animals to congregate more densely. Despite the war chest of vaccines designed to stop it and the near certain death of every organism infected by it, rabies persists.

In the United States, on average, fewer than two people a year die of rabies, about the same number as in Western Europe. Vaccination and animal control policies ensure that few, if any, of those cases come from dog bites. Worldwide, between 20,000 and 100,000 people die of rabies in a given year, most of them in developing countries, and some 10 million are treated annually for possible exposures, mostly from dog bites. Compared with the dangers of becoming infected with HIV, tuberculosis, or malaria, each of which strikes millions of people every year, the risk of contracting rabies is vanishingly small. But rabies has had far greater influence on culture and science than its current incidence might suggest. And its devastating effects assure that it is never far from people's minds. Rabies has the highest fatality rate of any known human infection.

Excerpted from "The Deadliest Virus," by Cynthia Mills, from the January/February 1997 issue of *THE SCIENCES*, reprinted by permission of The Sciences, 2 East 63rd Street, New York, NY 10021.

11. Rabies persists

   A. in spite of the vaccines designed to stop it.
   B. because of its highly adaptive nature.
   C. because people disrupt habitats, forcing animals to congregate more densely and allowing new hosts to emerge.
   D. A, B, and C

12. In the United States, the number of people who die of rabies every year is

   A. between 2,000 and 10,000.
   B. comparable to the number who die of rabies in Western Europe.
   C. increasing in spite of efforts to bring it under control.
   D. approaching the number in danger of becoming infected with malaria.

13. Which of these statements about rabies may be regarded as true, according to the passage you read?

A. It has the highest fatality rate of any known human infection.
B. Although frightening, rabies has had less influence on culture and science than its reputation might suggest.
C. Few cases of rabies in the United States and Western Europe, but most cases worldwide, come from dog bites.
D. Both A and C

14. Worldwide, the number of people treated annually for possible exposure to rabies is

A. between 20,000 and 100,000.
B. greater than the number infected with HIV.
C. 10 million.
D. None of the above

Passage 4:

Unlike an electron, a single red blood cell cannot go through two openings at once. Indeed, it is generally true that the physicist seeking to understand the circulation of the blood can ignore most of the perplexities of twentieth-century physics. Given the scale of the circulatory system and the speed of blood flow, neither quantum mechanics nor relativity applies. Instead the flow of blood through the heart and the vascular tree can be adequately described by the familiar mechanics of Newton and Galileo.

If the circulation of the blood obeys the laws of classical mechanics, however, this does not mean that it is simple. An early experimental model of the vascular tree was a system of glass tubes filled with water. But unlike water, blood is not an "ideal" fluid. Instead it is a suspension of cells that, under certain circumstances, can behave in non-Newtonian ways. Moreover, flow through the vascular tree is pulsatile rather than steady; blood vessels taper and are elastic rather than rigid; and flow in any part of the densely interconnected system is affected by flow in neighboring regions. When these factors and the fantastic geometrical complexity of the labyrinthine vascular system are taken into account, the equations of blood flow, while remaining classical in inspiration, quickly become too complex to be solved explicitly.

Confronted with a system of overwhelming complexity, scientists typically resort to the intelligent simplification, that is, to a model. The first mathematical model of the human circulation was the *windkessel*, or compression chamber, model developed by Otto Frank in 1899 to explain how pulsatile flow from the heart is converted into steadier flow in the peripheral circulation. Sophisticated analytical models, the descendants of the windkessel model, still provide insight into the functioning of the circulatory system. But they are increasingly supplemented by numerical models, which exploit the power of the computer to arrive at accurate approximations of values that satisfy systems of equations that would otherwise be unsolvable. The computer can also be used to produce stunning images that allow otherwise cryptic measurements or calculations to be grasped intuitively.

Excerpted from "The Biophysics of Stroke," by George J. Hademenos, *The American Scientist*, Vol. 85, p. 226, reprinted by permission of *American Scientist*, magazine of Sigma Xi, The Scientific Research Society.

15. Quantum physics and relativity may be ignored by the physicist seeking to understand the circulation of the blood because

   A. electrons cannot go through two openings at once in the vascular tree.
   B. the mechanics of Newton and Galileo do not apply.
   C. the scale of the circulatory system and the speed of blood flow can be adequately described by the mechanics of Newton and Galileo.
   D. blood is an "ideal" fluid.

16. An early experimental model of the vascular tree

   A. revealed that blood cannot behave in non-Newtonian ways.
   B. consisted of a system of glass tubes filled with water.
   C. was developed by Galileo.
   D. yielded equations that although complex, could be solved quickly and explicitly.

17. When scientists are confronted with a system of overwhelming complexity, they typically

   A. give up.
   B. resort to intelligent simplification, that is, to a model.
   C. adjust their most arbitrary assumptions accordingly.
   D. abandon the mechanics of Galileo and Newton.

18. Otto Frank developed the *windkessel* model in 1899 for the purpose of

A. explaining how pulsatile flow from the heart is converted into steadier flow in the peripheral circulation.

B. improving on previous mathematical models.

C. converting the flow of blood from the heart into steadier flow in the peripheral circulation of human subjects.

D. augmenting the mechanics of Galileo and Newton.

19. In the twentieth century

A. quantum physics and relativity have given us some useful insights into the functioning of the circulatory system.

B. the *windkessel* model is still in use.

C. computers have not proved as useful as physicists had hoped since many systems of equations remain unsolvable.

D. computers can be used to produce images that allow cryptic measurements or calculations to be grasped intuitively.

Passage 5:

A taxonomist viewing insects or crustaceans tends to see tough, jointed exoskeletons and elaborate limbs as their salient features—so salient, in fact, that the taxonomists who named the phylum to which these animals belong called it Arthropoda, or "jointed foot." The same biologist will also notice that the arthropod body plan is that of a modified worm, where the worm's more-or-less uniform series of segmented units becomes well differentiated along the length of the arthropod body. This gives arthropods distinct head, middle, and tail regions.

As neurobiologists considering evolution from simple to more complex animals, we are interested in the changes in the neural circuits serving locomotion and sensory coding that accompanied the transition from worm to arthropod. Such evolution is crucial to the emergence of advanced mobile animals. Because brains and body plans must have evolved in step from their simpler antecedents, comparative studies of neural development and of the mature nervous systems of animals promise to reveal much about arthropod evolution. In arthropods almost every nerve cell grows in a particular pattern and makes specific synaptic connections to form the elaborate neural circuits that give an animal its mobility and control; these features make each cell a recognizable identity.

Just as vertebrae and ribs are serially repeated, sets of neurons are repeated in each segment of an insect's body, or beneath each facet of the compound eye. Using identified neurons, anatomists can compare the development and structure of nervous systems from different arthropods much as they can compare vertebrate skeletons. In addition, we can record the electrical activity from a single neuron, which allows us to compare physiological function in different lineages. So far, most work has been done on insects, but comparisons can also be made between insects and crustaceans. Such comparisons tell biologists how these arthropods, with their jointed exoskeletons and specialized limbs, evolved from simpler ancestors and how they have subsequently diversified during evolutionary history.

Excerpted from "The Evolution of Anthropod Nervous Systems," by Daniel Ororio, Jonathan P. Bacon, and Paul M. Whitington, *The American Scientist*, Vol. 85, p. 244, reprinted by permission of *American Scientist*, magazine of Sigma Xi, The Scientific Research Society.

20. The passage suggests that

A. neurobiologists do not agree with taxonomists about the evolution of arthropods from worms.

B. the arthropod body plan is that of a modified worm.

C. since arthropods evolved from worms, they have no distinct head, middle, and tail regions.

D. neurobiologists consider the salient features of insects and crustaceans to be more clearly differentiated than those of arthropods.

21. As worms evolved into arthropods

A. their uniform series of segmented units became well differentiated.

B. the neural circuits serving locomotion and sensory coding changed.

C. they became advanced mobile animals.

D. All of the above

22. The name Arthropoda means

A. "jointed foot."

B. "wormlike."

C. "well-differentiated."

D. "mobile."

23. The phylum Arthropoda is distinguished by

   A. a lack of sets of repeated neurons.

   B. elaborate neural circuits allowing for mobility and control.

   C. a tough, jointed exoskeleton.

   D. Both B and C

24. Using identified neurons, anatomists can compare the development and structure of the nervous systems of different arthropods just as they can compare

   A. sets of nonrepeating neurons.

   B. vertebrate skeletons.

   C. exoskeletons and specialized limbs.

   D. worms and arthropods.

25. The passage suggests that neurobiologists are seeking to discover more about

   A. how arthropods evolved from simpler ancestors.

   B. how arthropods have diversified during their evolutionary history.

   C. how the neural circuits of insects and crustaceans function.

   D. All of the above

Passage 6:

Allergic drug reactions account for 5% to 20% of all observed adverse drug reactions. Adverse drug reactions have been reported to occur in as many as 30% of hospitalized patients, and 3% of all hospitalizations are a result of adverse drug reactions. In a computerized surveillance study of over 36,000 hospitalized patients, 731 adverse events were identified. Of those, 1% were categorized as severe, life threatening, and allergic in nature. The potential morbidity and mortality associated with allergic drug reactions is great even though these outcomes occur infrequently.

In order to appropriately diagnose and treat a patient experiencing an allergic reaction, it is necessary to be able to differentiate allergic reactions from other closely related adverse drug reactions. One method of classification divides adverse reactions into those that are "predictable, usually dose-dependent, and related to the pharmacologic actions of the drug," and those that are "unpredictable, often dose independent, and related to the individual's immunologic response or to genetic differences in susceptible patients." Under this classification scheme, drug allergy or drug hypersensitivity is an unpredictable adverse drug reaction that is immunologically mediated.

Excerpted with permission from "Chapter 6, Anaphylaxis and Drug Allergies," page 6-1, Applied Therapeutics: The Clinical Use of Drugs, Sixth Edition, edited by Lloyd Yee Young and Mary Anne Koda-Kimble, published by Applied Therapeutics, Inc., Vancouver, Washington, © 1995.

26. Which of the following is necessary in order to appropriately diagnose and treat a patient experiencing an allergic reaction to a drug?

A. A way to differentiate allergic reactions from other adverse drug reactions

B. Determination that the reaction is dose-dependent and related to the pharmacological actions of the drug

C. Access to appropriate statistics, such as computerized surveillance studies

D. Hospitalization

27. If an adverse reaction is not "predictable, usually dose-independent, and related to the pharmacologic actions of the drug," then it is likely to be

A. adverse but not allergic.

B. dose independent and unpredictable.

C. related to the individual's immunologic response.

D. Both B and C

28. Allergic drug reactions account for as many as what percent of all observed adverse drug reactions?

A. 1% to 5%

B. 5% to 20%

C. 30%

D. 1%

29. Of 731 adverse drug events identified in a surveillance study of over 36,000 patients, 1% were characterized as

A. dose-dependent.

B. allergic but not severe or life-threatening.

C. severe, life-threatening, and allergic in nature.

D. adverse but not allergic.

Passage 7:

You have seen the photographs, of course: An apple flaring on two sides as a bullet passes through it; tennis balls flattening themselves against rackets; jagged-edge balloons frozen in mid-pop; droplets in mid-drip; bubbles in mid-burst. They were the work of Harold E. Edgerton, an M.I.T. professor whose invention of the stroboscopic flash in the early 1930s made it possible, for the first time, to capture events as fleeting as a millionth of a second.

For decades chemists and solid-state physicists have yearned for a way of observing even more subtle alterations in matter: chemical reactions, or changes of state such as freezing or evaporation. Those changes depend on the breaking of bonds between atoms, a process that can take place in less than a picosecond—millions of times faster than anything Edgerton ever attempted. A fifth of a picosecond, for instance, is all the time it takes for photons entering your retina to trigger chemical changes in a pigment called rhodopsin—a reaction that makes it possible for you to read this article.

Lasers can flash that quickly. But laser light is too coarse a tool to give sharp closeup pictures of matter. Visible wavelengths are thousands of times longer than the space between the atoms in a solid material. Furthermore, visible light tends to interact with the fuzzy outer electron clouds of an atom—not with the tightly bound inner electrons that give a much better idea of where the atom is. For those reasons, physicists studying atomic structure have long relied on much shorter-wavelength radiation: X-rays. Stroboscopic X-ray crystallography, however, has been a long time coming. Now a team at Lawrence Berkeley National Laboratory in Berkeley, California, has taken a step in that direction by generating the shortest X-ray flash ever.

The main problem with X-rays is that their well known tendency to zip through materials makes them an optical nightmare. "You can't steer them the way you can light. It's difficult. You can't make a good mirror that operates at short wavelengths," says Robert W. Schoenlein, a staff scientist who coheaded the Lawrence Berkeley team. To point their X-rays in the right direction, Schoenlein and his colleagues generated them via Thomson scattering, an effect described early in this century by the English physicist J. J. Thomson. "Fast-moving particles such as electrons," Thomson said, "can transfer energy to photons, much as a Ping-Pong paddle energizes a ball." Thus, if you shoot a laser beam into a stream of high-velocity electrons, some of the photons in the beam may pick up enough energy to turn into X-rays. To produce X-ray flashes, some investigators fire a pulse of electrons head-on into a laser beam.

The shorter the pulse, the shorter the flash. So far, however, the X-ray flashes have been too long to be useful.

Excerpted from "Flash Point," by Robert J. Coontz Jr., from the January/February 1997 issue of *THE SCIENCES*, reprinted by permission of The Sciences, 2 East 63rd Street, New York, NY 10021.

30. The passage identifies Harold E. Edgerton as

   A. head of the research team at Lawrence Berkeley National Laboratory.
   B. an English physicist.
   C. an M.I.T. professor who invented the stroboscopic flash.
   D. the discoverer of X-rays in the early 1930s.

31. The time it takes for photons entering your retina to trigger chemical changes in a pigment called rhodopsin is

   A. about a picosecond.
   B. a millionth of a second.
   C. a single pulse.
   D. a fifth of a picosecond.

32. According to Robert W. Schoenlein, the main problem with X-rays is that

   A. they tend to zip through materials, making them an optical nightmare.
   B. they can't be steered the way light can.
   C. you can't make a good mirror that operates at short wavelengths.
   D. All of the above

33. Physicists studying atomic structure have relied on X-rays rather than lasers because

   A. lasers cannot flash quickly enough.
   B. laser light is too coarse a tool to give good close-up pictures of matter.
   C. visible light tends to interact with the fuzzy outer electron clouds of an atom.
   D. Both B and C

34. The main point of this passage is best summarized by which of the following statements?

A. Robert W. Schoenlein has invented a technique to transfer energy from electrons to photons, much as a Ping-Pong paddle energizes a ball.

B. Lasers have proved to be the most efficient way to produce sharp close-up pictures of matter.

C. Robert W. Schoenlein, a staff scientist at Lawrence Berkeley National Laboratory, and his team have succeeded in creating the shortest X-ray flashes ever.

D. Robert W. Schoenlein and his research team have succeeded in disproving the Thomson effect.

Passage 8:

Sulfasalazine, the most frequently prescribed drug for inflammatory bowel disease therapy, has been used commonly for 50 years for the induction of disease remission in patients with mild acute exacerbations of ulcerative colitis. Initial uncontrolled observations of its efficacy indicated that 80% to 90% of patients improved with the use of this agent. The first placebo-controlled trial using objective parameters of efficacy demonstrated that 80% of the treated group improved as compared to 35% receiving placebo. These data were confirmed subsequently, although improvement may not occur until after four weeks of therapy. Sulfasalazine, 250 to 500 mg four times a day, often is considered the drug of choice in ulcerative colitis exacerbation because its efficacy has been demonstrated and because it has less severe adverse effects than corticosteroids. However, controlled trials have shown that corticosteroids may be more prompt in onset of action than sulfasalazine, alone or in combination with corticosteroid, for the treatment of severe acute ulcerative colitis. While comparative efficacy trials are lacking, the combination of sulfasalazine and prednisone does not appear to be detrimental and often has been used in hope of alleviating patients' symptoms.

Excerpted with permission from "Chapter 24, Inflammatory Bowel Disease," page 24-3, Applied Therapeutics: The Clinical Use of Drugs, Sixth Edition, edited by Lloyd Yee Young and Mary Anne Koda-Kimble, published by Applied Therapeutics, Inc., Vancouver, Washington, © 1995.

35. The most frequently prescribed drug for inflammatory bowel disease therapy is

 A. prednisone.
 B. sulfasalazine.
 C. estrogen.
 D. All of the above

36. What percent of the patients in the uncontrolled observations
improved with sulfasalazine therapy?

 A. 50% to 60%
 B. 60% to 70%
 C. 70% to 80%
 D. 80% to 90%

37. What percent of the patients in the placebo group in the placebo-
controlled trial improved?

 A. 35%
 B. 45%
 C. 55%
 D. 65%

38. According to the passage, how many times per day is sulfasalazine
given?

 A. Four
 B. Five
 C. Six
 D. Eight

39. The combination of sulfasalazine and prednisone

 A. appears to be dangerous.
 B. offers hope.
 C. shows no benefit.
 D. A and C

Passage 9:

Angina pectoris can be defined as a sense of discomfort arising in the myocardium as a result of myocardial ischemia in the absence of infarction. Although angina usually implies severe chest pain or discomfort, its presentation is variable. At one extreme, angina may occur predictably with strenuous exercise; at the other, angina may develop unexpectedly with little or no exertion.

Patients who have a reproducible pattern of angina that is associated with a certain level of physical activity have *chronic stable angina* or exertional angina. In contrast, patients with unstable angina are experiencing new angina or a change in their angina intensity, frequency, or duration. Both chronic stable angina and unstable angina often reflect underlying atherosclerotic narrowing of coronary arteries. Classic Prinzmetal's *variant angina*, or vasospastic angina, occurs in patients without coronary heart disease and is due to a spasm of the coronary artery that decreases myocardial blood flow. When coronary vasospasm occurs at the site of a fixed atherosclerotic plaque, *mixed angina* can result.

Silent myocardial ischemia, which is a transient change in myocardial perfusion, function, or electrical activity, can be detected on an electro-cardiogram (ECG) in most angina patients. The patient, however, does not experience chest pain or other signs of angina [e.g., jaw pain, shortness of breath] during these episodes. Silent myocardial ischemia also can occur in patients with no angina history.

Excerpted with permission from "Chapter 13, Ischematic Heart Disease: Anginal Syndromes," pages 13-1 to 13-2, Applied Therapeutics: The Clinical Use of Drugs, Sixth Edition, edited by Lloyd Yee Young and Mary Anne Koda-Kimble, published by Applied Therapeutics, Inc., Vancouver, Washington, © 1995.

40. The term *angina* usually refers to

   A. headache.
   B. chest pain.
   C. athlete's foot.
   D. None of the above

41. Angina associated with physical activity is

   A. Prinzmetal's angina.
   B. variant angina.
   C. vasocolonic angina.
   D. stable angina.

42. Which type of angina occurs in patients without coronary heart disease?

   A. Variant angina
   B. Exertional angina
   C. Prinzmetal's variant angina
   D. None of the above

43. Silent myocardial ischemia

   A. is atherosclerotic plaque.
   B. has no consequences.
   C. is a permanent change in myocardial perfusion, function, or electrical activity.
   D. None of the above

44. Of the titles below, which would best describe the passage?

   A. Angina—the Silent Killer
   B. The Different Types of Angina
   C. Chest Pain
   D. Treating Chest Pain

Passage 10:

Many scientists would agree that prions (pronounced PREE-ons) are the most bizarre pathogenic substances ever discovered. The late renowned physician and researcher Dr. Lewis Thomas called them one of the Seven Wonders of the World. Biologists are still arguing as to their composition. Prions had been an elusive, controversial, and well-kept secret in the medical community but this is no longer true.

A new book, *Deadly Feasts*, written by Pulitzer Prize-winning author Richard Rhodes, reveals much of the mystery surrounding these strange and deadly agents. Rhodes believes prions will be responsible for the next worldwide plague. His concern is plausible; prions have been responsible for the deaths of more than 100,000 cows in Great Britain and other countries. The cattle were suspected of carrying bovine spongiform encephalopathy or BSE (also known as "mad cow disease"). This epidemic in English cattle raises concerns about whether Creutzfeldt-Jakob disease, the human counterpart of BSE, will also increase in incidence.

The known prion diseases are sometimes referred to as transmissible spongiform encephalopathies. They are so named because they frequently cause the brain to become riddled with holes. The diseases are distinguished by long incubation periods and failure to produce an inflammatory response.

Dr. Thomas's decision to place these agents on the Seven Wonders list was based on the fact that no nucleic acid had yet been found among the infectious material. Prions have been found to consist of protein and nothing else. (The word *prion* is derived from the words *proteinaceous* and *infectious*. The letters *o* and *i* were transposed by poetic license.) It has been generally accepted that conveyers of transmissible diseases require genetic material, composed of nucleic acid (DNA or RNA), in order to establish an infection in a host. Even viruses, which are among the simplest microbes, rely on such material to direct the synthesis of the proteins needed for survival and replication.

Prions appear to convert normal protein molecules into dangerous ones simply by inducing the benign molecules to change shape. Much of the infectious nature of a prion appears to depend on the similarity of prion protein (PrP) between species. The degree of similarity between bovine and human PrP may therefore be an important determinant of the risk of infection.

Excerpted with permission from "Prions, Bizarre Pathogens," by Max Sherman, R. Ph., *U.S. Pharmacist*, June, 1997, pages 54–61, © 1997.

45. The passage indicates that Creutzfeld-Jakob disease is

A. responsible for the deaths of 100,000 sheep.

B. a controversial and well-kept secret.

C. the human counterpart of BSE (bovine spongiform encephalopathy).

D. "mad cow disease."

46. Dr. Thomas decided to place prions on the Seven Wonders list because

A. prions have highly unusual DNA.

B. no nucleic acid was found among the infectious material.

C. prions have no proteins.

D. prions cause the brain to become riddled with holes.

47. Prions appear to convert normal protein molecules into dangerous ones by

  A. inducing benign molecules to change shape.
  B. using their DNA to direct the synthesis of dangerous proteins.
  C. using their RNA to direct the synthesis of dangerous proteins.
  D. Both B and C

48. The word *prion* is derived from

  A. *proteinaceous.*
  B. the name of Pulitzer Prize-winning author Richard Prion.
  C. *infectious.*
  D. Both A and C

49. The new book *Deadly Feasts* warns that

  A. prions will be responsible for the next worldwide plague.
  B. prions will wipe out cattle herds worldwide.
  C. prions will become our deadliest viruses.
  D. prions cannot be defeated until their DNA is understood.

50. The known prion diseases are characterized by

  A. long incubation periods.
  B. failure to produce an inflammatory response.
  C. frequently causing the brain to become riddled with holes.
  D. All of the above

READING COMPREHENSION ANSWER KEY

1. D	11. D	21. D	31. D	41. D
2. B	12. B	22. A	32. D	42. C
3. D	13. D	23. D	33. D	43. D
4. B	14. C	24. B	34. C	44. B
5. B	15. C	25. D	35. B	45. C
6. A	16. B	26. A	36. D	46. B
7. D	17. B	27. D	37. A	47. A
8. D	18. A	28. B	38. A	48. D
9. D	19. D	29. C	39. B	49. A
10. C	20. B	30. C	40. B	50. D

READING COMPREHENSION EXPLANATORY ANSWERS

The numbers in the left margin of the reprinted passages indicate the statements in which the answer to the questions can be found.

Passage 1:

In the past two decades, people living in the northeastern, north-central, and western United States have unwittingly entered a dangerous enzootic cycle—a cycle of disease that typically is restricted to wildlife. Wild mammals and birds host a wide variety of disease agents, with effects ranging from mild symptoms to mortality, but in most cases the pathogen affects only one or a few host species and never causes disease in humans. However, as a result of a complicated sequence of events, people have become frequent accidental hosts for ticks and the disease agents they carry,

1. including a corkscrew-shaped bacterium called *Borrelia burgdorferi*,
4. the agent of Lyme disease. As of 1995, cases of Lyme disease had been reported in 48 of the 50 states and appear to be increasing, both in numbers of people affected and in geographic distribution.

Where does this disease come from, why has it emerged so rapidly, and what can people do to reduce their risk of exposure? It is possible to address these questions not from a medical point of view, but rather from an ecological one. All living organisms—from the *B. burgdorferi* bacterium and the ticks it infects to the mice and deer on which the ticks feed—form an ecological relationship with

2. their habitats. Understanding the complex interactions between plant and animal species within those habitats may help people to predict the places where they are most likely to encounter disease-bearing ticks and become infected. Thus armed, individuals may ultimately be able to protect themselves from Lyme disease.

3. Currently, to prevent Lyme disease people wear protective clothing when they are in wooded areas and perform "tick checks" after leaving the woods. One underemphasized means to avoid exposure to Lyme disease, however, is avoiding the most heavily tick-infested habitats at the times of year when ticks are most

5. abundant or dangerous. Recent research performed in my laboratory, as well as in others, has suggested that such habitats can be predicted, often well in advance. Ultimately, it is the hope of ecologists studying this problem that we can use our expertise in pinpointing these habitats to warn the public away from areas that are likely to contain an abundance of disease-carrying ticks.

1. **Answer is D.** Answer A refers to the enzootic cycle (animal diseases present in a specific locality) in which wild mammals and birds (B) ordinarily participate. People living in specified areas (C) have become participants in this cycle, but the actual agent of Lyme disease is a microorganism, the bacterium *Borrelia burgdorferi* (D).

2. **Answer is B.** While A and D might well be sound ecological goals in other circumstances, when it comes to Lyme disease, ecologists are motivated by a desire to help people predict and avoid the places where they are likely to become infected (B). Although C is an important medical consideration, the development of a vaccine is not the province of ecologists.

3. **Answer is D.** The passage states that both B and C are protective measures. Answer A is not mentioned and is irrelevant.

4. **Answer is B.** Answer B is a true statement, taken directly from the passage. Answer A states the opposite of the truth, and C and D each combine a false statement with a true one.

5. **Answer is B.** Answer B states the main point of the passage. Answer A is mentioned as an often-used, rather than an under employed protective measure. Answers C and D are irrelevant.

Passage 2:

8.   To the average physician, Lyme disease is suspected when a patient arrives at a clinic or hospital complaining of a strange bull's-eye rash, known as erythema migrans, or EM, together with one or more flulike symptoms, such as fever, chills, muscle aches, or lethargy. The doctor will take a blood sample for laboratory confirmation, but will feel quite confident to make a diagnosis of Lyme disease after noting the telltale combination of symptoms, as well as the circumstances surrounding the infection. The patient will undoubtedly have been bitten by the black-legged tick *Ixodes scaplaris*, formerly called the deer tick, or a close relative, which transferred to him or her the *B. burgdorferi* bacterium. Most likely, the doctor will prescribe an oral course of antibiotics and will duly report the case to the county or state health department, which will include it in the morbidity statistics for Lyme disease.

Accurate diagnosis and effective treatment of Lyme disease are not always so straightforward, particularly in regions of the country newly invaded by the epidemic. In these regions, health care professionals and the public need to be educated about the confusing and generalized symptoms, the generally poor, but growing, accuracy of lab tests, and the efficacy of various antibiotic treatments. If

10. Lyme disease is left untreated for some time, *B. burgdorferi* may persist in the patient's tissues and can migrate to the central and peripheral nervous system or to joints and cause more severe late-stage symptoms, which include arthritis and neurological disorders, such as dizziness, memory loss and disorientation. Vaccines that protect against Lyme disease are now being field tested by pharmaceutical companies, but none has yet been approved by the Food and Drug Administration for public use. Even if an effective vaccine were certified and marketed, the primary means that individuals have of protecting themselves against the disease is avoiding the tick in the first place.

6. Answer is **A**. In order for the pathogen *B. burgdorferi* to pass from tick to human, the human must be bitten by the tick—in this case, the black-legged tick, *Ixodes scaplaris*. A tick-bearing mammal (B) might provide the tick, but not the bite. The microbe *B. burgdorferi* is not capable of biting, so C cannot be correct. Answer D is irrelevant (Lyme disease is not airborne).

7. Answer is **D**. The passage mentions both A and B, but not C.

8. Answer is **D**. Only the bull's-eye rash is called erythema migrans. Answer A is irrelevant; B refers to *B. burgdorferi*; C refers to *scaplaris*.

9. Answer is **D**. As stated in the passage, the physician will take a blood sample, prescribe antibiotics, and report the case (A, B, and C).

10. Answer is **C**. Answer A is not addressed in the paragraph. Answer B is false since leaving the disease untreated is not mentioned in the passage as having any effect on lab tests; D is neither stated nor implied in the passage. The result of leaving Lyme disease untreated is clearly described in C.

Passage 3:

Rabies is a master dissembler. No other disease so completely manipulates its stricken host while barely leaving a trace of its presence. And rabies is preeminently adaptive: even if one host species is eliminated, the virus resurfaces in another. It bides its time, shadowing its victims, waiting for new hosts to emerge as people disrupt habitats and force animals to congregate more densely. Despite the war chest of vaccines designed to stop it and the near-certain death of every organism infected by it, rabies persists.

In the United States, on average, fewer than two people a year die of rabies, about the same number as in Western Europe. Vaccination and animal control policies ensure that few, if any, of those cases come from dog bites. Worldwide, between 20,000 and 100,000 people die of rabies in a given year, most of them in developing countries, and some 10 million are treated annually for possible exposures, mostly from dog bites. Compared with the dangers of becoming infected with HIV, tuberculosis, or malaria, each of which strikes millions of people every year, the risk of contracting rabies is vanishingly small. But rabies has had far greater influence on culture and science than its current incidence might suggest. And its devastating effects assure that it is never far from people's minds. Rabies has the highest fatality rate of any known human infection.

11. **Answer is D.** Answers A, B, and C state facts taken directly from the passage.

12. **Answer is B.** Although you might be tempted to complete the statement with an incorrect figure (A), B is actually stated in the passage. Both C and D are false.

13. **Answer is D.** Both A and C are true; B is false and in fact contradicts a statement in the passage.

14. **Answer is C.** Only one specific figure can be correct in this instance, and the number of people treated for possible exposure is given in the passage as 10 million.

Passage 4:

Unlike an electron, a single red blood cell cannot go through two openings at once. Indeed, it is generally true that the physicist

15. seeking to understand the circulation of the blood can ignore most of the perplexities of twentieth century physics. Given the scale of the circulatory system and the speed of blood flow, neither quantum mechanics nor relativity applies. Instead the flow of blood through the heart and the vascular tree can be adequately described by the familiar mechanics of Newton and Galileo.

16. If the circulation of the blood obeys the laws of classical mechanics, however, this does not mean that it is simple. An early experimental model of the vascular tree was a system of glass tubes filled with water. But unlike water, blood is not an "ideal" fluid. Instead it is a suspension of cells that, under certain circumstances, can behave in non-Newtonian ways. Moreover, flow through the vascular tree is pulsatile rather than steady; blood vessels taper and are elastic rather than rigid; and flow in any part of the densely interconnected system is affected by flow in neighboring regions. When these factors and the fantastic geometrical complexity of the labyrinthine vascular system are taken into account, the equations of blood flow, while remaining classical in inspiration, quickly become too complex to be solved explicitly.

17. Confronted with a system of overwhelming complexity, scientists typically resort to the intelligent simplification, that is, to a
18. model. The first mathematical model of the human circulation was the *windkessel,* or compression chamber, model developed by Otto Frank in 1899 to explain how pulsatile flow from the heart is converted into steadier flow in the peripheral circulation. Sophisticated analytical models, the descendants of the windkessel model, still provide insight into the functioning of the circulatory system. But they are increasingly supplemented by numerical models, which exploit the power of the computer to arrive at accurate approximations of values that satisfy systems of equations that

19. would otherwise be unsolvable. The computer can also be used to produce stunning images that allow otherwise cryptic measurements or calculations to be grasped intuitively.

15. Answer is **C**. The passage states that the mechanics of Newton and Galileo are adequate for describing the circulatory system and blood flow. Answer A is irrelevant; B and D contradict information given in the passage.

16. Answer is **B**. As described in the passage, an early experimental model was a system of glass tubes filled with water. Answer A is irrelevant; C is false; and D is both false and absurd.

17. Answer is **B**. According to the passage, scientists are likely to turn to a model when confronted with a system of overwhelming complexity. Answers A and D are decidedly untrue; in fact, D contradicts information given in the passage.

18. Answer is **A**. As stated in the passage, Frank developed his *windkessel* model of the circulatory system to explain how pulsatile flow from the heart is converted into steadier flow in the peripheral circulation. Since he made use of the model, not human subjects, the answer cannot be C (which is a nonsense statement anyway). His was the first mathematical model, so B cannot be correct, and Frank was not attempting to augment the mechanics of Galileo and Newton (D).

19. Answer is **D**. As the passage indicates, quantum physics and relativity are not relevant to the study of the circulatory system, so A cannot be the correct answer. Nor is B correct, since the *windkessel* dates back to 1899 and is no longer in use. Answer C contradicts information stated in the passage. Only D actually occurs as a statement in the passage.

Passage 5:

A taxonomist viewing insects or crustaceans tends to see tough, jointed exoskeletons and elaborate limbs as their salient features—so salient, in fact, that the taxonomists who named the phylum to which these animals belong called it Arthropoda, or "jointed foot." The same biologist will also notice that the arthropod body plan is that of a modified worm, where the worm's more-or-less uniform series of segmented units becomes well differentiated along the length of the arthropod body. This gives arthropods distinct head, middle, and tail regions.

As neurobiologists considering evolution from simple to more complex animals, we are interested in the changes in the neural circuits serving locomotion and sensory coding that accompanied the transition from worm to arthropod. Such evolution is crucial to the emergence of advanced mobile animals. Because brains and body plans must have evolved in step from their simpler antecedents, comparative studies of neural development and of the mature nervous

20.

21.

22.

23.

systems of animals promise to reveal much about arthropod evolution.

23. In arthropods almost every nerve cell grows in a particular pattern and makes specific synaptic connections to form the elaborate neural circuits that give an animal its mobility and control; these features make each cell a recognizable identity.

Just as vertebrae and ribs are serially repeated, sets of neurons are repeated in each segment of an insect's body, or beneath each

24. facet of the compound eye. Using identified neurons, anatomists can compare the development and structure of nervous systems from different arthropods much as they can compare vertebrate skeletons. In addition, we can record the electrical activity from a single neuron, which allows us to compare physiological function in different lineages. So far, most work has been done on insects, but comparisons can also be made between insects and crustaceans.

25. Such comparisons tell biologists how these arthropods, with their jointed exoskeletons and specialized limbs, evolved from simpler ancestors and how they have subsequently diversified during evolutionary history.

20. Answer is **B**. The passage states that the arthropod body plan is that of a modified worm (B). A contradicts information given in the passage, as does C; D is a nonsense statement since insects and crustaceans are arthropods.

21. Answer is **D**. The passage lists A, B, and C as changes that took place as worms evolved into arthropods.

22. Answer is **A**. As the passage states, *arthropod* means "jointed foot." Answers B, C, and D are false.

23. Answer is **D**. Answer A contradicts information given in the passage, but both B and C are accurate.

24. Answer is **B**. The passage draws an analogy between the work done by anatomists who compare neurons to learn more about the development and structure of the nervous systems of different arthropods and the work done by anatomists who compare the skeletons of different vertebrates. Answers A, C, and D do not make sense in the context of the passage.

25. Answer is **D**. The passage directly mentions A, B, and C as subjects that neurobiologists are seeking to discover more about.

Passage 6:

26. In order to appropriately diagnose and treat a patient experiencing an allergic reaction, it is necessary to be able to differentiate allergic reactions from other closely related adverse drug reactions.

27. One method of classification divides adverse reactions into those that are "predictable, usually dose-dependent, and related to the pharmacologic actions of the drug," and those that are "unpredictable, often dose independent, and are related to the individual's immunologic response or to genetic differences in susceptible patients." Under this classification scheme, drug allergy or drug hypersensitivity is an unpredictable adverse drug reaction that is immunologically mediated.

28. Allergic drug reactions account for 5% to 20% of all observed adverse drug reactions. Adverse drug reactions have been reported to occur in as many as 30% of hospitalized patients, and 3% of all hospitalizations are a result of adverse drug reactions. In a computerized surveillance study of over 36,000 hospitalized patients, 731 adverse events were identified. Of those, 1% were categorized as severe, life threatening, and allergic in nature. The potential morbidity and mortality associated with allergic drug reactions is great even though these outcomes occur infrequently.

29.

---

26. Answer is A. As the passage states, allergic reactions must be differentiated from other closely related adverse drug reactions. Answer B describes reactions that are typically adverse but not allergic, and C is irrelevant to diagnosing and treating allergic drug reactions appropriately. While some allergic reactions may require hospitalization (D), this is not necessary to diagnose appropriately and treat all allergic reactions to drugs.

27. Answer is D. Both B and C appear in the passage.

28. Answer is B. According to the passage, 5% to 20% of all observed drug reactions represent allergic drug reactions.

29. Answer is C. That 1% of the 731 adverse drug events were characterized as severe, life-threatening, and allergic in nature is stated in the passage (C). Answer B is only partially true, since the allergic reactions identified *were* of a severe and life-threatening nature. Both A and D refer to adverse reactions that are not classified as allergic.

Passage 7

You have seen the photographs, of course: An apple flaring on two sides as a bullet passes through it; tennis balls flattening themselves against rackets; jagged-edge balloons frozen in mid-pop; droplets in mid-drip; bubbles in mid-burst. They were the work of Harold E. Edgerton, an M.I.T. professor whose invention of the stroboscopic flash in the early 1930s made it possible, for the first time, to capture events as fleeting as a millionth of a second.

30.

For decades chemists and solid-state physicists have yearned for a way of observing even more subtle alterations in matter: chemical reactions, or changes of state such as freezing or evaporation. Those changes depend on the breaking of bonds between atoms, a process that can take place in less than a picosecond—millions of times faster than anything Edgerton ever attempted. A fifth of a picosecond, for instance, is all the time it takes for photons entering your retina to trigger chemical changes in a pigment called rhodopsin—a reaction that makes it possible for you to read this article.

31.

Lasers can flash that quickly. But laser light is too coarse a tool to give sharp closeup pictures of matter. Visible wavelengths are thousands of times longer than the space between the atoms in a solid material. Furthermore, visible light tends to interact with the fuzzy outer electron clouds of an atom—not with the tightly bound inner electrons that give a much better idea of where the atom is. For those reasons, physicists studying atomic structure have long relied on much shorter-wavelength radiation: X-rays. Stroboscopic X-ray crystallography, however, has been a long time coming. Now a team at Lawrence Berkeley National Laboratory in Berkeley, California, has taken a step in that direction by generating the shortest X-ray flash ever.

33.

The main problem with X-rays is that their well known tendency to zip through materials makes them an optical nightmare. "You can't steer them the way you can light. It's difficult. You can't make a good mirror that operates at short wavelengths," says Robert W. Schoenlein, a staff scientist who coheaded the Lawrence Berkeley team. To point their X-rays in the right direction, Schoenlein and his colleagues generated them via Thomson scattering, an effect described early in this century by the English physicist J. J. Thomson. "Fast-moving particles such as electrons," Thomson said, "can transfer energy to photons, much as a Ping-Pong paddle energizes a ball." Thus, if you shoot a laser beam into a stream of high-velocity electrons, some of the photons in the beam may pick up enough energy to turn into X-rays. To produce X-ray flashes, some investigators fire a pulse of electrons head-on into a laser beam. The shorter the pulse, the shorter the flash. So far, however, the X-ray flashes have been too long to be useful.

34.

32.

34.

30. Answer is **C**. The passage identifies Harold E. Edgerton as an M.I.T. professor who invented the stroboscopic flash.

31. Answer is **D**. A precise figure is required here. According to the passage, the correct answer is a fifth of a picosecond.

32. Answer is **D**. The author of the passage states A, and Schoenlein is quoted in the passage as complaining about B and C.

33. Answer is **D**. The passage reports that physicists have had problems with both B and C, but not A, since lasers do flash quickly enough.

34. Answer is **C**. The main thrust of the passage is that Shoenlein and his team have created the shortest X-ray flashes ever (even if they are still not short enough to be truly useful). Answer A is false, since this technique was described early in this century by the English physicist J. J. Thomson. Answer B contradicts information given in the passage, and D is untrue because Schoenlein's research depends on the Thomson effect.

Passage 8:

35. Sulfasalazine, the most frequently prescribed drug for inflammatory bowel disease therapy, has been used commonly for 50 years for the induction of disease remission in patients with mild acute exacerbations of ulcerative colitis. Initial uncontrolled observations of its efficacy indicated that 80% to 90% of patients

36. improved with the use of this agent. The first placebo-controlled trial using objective parameters of efficacy demonstrated that 80% of the treated group improved as compared to 35% receiving placebo. These data were confirmed subsequently, although improvement

37. may not occur until after four weeks of therapy. Sulfasalazine, 250 to 500 mg four times a day, often is considered the drug of choice in ulcerative colitis exacerbation because its efficacy has been

38. demonstrated and because it has less severe adverse effects than corticosteroids. However, controlled trials have shown that corticosteroids may be more prompt in onset of action than sulfasalazine, alone or in combination with corticosteroid, for the treatment of severe acute ulcerative colitis. While comparative efficacy trials

39. are lacking, the combination of sulfasalazine and prednisone does not appear to be detrimental and often has been used in hope of alleviating patients' symptoms.

35. <u>Answer is **B**</u>. Although prednisone (A) is used to treat inflammatory bowel disease, the first sentence of the passage states clearly that the most frequently prescribed drug for inflammatory bowel disease therapy is sulfasalazine. Ulcerative colitis (C) is a type of inflammatory bowel disease.

36. <u>Answer is **D**</u>. This percentage is given in the passage.

37. <u>Answer is **A**</u>. This percentage is given in the passage.

38. <u>Answer is **A**</u>. Sulfasalazine is given four times per day at doses of 250–500 mg.

39. <u>Answer is **B**</u>. The passage clearly states that the combination of sulfasalazine and prednisone does not appear to be detrimental (dangerous, A) and often has been used in hope of alleviating patients' symptoms.

Passage 9:

Angina pectoris can be defined as a sense of discomfort arising in the myocardium as a result of myocardial ischemia in the absence

40. of infarction. Although angina usually implies severe chest pain or discomfort, its presentation is variable. At one extreme, angina may occur predictably with strenuous exercise; at the other, angina may develop unexpectedly with little or no exertion.

41. Patients who have a reproducible pattern of angina that is associated with a certain level of physical activity have *chronic stable angina* or exertional angina. In contrast, patients with unstable angina are experiencing new angina or a change in their angina intensity, frequency, or duration. Both chronic stable angina and unstable angina often reflect underlying atherosclerotic narrowing of

42. coronary arteries. Classic Prinzmetal's *variant angina*, or vasospastic angina, occurs in patients without coronary heart disease and is due to a spasm of the coronary artery that decreases myocardial blood flow. When coronary vasospasm occurs at the site of a fixed atherosclerotic plaque, mixed angina can result.

43. *Silent myocardial ischemia*, which is a transient change in myocardial perfusion, function, or electrical activity, can be detected on an electrocardiogram (ECG) in most angina patients. The patient, however, does not experience chest pain or other signs of angina [e.g., jaw pain, shortness of breath] during these episodes. Silent myocardial ischemia also can occur in patients with no angina history.

40. Answer is **B**. Although a headache (A) may accompany chest pain (B), angina usually implies severe chest pain. Answer C is absurd in the context of the passage.

41. Answer is **D**. Prinzmetal's and variant angina (A and B) are due to a spasm of the coronary artery. There is no such disorder as vasocolonic angina. Angina that is associated with a certain level of physical activity is called stable angina or exertional angina.

42. Answer is **C**. The passage states that Prinzmetal's variant angina occurs in patients without coronary heart disease. Answers A, B, and D are untrue.

43. Answer is **D**. Statement C is incorrect because silent myocardial ischemia is a *transient* (not permanent) change in myocardial perfusion, function, or electrical activity. Silent myocardial ischemia is not atherosclerotic plaque (A), although atherosclerotic plaque may cause ischemia. Myocardial ischemia can cause serous damage (consequences, B). Answers A, B, and C are all false.

44. Answer is **B**. Since the passage does not discuss the mortality rates associated with angina or the treatment of chest pain, answers A and D are incorrect. Chest pain (C) is too broad a title for this passage. Answer B, The Different Types of Angina, best describes the focus of this passage.

Passage 10:

Many scientists would agree that prions (pronounced PREE-ons) are the most bizarre pathogenic substances ever discovered. The late, renowned physician and researcher Dr. Lewis Thomas called them one of the Seven Wonders of the World. Biologists are still arguing as to their composition. Prions had been an elusive, controversial, and well-kept secret in the medical community but this is no longer true.

49.   A new book, *Deadly Feasts*, written by Pulitzer Prize-winning author Richard Rhodes, reveals much of the mystery surrounding these strange and deadly agents. Rhodes believes prions will be responsible for the next worldwide plague. His concern is plausible; prions have been responsible for the deaths of more than 100,000 cows in Great Britain and other countries. The cattle were suspected of carrying bovine spongiform encephalopathy or BSE

45. (also known as "mad cow disease"). This epidemic in English cattle raises concerns about whether Creutzfeldt-Jakob disease, the human counterpart of BSE, will also increase in incidence.

The known prion diseases are sometimes referred to as trans-

50. missible spongiform encephalopathies. They are so named because they frequently cause the brain to become riddled with holes. The diseases are distinguished by long incubation periods and failure to produce an inflammatory response.

46. Dr. Thomas's decision to place these agents on the Seven Wonders list was based on the fact that no nucleic acid had yet been found among the infectious material. Prions have been found to consist

48. of protein and nothing else. (The word *prion* is derived from the words *proteinaceous* and *infectious*. The letters *o* and *i* were transposed by poetic license.) It has been generally accepted that conveyers of transmissible diseases require genetic material, composed of nucleic acid (DNA or RNA), in order to establish an infection in a host. Even viruses, which are among the simplest microbes, rely on such material to direct the synthesis of the proteins needed for survival and replication.

47. Prions appear to convert normal protein molecules into dangerous ones simply by inducing the benign molecules to change shape. Much of the infectious nature of a prion appears to depend on the similarity of prion protein (PrP) between species. The degree of similarity between bovine and human PrP may therefore be an important determinant of the risk of infection.

45. Answer is **C**. Creutzfeldt-Jakob disease is the human counterpart of BSE, according to the passage. Answer A is false (prions killed more than 100,000 cows, not sheep, according to the passage). Answer B refers to prions in general rather than to Creutzfeld-Jakob disease; D is BSE, a disease of animals.

46. Answer is **B**. Prions are regarded as an oddity because they have no nucleic acid and consist only of protein. Both A and C, therefore, are false. D is definitely a result of diseases caused by prions but is not the reason that Thomas placed them on the Seven Wonders list.

47. Answer is **A**. That prions appear to induce benign molecules to change shape is the only true statement. Since prions have no nucleic acid, they have neither RNA nor DNA, thereby ruling out B, C, and D.

48. Answer is **D**. The word *prion* is formed from two adjectives, *proteinaceous* and *infectious*. "Richard Prion" is not mentioned in the passage although the passage states that Richard Rhodes is the Pulitzer Prize-winning author of *Deadly Feasts*.

49. Answer is **A**. The passage warns that prions will be responsible for the next worldwide plague. While theoretically possible, B is not mentioned in the passage; C is clearly false (prions are not viruses), and D is false as well (prions have no DNA).

50. Answer is **D**. Prion diseases are characterized by A, B, and C.

Practice PCAT 1

This sample PCAT is not a copy of an actual PCAT, but it has been designed to closely represent the types of questions that may be included in an actual exam. As in the actual PCAT, this test has five separate sections—Verbal Ability, Biology, Chemistry, Quantitative Ability, and Reading Comprehension. The actual PCAT may have an additional experimental section that consists of questions that are being tested for use on future exams. Because the experimental questions do not count toward your actual PCAT score, there are no equivalent questions included in this sample PCAT.

You may find it best to proceed with this practice exam as if you were taking the actual PCAT by adhering to the time allowed for each section in the table below. Your overall strategy should be to answer every question in the time allotted, while getting as many correct answers as possible. Do not leave any questions unanswered, as there will be no penalty for guessing on the actual PCAT. Your score on this sample PCAT will give you a good idea of the subject areas you need to study further. By timing yourself on the sample PCAT, you will also learn whether you need to increase your speed or slow down when you take the actual PCAT.

Section	Time Allowed*
Verbal Ability	30 minutes
Biology	45 minutes
Chemistry	50 minutes
Quantitative Ability	45 minutes
Reading Comprehension	45 minutes
Experimental Questions	45 minutes

*The times listed are an approximation of possible test section durations. Your actual test may vary slightly from these times.

After completing the sample PCAT, you may grade your exam by using the answer key. Regardless of your score on the sample PCAT, it will benefit you to review all the explanatory answers at the end of the sample PCAT. If your answer to a question was incorrect, the explanation may help you understand where you went wrong. If your answer was correct, the explanation may broaden your understanding of the topic area being tested.

Before starting the exam, please refresh your memory on the test taking strategies discussed earlier in this book. Good luck on the examination.

PRACTICE PCAT 1 ANSWER SHEET

Verbal Ability

#					#					#					#				
1	Ⓐ Ⓑ Ⓒ Ⓓ				11	Ⓐ Ⓑ Ⓒ Ⓓ				21	Ⓐ Ⓑ Ⓒ Ⓓ				41	Ⓐ Ⓑ Ⓒ Ⓓ			
2	Ⓐ Ⓑ Ⓒ Ⓓ				12	Ⓐ Ⓑ Ⓒ Ⓓ				22	Ⓐ Ⓑ Ⓒ Ⓓ				42	Ⓐ Ⓑ Ⓒ Ⓓ			
3	Ⓐ Ⓑ Ⓒ Ⓓ				13	Ⓐ Ⓑ Ⓒ Ⓓ				23	Ⓐ Ⓑ Ⓒ Ⓓ				43	Ⓐ Ⓑ Ⓒ Ⓓ			
4	Ⓐ Ⓑ Ⓒ Ⓓ				14	Ⓐ Ⓑ Ⓒ Ⓓ				24	Ⓐ Ⓑ Ⓒ Ⓓ				44	Ⓐ Ⓑ Ⓒ Ⓓ			
5	Ⓐ Ⓑ Ⓒ Ⓓ				15	Ⓐ Ⓑ Ⓒ Ⓓ				25	Ⓐ Ⓑ Ⓒ Ⓓ				45	Ⓐ Ⓑ Ⓒ Ⓓ			
6	Ⓐ Ⓑ Ⓒ Ⓓ				16	Ⓐ Ⓑ Ⓒ Ⓓ				26	Ⓐ Ⓑ Ⓒ Ⓓ				46	Ⓐ Ⓑ Ⓒ Ⓓ			
7	Ⓐ Ⓑ Ⓒ Ⓓ				17	Ⓐ Ⓑ Ⓒ Ⓓ				27	Ⓐ Ⓑ Ⓒ Ⓓ				47	Ⓐ Ⓑ Ⓒ Ⓓ			
8	Ⓐ Ⓑ Ⓒ Ⓓ				18	Ⓐ Ⓑ Ⓒ Ⓓ				28	Ⓐ Ⓑ Ⓒ Ⓓ				48	Ⓐ Ⓑ Ⓒ Ⓓ			
9	Ⓐ Ⓑ Ⓒ Ⓓ				19	Ⓐ Ⓑ Ⓒ Ⓓ				29	Ⓐ Ⓑ Ⓒ Ⓓ				49	Ⓐ Ⓑ Ⓒ Ⓓ			
10	Ⓐ Ⓑ Ⓒ Ⓓ				20	Ⓐ Ⓑ Ⓒ Ⓓ				30	Ⓐ Ⓑ Ⓒ Ⓓ				50	Ⓐ Ⓑ Ⓒ Ⓓ			

Biology

#		#		#		#	
51	Ⓐ Ⓑ Ⓒ Ⓓ	61	Ⓐ Ⓑ Ⓒ Ⓓ	71	Ⓐ Ⓑ Ⓒ Ⓓ	91	Ⓐ Ⓑ Ⓒ Ⓓ
52	Ⓐ Ⓑ Ⓒ Ⓓ	62	Ⓐ Ⓑ Ⓒ Ⓓ	72	Ⓐ Ⓑ Ⓒ Ⓓ	92	Ⓐ Ⓑ Ⓒ Ⓓ
53	Ⓐ Ⓑ Ⓒ Ⓓ	63	Ⓐ Ⓑ Ⓒ Ⓓ	73	Ⓐ Ⓑ Ⓒ Ⓓ	93	Ⓐ Ⓑ Ⓒ Ⓓ
54	Ⓐ Ⓑ Ⓒ Ⓓ	64	Ⓐ Ⓑ Ⓒ Ⓓ	74	Ⓐ Ⓑ Ⓒ Ⓓ	94	Ⓐ Ⓑ Ⓒ Ⓓ
55	Ⓐ Ⓑ Ⓒ Ⓓ	65	Ⓐ Ⓑ Ⓒ Ⓓ	75	Ⓐ Ⓑ Ⓒ Ⓓ	95	Ⓐ Ⓑ Ⓒ Ⓓ
56	Ⓐ Ⓑ Ⓒ Ⓓ	66	Ⓐ Ⓑ Ⓒ Ⓓ	76	Ⓐ Ⓑ Ⓒ Ⓓ	96	Ⓐ Ⓑ Ⓒ Ⓓ
57	Ⓐ Ⓑ Ⓒ Ⓓ	67	Ⓐ Ⓑ Ⓒ Ⓓ	77	Ⓐ Ⓑ Ⓒ Ⓓ	97	Ⓐ Ⓑ Ⓒ Ⓓ
58	Ⓐ Ⓑ Ⓒ Ⓓ	68	Ⓐ Ⓑ Ⓒ Ⓓ	78	Ⓐ Ⓑ Ⓒ Ⓓ	98	Ⓐ Ⓑ Ⓒ Ⓓ
59	Ⓐ Ⓑ Ⓒ Ⓓ	69	Ⓐ Ⓑ Ⓒ Ⓓ	79	Ⓐ Ⓑ Ⓒ Ⓓ	99	Ⓐ Ⓑ Ⓒ Ⓓ
60	Ⓐ Ⓑ Ⓒ Ⓓ	70	Ⓐ Ⓑ Ⓒ Ⓓ	80	Ⓐ Ⓑ Ⓒ Ⓓ	100	Ⓐ Ⓑ Ⓒ Ⓓ
				81	Ⓐ Ⓑ Ⓒ Ⓓ		
				82	Ⓐ Ⓑ Ⓒ Ⓓ		
				83	Ⓐ Ⓑ Ⓒ Ⓓ		
				84	Ⓐ Ⓑ Ⓒ Ⓓ		
				85	Ⓐ Ⓑ Ⓒ Ⓓ		
				86	Ⓐ Ⓑ Ⓒ Ⓓ		
				87	Ⓐ Ⓑ Ⓒ Ⓓ		
				88	Ⓐ Ⓑ Ⓒ Ⓓ		
				89	Ⓐ Ⓑ Ⓒ Ⓓ		
				90	Ⓐ Ⓑ Ⓒ Ⓓ		

Chemistry

#		#		#		#	
101	Ⓐ Ⓑ Ⓒ Ⓓ	113	Ⓐ Ⓑ Ⓒ Ⓓ	125	Ⓐ Ⓑ Ⓒ Ⓓ	149	Ⓐ Ⓑ Ⓒ Ⓓ
102	Ⓐ Ⓑ Ⓒ Ⓓ	114	Ⓐ Ⓑ Ⓒ Ⓓ	126	Ⓐ Ⓑ Ⓒ Ⓓ	150	Ⓐ Ⓑ Ⓒ Ⓓ
103	Ⓐ Ⓑ Ⓒ Ⓓ	115	Ⓐ Ⓑ Ⓒ Ⓓ	127	Ⓐ Ⓑ Ⓒ Ⓓ	151	Ⓐ Ⓑ Ⓒ Ⓓ
104	Ⓐ Ⓑ Ⓒ Ⓓ	116	Ⓐ Ⓑ Ⓒ Ⓓ	128	Ⓐ Ⓑ Ⓒ Ⓓ	152	Ⓐ Ⓑ Ⓒ Ⓓ
105	Ⓐ Ⓑ Ⓒ Ⓓ	117	Ⓐ Ⓑ Ⓒ Ⓓ	129	Ⓐ Ⓑ Ⓒ Ⓓ	153	Ⓐ Ⓑ Ⓒ Ⓓ
106	Ⓐ Ⓑ Ⓒ Ⓓ	118	Ⓐ Ⓑ Ⓒ Ⓓ	130	Ⓐ Ⓑ Ⓒ Ⓓ	154	Ⓐ Ⓑ Ⓒ Ⓓ
107	Ⓐ Ⓑ Ⓒ Ⓓ	119	Ⓐ Ⓑ Ⓒ Ⓓ	131	Ⓐ Ⓑ Ⓒ Ⓓ	155	Ⓐ Ⓑ Ⓒ Ⓓ
108	Ⓐ Ⓑ Ⓒ Ⓓ	120	Ⓐ Ⓑ Ⓒ Ⓓ	132	Ⓐ Ⓑ Ⓒ Ⓓ	156	Ⓐ Ⓑ Ⓒ Ⓓ
109	Ⓐ Ⓑ Ⓒ Ⓓ	121	Ⓐ Ⓑ Ⓒ Ⓓ	133	Ⓐ Ⓑ Ⓒ Ⓓ	157	Ⓐ Ⓑ Ⓒ Ⓓ
110	Ⓐ Ⓑ Ⓒ Ⓓ	122	Ⓐ Ⓑ Ⓒ Ⓓ	134	Ⓐ Ⓑ Ⓒ Ⓓ	158	Ⓐ Ⓑ Ⓒ Ⓓ
111	Ⓐ Ⓑ Ⓒ Ⓓ	123	Ⓐ Ⓑ Ⓒ Ⓓ	135	Ⓐ Ⓑ Ⓒ Ⓓ	159	Ⓐ Ⓑ Ⓒ Ⓓ
112	Ⓐ Ⓑ Ⓒ Ⓓ	124	Ⓐ Ⓑ Ⓒ Ⓓ	136	Ⓐ Ⓑ Ⓒ Ⓓ	160	Ⓐ Ⓑ Ⓒ Ⓓ
				137	Ⓐ Ⓑ Ⓒ Ⓓ		
				138	Ⓐ Ⓑ Ⓒ Ⓓ		
				139	Ⓐ Ⓑ Ⓒ Ⓓ		
				140	Ⓐ Ⓑ Ⓒ Ⓓ		
				141	Ⓐ Ⓑ Ⓒ Ⓓ		
				142	Ⓐ Ⓑ Ⓒ Ⓓ		
				143	Ⓐ Ⓑ Ⓒ Ⓓ		
				144	Ⓐ Ⓑ Ⓒ Ⓓ		
				145	Ⓐ Ⓑ Ⓒ Ⓓ		
				146	Ⓐ Ⓑ Ⓒ Ⓓ		
				147	Ⓐ Ⓑ Ⓒ Ⓓ		
				148	Ⓐ Ⓑ Ⓒ Ⓓ		

Quantitative Ability

161 (A)(B)(C)(D)	174 (A)(B)(C)(D)	187 (A)(B)(C)(D)	200 (A)(B)(C)(D)	213 (A)(B)(C)(D)
162 (A)(B)(C)(D)	175 (A)(B)(C)(D)	188 (A)(B)(C)(D)	201 (A)(B)(C)(D)	214 (A)(B)(C)(D)
163 (A)(B)(C)(D)	176 (A)(B)(C)(D)	189 (A)(B)(C)(D)	202 (A)(B)(C)(D)	215 (A)(B)(C)(D)
164 (A)(B)(C)(D)	177 (A)(B)(C)(D)	190 (A)(B)(C)(D)	203 (A)(B)(C)(D)	216 (A)(B)(C)(D)
165 (A)(B)(C)(D)	178 (A)(B)(C)(D)	191 (A)(B)(C)(D)	204 (A)(B)(C)(D)	217 (A)(B)(C)(D)
166 (A)(B)(C)(D)	179 (A)(B)(C)(D)	192 (A)(B)(C)(D)	205 (A)(B)(C)(D)	218 (A)(B)(C)(D)
167 (A)(B)(C)(D)	180 (A)(B)(C)(D)	193 (A)(B)(C)(D)	206 (A)(B)(C)(D)	219 (A)(B)(C)(D)
168 (A)(B)(C)(D)	181 (A)(B)(C)(D)	194 (A)(B)(C)(D)	207 (A)(B)(C)(D)	220 (A)(B)(C)(D)
169 (A)(B)(C)(D)	182 (A)(B)(C)(D)	195 (A)(B)(C)(D)	208 (A)(B)(C)(D)	221 (A)(B)(C)(D)
170 (A)(B)(C)(D)	183 (A)(B)(C)(D)	196 (A)(B)(C)(D)	209 (A)(B)(C)(D)	222 (A)(B)(C)(D)
171 (A)(B)(C)(D)	184 (A)(B)(C)(D)	197 (A)(B)(C)(D)	210 (A)(B)(C)(D)	223 (A)(B)(C)(D)
172 (A)(B)(C)(D)	185 (A)(B)(C)(D)	198 (A)(B)(C)(D)	211 (A)(B)(C)(D)	224 (A)(B)(C)(D)
173 (A)(B)(C)(D)	186 (A)(B)(C)(D)	199 (A)(B)(C)(D)	212 (A)(B)(C)(D)	225 (A)(B)(C)(D)

Reading Comprehension

226 (A)(B)(C)(D)	235 (A)(B)(C)(D)	244 (A)(B)(C)(D)	253 (A)(B)(C)(D)	262 (A)(B)(C)(D)
227 (A)(B)(C)(D)	236 (A)(B)(C)(D)	245 (A)(B)(C)(D)	254 (A)(B)(C)(D)	263 (A)(B)(C)(D)
228 (A)(B)(C)(D)	237 (A)(B)(C)(D)	246 (A)(B)(C)(D)	255 (A)(B)(C)(D)	264 (A)(B)(C)(D)
229 (A)(B)(C)(D)	238 (A)(B)(C)(D)	247 (A)(B)(C)(D)	256 (A)(B)(C)(D)	265 (A)(B)(C)(D)
230 (A)(B)(C)(D)	239 (A)(B)(C)(D)	248 (A)(B)(C)(D)	257 (A)(B)(C)(D)	266 (A)(B)(C)(D)
231 (A)(B)(C)(D)	240 (A)(B)(C)(D)	249 (A)(B)(C)(D)	258 (A)(B)(C)(D)	267 (A)(B)(C)(D)
232 (A)(B)(C)(D)	241 (A)(B)(C)(D)	250 (A)(B)(C)(D)	259 (A)(B)(C)(D)	268 (A)(B)(C)(D)
233 (A)(B)(C)(D)	242 (A)(B)(C)(D)	251 (A)(B)(C)(D)	260 (A)(B)(C)(D)	269 (A)(B)(C)(D)
234 (A)(B)(C)(D)	243 (A)(B)(C)(D)	252 (A)(B)(C)(D)	261 (A)(B)(C)(D)	270 (A)(B)(C)(D)

VERBAL ABILITY

50 Questions (#1–#50)

<u>Directions:</u> Choose the word that means the **opposite** or most nearly the opposite of the given word. You have 30 minutes to complete this section.

1. RETREAT

A. Advance
B. Reinstall
C. Link
D. Stare

2. ABOLISH

A. Forsake
B. Establish
C. Count
D. Accord

3. BRILLIANT

A. Expensive
B. Brittle
C. Small
D. Dull

4. EXAGGERATE

A. Eternal
B. Immoral
C. Diminish
D. Forget

5. PRESERVE

A. Discontinue
B. Praise
C. Restrict
D. Relent

6. RELISH

A. Set
B. Disfavor
C. Count
D. Perfect

7. ABANDON

A. Desert
B. Establish
C. Fix
D. Retain

8. SUBORDINATE

A. Superior
B. Large
C. Lonely
D. Far

9. SUMMIT

A. Base
B. Confident
C. Surpass
D. Sway

10. DESOLATE

A. Smooth
B. Tiny
C. Crowded
D. Transparent

11. UNCIVIL
   A. Imbalanced
   B. Polite
   C. Reside
   D. Resourceful

12. PROSAIC
   A. Tender
   B. Solid
   C. Large
   D. Imaginative

13. SILKY
   A. Smooth
   B. Patina
   C. Abrasive
   D. Sensory

14. IRIDESCENT
   A. Shallow
   B. Dense
   C. Colorless
   D. Dull

15. DISTEND
   A. Expand
   B. Contract
   C. Negotiate
   D. Wither

16. IMPRECATE
   A. Join
   B. Bless
   C. Blame
   D. Deny

17. REVEAL
   A. Closure
   B. Divulge
   C. Proclaim
   D. Hide

18. FUNDAMENTAL
   A. Superficial
   B. Aggravating
   C. Hidden
   D. Divergent

19. AVID
   A. Eager
   B. Embrace
   C. Averse
   D. Decrepit

20. DRUDGERY
   A. Fun
   B. Meaningful
   C. Helpful
   D. Easy

21. ANIMATED
   A. Lively
   B. Fast
   C. Subdued
   D. Kind

22. SIMULTANEOUS
   A. Fixed
   B. Diverse
   C. Asynchronous
   D. Plentiful

23. UNINTENDED

A. Annulled
B. Accidental
C. Planned
D. Motif

24. BLEAK

A. Lacking
B. Weathered
C. Distempered
D. Encouraging

25. DWINDLE

A. Trickle
B. Increase
C. Foment
D. Denature

Directions: Select the word that **best** completes the analogy.

26. FENCE : ENCLOSE :: DAUB :

A. Foil
B. Detain
C. Smear
D. Dry

27. PLACATE : PACIFY :: CONFIRM :

A. Ratify
B. Invalidate
C. Comply
D. Reply

28. MELT : FREEZE :: PLAY :

A. Sunshine
B. Work
C. Game
D. Performance

29. BOLD : COWARDLY :: OBLIQUE :

A. Triangle
B. Devious
C. Straight
D. Timidity

30. VIRUS : COLD :: DEITY :

A. Miracle
B. Transcendent
C. Ubiquitous
D. Prayer

31. RIM : VOLCANO :: MARGIN :

A. Wound
B. Edge
C. Probability
D. Erupt

32. BOOK : CHAPTER :: CONCERTO :

A. Oboe
B. Movement
C. Applause
D. Strings

33. SMALL INTESTINE : DUODENUM :: HAND :

A. Finger
B. Echidna
C. Knee
D. Elbow

34. RASPBERRY : KIWI FRUIT :: ROMAINE :

A. Papaya
B. Horseradish
C. Boston lettuce
D. Tuber

35. NEEDLE : SEW :: HOSE :

A. Lawn
B. Down
C. Garter
D. Siphon

36. UMBRELLA : PEDESTRIAN :: ROOF :

A. House
B. Stationary
C. Dome
D. Downpour

37. RECYCLE : PAPER :: INCUBATE :

A. Hatch
B. Egg
C. Sit on
D. Return

38. DRINK : JUICE :: MOW :

A. Perspire
B. Shade
C. Lawn
D. Lemonade

39. THEORY : REFUTE :: PRESIDENT :

A. Impeach
B. Elect
C. Veto
D. Obscure

40. ITHACA : ODYSSEUS :: KANSAS :

A. Cyclops
B. Dorothy
C. Ruby slippers
D. Glenda

41. EAR : CORN :: BOLL :

A. Weevil
B. Stem
C. Pod
D. Cotton

42. DEBRIS : COMPOST :: RESIN :

A. Tar
B. Amber
C. Industry
D. Pitch-blende

43. SEAL : ROTUND :: CHEETAH :

A. Fast
B. Mammal
C. Protected
D. Sleek

44. COLD : FLU :: RECESSION :

A. Temperature
B. Danger
C. Depression
D. Glacier

45. SEEP : SEEPED :: SWEEP :

A. Seeping
B. Swept
C. Broom
D. Tea

46. ON : COMMENT :: OUT:

   A. Direction
   B. Pool
   C. Eke
   D. Down

47. PHARMACIST : PHARMACY ::
   DIPLOMAT :

   A. Ambassador
   B. Embassy
   C. Immunity
   D. Foreign

48. PAINTER : PALETTE :: COOK :

   A. Spices
   B. Chef
   C. Spatula
   D. Bake

49. SENTENCE : ELLIPSIS :: SPEECH :

   A. Applause
   B. Pause
   C. Finale
   D. Silence

50. HAT : PANAMA :: SHARK :

   A. Predator
   B. Skin
   C. Cichlid
   D. Mako

STOP

End of Verbal Ability section. If you have any time left, you may go over your work in this section only.

BIOLOGY

50 Questions (#51–#100)

Directions: Choose the **best** answer to each of the following questions. You have 45 minutes to complete this section.

51. Which of the following statements is FALSE concerning Monera?

A. These organisms are of eukaryotic origin.

B. These organisms are mostly single celled.

C. These organisms are surrounded by a cell wall.

D. These organisms are mostly bacteria.

52. Living organisms can be grouped into five categories called

A. divisions.

B. phylums.

C. kingdoms.

D. organs.

Use **Figure 1** to answer questions 53 and 54.

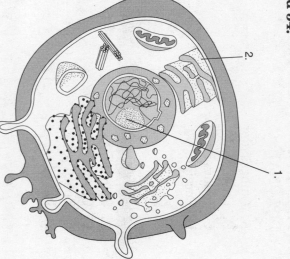

Figure 1.

53. In Figure 1, number 1 is pointing to what part of the animal cell?

A. Nucleolus

B. Nuclear envelope

C. Ribosomes

D. Nucleus

54. In Figure 1, number 2 is pointing to what part of the animal cell?

A. Golgi complex

B. Smooth endoplasmic reticulum

C. Mitochondrion

D. Nucleus

Use Figure 2 to answer questions 55 and 56.

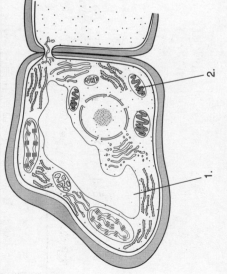

Figure 2.

55. In Figure 2, number 1 is pointing to what part of the plant cell?

   A. Mitochondrion
   B. Chloroplast
   C. Leucoplast
   D. Vacuole

56. In Figure 2, number 2 is pointing to what part of the plant cell?

   A. Mitochondrion
   B. Chloroplast
   C. Nucleus
   D. Leucoplast

57. Cells that are used to filter the respiratory tract are able to ambulate because of

   A. flagella.
   B. cilia.
   C. the Golgi apparatus.
   D. basal bodies.

58. If a cell is placed in hypotonic solution, the cell will

   A. swell.
   B. shrivel.
   C. disappear.
   D. remain unchanged.

59. Factors that determine a given trait are called

   A. alleles.
   B. genes.
   C. the genotype.
   D. the phenotype.

60. The actual alleles carried by an individual are called

   A. genes.
   B. chromosomes.
   C. the genotype.
   D. the phenotype.

61. The chromosome set in Klinefelter's syndrome is

   A. XYY.
   B. YXX.
   C. YYY.
   D. XXY.

62. A microorganism that obtains its carbon, as well as its energy, from organic compounds is called

   A. an autotroph.
   B. a heterotroph.
   C. a heterozygote.
   D. a homozygote.

63. The last stage in cell division is

A. prophase.
B. interphase.
C. telophase.
D. anaphase.

64. If A represents blue (dominant color) and a represents red (recessive color), which of the following crosses would be expected to result in 50% red offspring?

A. Aa × aa
B. AA × aa
C. Aa × Aa
D. Aa × AA

65. If A represents blue (dominant color) and a represents red (recessive color), which of the following crosses would be expected to result in 25% red offspring?

A. Aa × aa
B. AA × aa
C. Aa × Aa
D. Aa × AA

66. Which of the following respond(s) to dim light for black and white vision?

A. Cones
B. Rods
C. Iris
D. Cornea

67. Normal red blood cells have an average life span of

A. 30 days.
B. 60 days.
C. 120 days.
D. 180 days.

68. Impulses are picked up by which part of the neurons?

A. Axon
B. Cell body
C. Dendrites
D. Cell

69. The signal conduction region of the neurons is the

A. axon.
B. cell body.
C. dendrites.
D. cell.

70. Which of the following modifies materials synthesized in the rough and smooth endoplasmic reticulum?

A. Plastids
B. Golgi apparatus
C. Ribosomes
D. Mitochondria

71. In mitosis, at what stage does cytokinesis begin?

A. Interphase
B. Metaphase
C. Prophase
D. Anaphase

72. During which phase of the mitosis cell cycle does the cell grow?

A. Interphase
B. Metaphase
C. Prophase
D. Anaphase

73. Which of the following transports specific amino acids to specific sites on the mRNA?

   A. Codon
   B. tRNA
   C. mRNA
   D. Cytocell

74. In oogenesis, the haploid egg that is fertilized by a sperm is the

   A. ovum.
   B. gamete.
   C. spermocyte.
   D. neocyte.

75. A major function of white blood cells is to fight

   A. insulin resistance.
   B. infections.
   C. anemias.
   D. pain.

76. Which of the following is NOT true concerning the hypothalamus?

   A. It regulates body temperature.
   B. It regulates water and electrolyte balance.
   C. It regulates hunger and control of gastrointestinal activity.
   D. It regulates the rate and depth of breathing.

77. The temporal lobe

   A. interprets some sensory experiences and stores memories of both auditory and visual experiences.
   B. integrates eye movements by directing and focusing the eye.
   C. A and B
   D. Neither A nor B

78. Lobes of the cerebrum include all of the following EXCEPT

   A. frontal.
   B. permatoral.
   C. temporal.
   D. parietal.

79. Which of the following hormones is NOT secreted by the pituitary gland?

   A. Growth hormone
   B. Prolactin
   C. Antidiuretic hormone
   D. Insulin

80. The adrenal cortex secretes steroid hormones called

   A. cholesterol.
   B. stress hormones.
   C. corticosteriods.
   D. All of the above

81. The islet of Langerhans secretes

   A. insulin.
   B. gastrin.
   C. pepsinogen.
   D. A and C

82. Insulin

A. promotes cellular uptake of glucose and formation of glycogen and fat.

B. stimulates hydrolysis of glycogen and fat.

C. inhibits cellular uptake of glucose and formation of glycogen and fat.

D. None of the above

83. The heart wall is composed of three distinct layers. Which of the following is NOT a layer?

A. Epicardium

B. Asocardium

C. Myocardium

D. Endocardium

84. Blood from the right atrium passes through the _____ to fill the right ventricle.

A. bicuspid valve

B. tricuspid valve

C. centric valve

D. None of the above

85. In the cardiac cycle, the relaxation of the heart is referred to as

A. systole.

B. diastole.

C. cardiac rate.

D. systemic relaxation.

86. The superficial protective layer of the skin is the

A. dermis.

B. hypodermis.

C. epidermis.

D. None of the above

87. Which of the following is NOT a function of the skeletal system?

A. Hemopoiesis

B. Mineral storage

C. Secretion of hydrochloric acid

D. Body movement

88. Urea is

A. the waste product of amino acid metabolism that is formed in the liver and excreted in normal adult human urine.

B. the waste product of amino acid formation that is formed in the kidney and excreted in normal adult human urine.

C. an essential amino acid.

D. None of the above

89. Aldosterone

A. promotes potassium retention and sodium loss.

B. promotes sodium retention and potassium loss.

C. A and B

D. Neither A nor B

90. What is the functional unit of the kidney?

A. Urinary tubules

B. Glomerular capsule

C. Loop of Henle

D. Nephron

91. Which of the following is the largest?

   A. Liver
   B. Heart
   C. Pancreas
   D. Brain

92. Bile is produced in the

   A. pancreas.
   B. kidney.
   C. liver.
   D. gallbladder.

93. Parietal cells in the stomach secrete

   A. hydrochloric acid.
   B. intrinsic factor.
   C. A and B
   D. Neither A nor B

94. The function of cellular respiration is to produce

   A. ATP.
   B. cAMP.
   C. glucose.
   D. lactic acid.

95. In aerobic cellular respiration, most of the ATP is synthesized during

   A. the Krebs cycle.
   B. electron transport.
   C. electron oxidation:
   D. the citric acid cycle.

96. In plant cells, light reactions of photo-synthesis occur in the

   A. chloroplast.
   B. mitochondria.
   C. nucleus.
   D. chloromast.

97. A normal cell spends approximately 90% of its time in

   A. prophase.
   B. metaphase.
   C. interphase.
   D. anaphase.

98. Which of the following is NOT a carbohydrate?

   A. Sugars
   B. Lipids
   C. Starches
   D. Cellulose

99. The fat-soluble vitamins include:

   A. Vitamin A
   B. Vitamin G
   C. Vitamin R
   D. Vitamin B

100. Cell membranes are composed of

   A. phospholipids.
   B. proteins.
   C. A and B
   D. Neither A nor B

STOP

End of Biology section. If you have any time left, you may go over your work in this section only.

CHEMISTRY

60 Questions (#101–#160)

Directions: Choose the **best** answer to each of the following questions. You will have 50 minutes to complete this section.

101. Atoms of the same element having different numbers of neutrons are called

A. isotopes.
B. isomers.
C. allotropes.
D. diastereomers.

102. The name of the compound symbolized as $KHCO_3$ is

A. sodium hydrogen carbonate.
B. potassium bicarbonate.
C. potassium carbonic acid.
D. sodium carbonate.

103. Which of the following solutions is a good conductor of electricity?

A. Sugar dissolved in water
B. Table salt dissolved in water
C. Ethanol dissolved in water
D. Oxygen dissolved in water

104. In the following reaction, 42.5 g of NH_3 are reacted with 48.0 g of O_2. How many grams of nitrous oxide, NO, are produced? (O = 16 amu, N = 14 amu, H = 1 amu)

$$4NH_3 + 5O_2 \longrightarrow 4NO + 6H_2O$$

A. 60
B. 45
C. 36
D. 75

105. In the following reaction:

$$CS_2 + 2O_2 \longrightarrow CO_2 + 2SO_2$$

38.0 grams of CS_2 (carbon disulfide) are reacted with excess O_2 to produce 32.0 grams of SO_2. What is the percent yield of this reaction? (S = 32 amu, O = 16 amu, C = 12 amu, H = 1 amu)

A. 50
B. 25
C. 38
D. 13

106. What is the molarity (M) of a solution prepared by dissolving 18.0 grams of sugar, $C_6H_{12}O_6$, in 500 milliliters of solution? (O = 16 amu, C = 12 amu, H = 1 amu)

A. 0.130
B. 0.230
C. 0.200
D. 0.910

107. How many milliliters of 5.0 M NaOH solution must be used to prepare 250 milliliters of 2.5M solution?

A. 125
B. 36
C. 500
D. 50

108. What is the density, in grams per liter, of oxygen gas, O_2, if the pressure is 1.0 atmospheres and the temperature is 47°C? ($O = 16$ amu, $R = 0.082$ L-atm/K-mole)

   A. 1.2
   B. 8.3
   C. 4.2
   D. 0.6

109. A sample of gas contains approximately 84 grams nitrogen, N_2, and 64 grams oxygen, O_2. What is the partial pressure, in atmospheres, of nitrogen if the total pressure of the air is 1.6 atmospheres? ($O = 16$ amu, $N = 14$ amu)

   A. 0.91
   B. 1.05
   C. 0.96
   D. 1.09

110. The specific heat of copper, Cu, is 0.385 joule per gram–°C. What is the heat capacity, in joules per gram–°C of 10.0 grams of copper?

   A. 5.24
   B. 1.14
   C. 3.85
   D. 8.19

111. The wavelength of a light wave is 300 nanometers. What is its frequency, in cycles per second? (The speed of light is 3.00×10^8 m/s.)

   A. 1.0×10^{15}
   B. 1.0×10^{14}
   C. 1.0×10^{-15}
   D. 1.0×10^{-13}

112. Gamma rays have

   A. low energy, long wavelength, and high frequency.
   B. high energy, long wavelength, and low frequency.
   C. low energy, short wavelength, and high frequency.
   D. high energy, short wavelength, and high frequency.

113. Atoms or ions of elements having the same number of electrons are said to be

   A. allotropic.
   B. isotopes.
   C. isomers.
   D. isoelectronic.

114. Which of the following is a basic oxide?

   A. CO_2
   B. K_2O
   C. SO_2
   D. P_2O_5

115. Hydrogen bonding can exist between molecules of all the following EXCEPT

   A. H_2O
   B. CH_4
   C. CH_3OH
   D. NH_3

116. Which of the following liquids at room temperature has the highest vapor pressure?

   A. Water, boiling point, 100°C
   B. Ethyl ether, boiling point, 34.6°C
   C. Benzene, boiling point, 80.1°C
   D. Acetone, boiling point, 56°C

117. The conversion of a gas into a liquid is called

  A. sublimation.
  B. evaporation.
  C. condensation.
  D. freezing.

118. Gases are usually most soluble in liquids with

  A. low temperature.
  B. high temperature.
  C. low pressure.
  D. high agitation.

119. Which one of the following methods of reporting concentration is temperature dependent?

  A. Grams
  B. Molarity
  C. Mole fraction
  D. Percentage by weight

120. The following reactions have equilibrium constants as indicated below:

$$A + B \longleftrightarrow C + D \quad K^1$$
$$E + F \longleftrightarrow G + H \quad K^2$$

The reactions are added to give the following overall reaction. What will be the overall equilibrium constant for the new equation?

$$A + B + E + F \longleftrightarrow C + D + G + H$$

  A. $K^1 + K^2$
  B. $(K^1)(K^2)$
  C. K^1/K^2
  D. K^2/K^1

121. What is the atomic weight of the element $^{35}_{21} X$?

  A. 35
  B. 21
  C. 14
  D. 28

122. Which substance is a weak acid?

  A. HNO_2
  B. HI
  C. H_2SO_4
  D. $HClO_4$

123. Which acid is NOT a strong acid?

  A. HF
  B. HNO_3
  C. HCl
  D. HBr

124. In which of the following are the acids listed correctly in decreasing order of strength (i.e., the strongest acid is first and the weakest acid last)?

  A. $HF > HCl > HBr > HI$
  B. $HI > HBr > HCl > HF$
  C. $HBr > HCl > HI > HF$
  D. $HCl > HBr > HI > HF$

125. Which of the following can be a buffer solution?

  A. H_2SO_4, Na_2SO_4
  B. H_2SO_4
  C. CH_3COOH
  D. CH_3COOH, CH_3COONa

126. Which of the following is an alpha particle?

A. ^1_1H

B. ^1_0n

C. $^0_{-1}e$

D. ^4_2He

127. The following reaction:

$^{90}_{38}Sr \longrightarrow {}^{90}_{39}Y + ?$

can be balanced by adding

A. ^1_1H.

B. ^1_0n.

C. $^0_{-1}e$.

D. ^4_2He.

128. Which of the following is a statement of the first law of thermodynamics?

A. Entropy for a crystalline substance is zero at absolute zero temperature.

B. Energy can be converted from one form to another but is neither created nor destroyed.

C. Entropy increases in spontaneous reactions and remains the same in equilibrium systems.

D. The Gibbs free energy is a measure of the spontaneity of a reaction.

129. If the Gibbs free energy for a certain reaction has a negative value, which of the following statements is true?

A. The reaction does not take place.

B. The reaction system is at equilibrium.

C. The reaction is nonspontaneous.

D. The reaction is spontaneous.

130. When the solution of a complex ion appears red, what is the color of the wavelength of light absorbed?

A. Yellow

B. Violet

C. Green

D. Blue

131. What is the general formula for an alkyne?

A. C_nH_{2n+2}

B. C_nH_{2n}

C. C_nH_n

D. C_nH_{2n-2}

132. What is the general formula for a cycloalkane?

A. C_nH_{2n+2}

B. C_nH_{2n}

C. C_nH_n

D. C_nH_{2n-2}

133. Which of the following formulas represents a compound capable of forming isomers?

A. C_2H_6
B. C_3H_6
C. C_2H_6O
D. CH_3Cl

134. The name the compound symbolized as $CH_3CH_2COOCH_3$ is

A. methyl ethyl ester.
B. methyl propanoate.
C. ethyl ethanoate.
D. methyl propyl ether.

135. The reaction of Br_2 with C_2H_6 to produce C_2H_5Br and HBr in the presence of ultraviolet light or heat is an example of

A. a nucleophilic substitution reaction.
B. a free radical substitution reaction.
C. an electrophilic addition reaction.
D. an electrophilic elimination reaction.

136. The reaction of Br_2 with C_2H_4 to produce $C_2H_4Br_2$ is an example of

A. a nucleophilic substitution reaction.
B. a free radical reaction.
C. an electrophilic addition reaction.
D. an electrophilic elimination reaction.

137. Two molecules that are nonsuperimposable mirror images of each other are called

A. diastereomers.
B. enantiomers.
C. the same compound.
D. geometric isomers.

138. What is the name of the compound whose structure is shown below?

$$CH_3 - CH_2 - CH_2 - CH - CH - CH - CH_3$$
$$\quad\quad\quad\quad\quad\quad\quad | \quad\quad | \quad\quad\quad |$$
$$\quad\quad\quad\quad\quad\quad Cl \quad CH_3 \quad CH_2 - CH_3$$

A. 5-Chloro-3,4-dimethyloctane
B. 4-Chloro-2-ethyl-3-methylheptane
C. 4-Chloro-6-ethyl-5-methylheptane
D. 4-Chloro-5,6-dimethyloctane

139. The reaction of an acyl chloride and an amine yields an

A. amide.
B. ester.
C. acid anhydride.
D. alkyl chloride.

140. Complete catalytic hydrogenation of benzene yields

A. 1-cyclohexene.
B. 1,3-cyclohexadiene.
C. cyclohexane.
D. methylcyclopentane.

141. Which of the following functional groups is commonly present in lipids?

A. Alcohols
B. Esters
C. Alkyl halides
D. Carboxylic acids

142. The reaction of an alcohol with a carboxylic acid will produce

A. an aldehyde.
B. a ketone.
C. an ester.
D. an alcohol.

143. What functional group is most commonly present in proteins?

    A. Alcohol
    B. Amide
    C. Ester
    D. Ketone

144. What functional group is most commonly present in carbohydrates?

    A. Alcohol
    B. Amide
    C. Alkyl halide
    D. Alkyne

145. Which of the following statements about benzene is INCORRECT?

    A. The benzene molecule has 120° bond angles.
    B. All bonds in benzene are equivalent in length.
    C. Hybridization of the carbon atoms is sp^2.
    D. The benzene molecule is planar.

146. How many minutes are there in 1 week?

    A. 2.80×10^4
    B. 2.00×10^4
    C. 1.01×10^4
    D. 1.80×10^4

147. The name of the following compound:

$$CH_3CH_2CHCH_2COOH$$
$$|$$
$$CH_3$$

is

    A. 3-methylpentanoic acid.
    B. 2-methylpentanoic acid.
    C. 2-methylbutanoic acid.
    D. 3-methylbutanoic acid.

148. Each of the compounds shown below has the same molecular weight. However, they have different boiling temperatures.

$$CH_3CH_2OCH_2CH_3$$
ethyl ether

$$CH_3CH_2CH_2CH_2OH$$
1-butanol

$$CH_3CH_2CHOH$$
$$|$$
$$CH_3$$
2-butanol

In which of the following are the compounds listed correctly in decreasing order of boiling point, with the compound of highest boiling point first and the one of lowest boiling point last?

    A. Ethyl ether > 1-butanol > 2-butanol
    B. 2-Butanol > 1-butanol > ethyl ether
    C. 1-Butanol > 2-butanol > ethyl ether
    D. Ethyl ether > 2-butanol > 1-butanol

149. The reaction of Br_2 with C_2H_6 to produce C_2H_5Br and HBr in the presence of ultraviolet light or heat is an example of

    A. a nucleophilic substitution reaction.
    B. a free-radical substitution reaction.
    C. an electrophilic addition reaction.
    D. an electrophilic elimination reaction.

150. The reaction of Br_2 with C_2H_4 to produce $C_2H_4Br_2$ is an example of

   A. a nucleophilic substitution reaction.
   B. a free-radical reaction.
   C. an electrophilic addition reaction.
   D. an electrophilic elimination reaction.

151. Two molecules that are nonsuperimposable mirror images of each other are called

   A. diastereomers.
   B. enantiomers.
   C. the same compound.
   D. geometric isomers.

152. Oxidation of an aldehyde produces

   A. a ketone.
   B. an alcohol.
   C. a carboxylic acid.
   D. an amide.

153. Dehydration of an alcohol produces

   A. a ketone.
   B. an alkene.
   C. an aldehyde.
   D. an alkyl halide.

154. A sample of metal weighing 6.0 grams is placed in a graduated cylinder containing 16 milliliters of water. The volume of water increases to 20 milliliters. What is the density, in grams per milliliter, of the metal?

   A. 1.30
   B. 1.50
   C. 2.0
   D. 2.5

155. Given the following equation:

$$°C = \frac{5°C}{9°F}(°F - 32)$$

convert 10°F to °C.

   A. -12
   B. -23
   C. 10
   D. 14

156. How many neutrons does the atom $_{21}^{35}X$, of the element X, contain?

   A. 21
   B. 35
   C. 14
   D. 28

157. What is the final volume in milliliters of a solution prepared by dissolving 18 grams of sugar, $C_6H_{12}O_6$, in sufficient water to produce a 0.5 M solution? (O = 16 amu, C = 12 amu, H = 1 amu)

   A. 36
   B. 100
   C. 200
   D. 52

158. The reaction of a neutron with a uranium-235 nucleus to generate a strontium atom, a xenon atom, and three neutrons as shown in the equation below is known as

$$_{92}^{235}U + _0^1n \longrightarrow _{38}^{90}Sr + _{54}^{143}Xe + 3_0^1n$$

   A. radioactive decay
   B. nuclear fusion
   C. carbon dating
   D. nuclear fission

159. All radioactive decay occurs according to

A. zero order kinetics
B. first order kinetics
C. second order kinetics
D. third order kinetics

160. The most dangerous type of nuclear radiation on the human body is

A. alpha particles
B. beta particles
C. gamma rays
D. sigma rays

STOP

End of Chemistry section. If you have any time left, you may go over your work in this section only.

QUANTITATIVE ABILITY
65 Questions (#161–#225)

Directions: Choose the **best** answer to each of the following questions. You will have 45 minutes to complete this section.

161. $7^0 \times 5 =$

A. 35
B. 350
C. 7
D. 5

162. $\frac{7}{20} =$

A. 20%
B. 25%
C. 30%
D. 35%

163. What is the circumference of the circle shown below?

$\pi = 3.14, r = 3$

A. 18.84
B. 28.26
C. 35.16
D. 52.17

164. A plane traveling at 300 miles per hour is 100 miles from its landing site at 2:30 P.M. At what time will it land at the airport?

A. 2:50 P.M.
B. 3:10 P.M.
C. 3:50 P.M.
D. 4:00 P.M.

165. $\frac{3}{9} =$

A. 22%
B. 33%
C. 44%
D. 48%

166. $\frac{8}{16} =$

A. 40%
B. 50%
C. 60%
D. 70%

167. A truck is 50 miles from its destination at 2:00 P.M. At what speed must the truck travel to arrive by 2:40 P.M.?

A. 50 mph
B. 75 mph
C. 90 mph
D. 100 mph

168. $10^4 + 9^3 =$

- **A.** 1,729
- **B.** 10,729
- **C.** 100,729
- **D.** 1,379

169. $10^3 \times 2^3 =$

- **A.** 80
- **B.** 800
- **C.** 8,000
- **D.** 80,000

170. $\dfrac{19}{20} =$

- **A.** 80%
- **B.** 85%
- **C.** 90%
- **D.** 95%

171. In the figure shown below *ABCD* is a parallelogram, and *AE* = *ED*. What is the ratio of the area of triangle *ABE* to the area of the parallelogram?

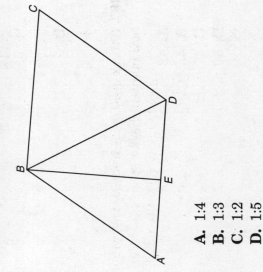

- **A.** 1:4
- **B.** 1:3
- **C.** 1:2
- **D.** 1:5

172. 19% of 50 =

- **A.** 8.3
- **B.** 9.5
- **C.** 10.3
- **D.** 11.2

173. $6^3 + 4^2 =$

- **A.** 44
- **B.** 136
- **C.** 224
- **D.** 232

174. $0.50^2 + \dfrac{1}{4} =$

- **A.** 0.25
- **B.** 0.40
- **C.** 0.5
- **D.** 1

175. If $\dfrac{2}{5}$ of a basket can be filled in 1 minute, how many minutes will be required to fill the rest of the basket?

- **A.** 1.5
- **B.** 2.25
- **C.** 2.5
- **D.** 2.75

176. During an 8-hour flight, a plane flew at 300 miles per hour for the first hour, at 500 miles per hour for the next 6 hours, and at 100 miles per hour for the last hour. How many miles long was the flight?

- **A.** 3,400
- **B.** 1,800
- **C.** 2,500
- **D.** 4,000

177. log 0.1 =

A. −2
B. −1
C. 0
D. 1

178. log 0.0001 =

A. −4
B. −3
C. 0
D. 1

179. log (5 • 3)

A. (log 5) • (log 3)
B. (log 5) + 3
C. (log 5) + (log 3)
D. (log 3) + 5

180. 160 pounds are equivalent to how many kilograms?

A. 72.7
B. 80.3
C. 83.4
D. 89.6

181. 70 kilograms are equivalent to how many pounds?

A. 140
B. 154
C. 164
D. 168

182. What is the slope of a line through points (2,3) and (4,6)?

A. 15
B. 10
C. 5
D. 1.5

183. In the figure below, if CD = DE and the area of triangle BDE is 16, what is the area of square ABCD?

A. 64
B. 32
C. 16
D. 8

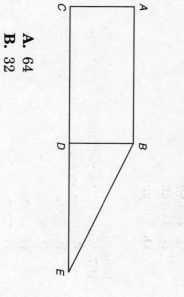

184. If a coin is tossed four times, what is the probability that the outcome will be all heads?

A. $\frac{1}{16}$

B. $\frac{1}{4}$

C. $\frac{1}{2}$

D. $\frac{1}{8}$

185. 120 centimeters are equivalent to how many inches?

A. 42
B. 45
C. 47
D. 50

186. 54 inches =

    A. 130 cm

    B. 137 cm

    C. 140 cm

    D. 143 cm

187. What is the perimeter of a square that has an area of 144 square meters?

    A. 12 m

    B. 24 m

    C. 48 m

    D. 96 m

188. $\dfrac{2}{5} \div 2 =$

    A. $\dfrac{4}{5}$

    B. $\dfrac{2}{5}$

    C. $\dfrac{1}{5}$

    D. None of the above

189. $\dfrac{2}{27} \div 3 =$

    A. 0.025

    B. 0.25

    C. 1.23

    D. None of the above

190. A graph of which line would be parallel to the x-axis?

    A. $y = 4$

    B. $x = 3$

    C. $x = 1 - y$

    D. $y = 1 + x$

191. $\dfrac{3}{4} \div \dfrac{1}{5} =$

    A. $5\dfrac{3}{4}$

    B. $1\dfrac{3}{20}$

    C. $3\dfrac{3}{4}$

    D. None of the above

192. Find the mode of the following data set: 3, 6, 29, 8, 6, 4, 2, 6, 8, 6, 9, 3.

    A. 3

    B. 6

    C. 9

    D. 29

193. $\sqrt[3]{64} =$
A. 2
B. 3
C. 4
D. 5

194. $\sqrt[3]{8} =$
A. 2
B. 3
C. 4
D. 5

195. Right triangles ABC and DEF, shown below, are similar. How long is DE?

A. 4
B. 6
C. 9
D. 12

196. $\frac{3}{10} =$
A. 15%
B. 20%
C. 30%
D. 50%

197. $\sqrt[3]{1,000} =$
A. 10
B. 100
C. 0.10
D. None of the above

198. $\sqrt{20} + \sqrt{125} =$
A. $7\sqrt{5}$
B. $5\sqrt{5}$
C. $10\sqrt{5}$
D. $8\sqrt{5}$

199. $x^3 + 123 = 1{,}123; x =$
A. 8
B. 9
C. 10
D. None of the above

200. Which of the following is a solution for x in the equation, $2x^2 = 200$?
A. 8
B. 9
C. 10
D. None of the above

201. $12x - 16 = 944; x =$
A. 50
B. 75
C. 80
D. 97

202. $3x = \frac{1}{2}; x =$

A. $\frac{1}{3}$

B. $\frac{2}{3}$

C. $\frac{1}{6}$

D. None of the above

203. A line contains points (4,2) and (5,3). What is the slope of this line?

A. 3

B. $\frac{1}{2}$

C. 1

D. $-\frac{1}{2}$

204. $\sqrt{0.36} \cdot 10^4 =$

A. 64

B. 6,000

C. 600

D. 360

205. A coin has been tossed four times, and heads has come up each time. What is the probability of heads on the fifth toss?

A. $\frac{1}{2}$

B. $\frac{1}{16}$

C. $\frac{1}{5}$

D. $\frac{2}{5}$

206. If 12 grams of powder X are required to make 100 milliliters of product, how many grams of powder X are needed to make 250 milliliters of product?

A. 15

B. 20

C. 30

D. 50

207. If a patient takes 1 tablespoonful of medicine three times daily, how many milliliters equals a 7-day supply for this person? (1 tbsp = 15 mL).

A. 300

B. 315

C. 330

D. 350

208. If a patient is receiving 200 micrograms of X tablets, and X tablets is equivalent to 77% of X injection, what is the equivalent injection dose for this patient?

A. 77 milligrams

B. 154 micrograms

C. 154 milligrams

D. 165 micrograms

209. $|{-120}| - 120 =$

   A. 240
   B. 120
   C. 0
   D. −120

210. 128 ounces is equivalent to how many pounds?

   A. 6
   B. 7
   C. 8
   D. 9

211. $0.05(10^3) =$

   A. 50
   B. 500
   C. 5,000
   D. 50,000

212. $4! =$

   A. 96
   B. 24
   C. 6
   D. 2

213. $6! =$

   A. 720
   B. 144
   C. 100
   D. 18

214. 50% of 100 = 25% of

   A. 500
   B. 250
   C. 200
   D. 150

215. What is the formula for finding the area of the figure shown below?

   A. $2\pi a^2$
   B. $2a^2 + \dfrac{\pi a^2}{2}$
   C. $2a^2 + \pi a^2$
   D. $2\pi^2$

216. $x^3 = 729;\ x =$

   A. 6
   B. 7
   C. 8
   D. 9

217. $3x - 4 = 20;\ x =$

   A. 5
   B. 6
   C. 7
   D. 8

218. $\dfrac{2}{3} + \dfrac{1}{5} =$

   A. 0.42
   B. 0.50
   C. 0.87
   D. 1.30

219. What is the area of the circle shown below?

$$\pi = 3.14, \ r = 4$$

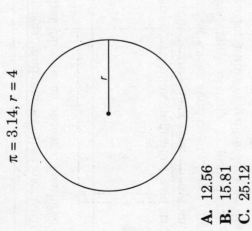

A. 12.56
B. 15.81
C. 25.12
D. 50.24

220. Which of the following is a solution for the equation $x^2 + 50 = 131$?

A. 5
B. 7
C. 9
D. 12

221. $\dfrac{5}{8} + \dfrac{2}{3} =$

A. 1.29
B. 2.01
C. 2.30
D. 2.55

222. 40% of 160 =

A. 50
B. 54
C. 60
D. 64

223. 1% of 50 =

A. 1
B. 0.5
C. 0.25
D. 0.35

224. 10% of 220 =

A. 2.2
B. 22
C. 222
D. 242

225. 5% of 200 =

A. 1
B. 2.5
C. 5
D. 10

STOP

End of Quantitative Ability section. If you have any time left, you may go over your work in this section only.

READING COMPREHENSION

45 Questions (#226–#270)

Directions: Read each of the following passages, and choose the one best answer to each of the questions that follow each passage. You have 45 minutes to complete this section.

Passage 1

Although phenytoin may be used to treat cardiac arrhythmias, migraines, and trigeminal neuralgia, the primary use of phenytoin is to treat seizure disorders. Phenytoin, one of the most important agents used to manage seizures, works similarly to those of other hydantoin-derivative anticonvulsants. It decreases seizure activity by stabilizing neuronal membranes and by increasing efflux or decreasing influx of sodium ions across cell membranes in the motor cortex during generation of nerve impulses. Phenytoin is commercially available as oral suspension, tablets, and capsules. It is also available as an injection. The dosage of phenytoin varies according to the frequency of seizures, the type of seizures, and the patient's tolerance for phenytoin. Therefore, it is extremely important to monitor the patient for seizure activity as well as to monitor phenytoin serum concentrations. Phenytoin has a narrow therapeutic window and monitoring of serum concentrations is necessary. Therapeutic serum concentrations of phenytoin are usually 10–20 mcg per mL (millimeter) and depend on the assay method used. Serum concentrations above 20 mcg per mL often result in toxicity. Adverse reactions associated with dose related toxicities include blurred vision, lethargy, rash, fever, slurred speech, nystagmus, and confusion. In some patients, seizure control is not achieved when plasma concentrations are within the therapeutic concentration range and therefore clinical response of the patient is more meaningful than plasma concentrations. Generally, therapeutic steady state serum concentrations are achieved within 30 days of therapy with an oral dosage of 300 mg daily in adults. Following an intravenous administration of 1000–1500 mg, at a rate not exceeding 50 mg per minute, therapeutic concentrations can be attained within 2 hours. Rapid administration of intravenous phenytoin may result in adverse effects such as decreased blood pressure and other cardiac complications. The use of phenytoin has been associated with osteomalacia, thrombocytopenia, and gastrointestinal upset.

226. According to the passage, which of the following is treated with phenytoin?

A. Trigeminal neuralgia
B. Arthritis
C. Osteomalacia
D. Nystagmus

227. The primary use of phenytoin is to treat

A. cardiac arrhythmias.
B. migraines.
C. seizure disorders.
D. arthritis.

228. Which of the following best represents the mechanism of action of phenytoin in treating seizures?

A. Increases neuronal activity
B. Excites peripheral impulses to excite neuronal activity
C. Stabilizes neuronal membranes and decreases seizure activity by decreasing the entrance of sodium ions across the cell membranes in the motor cortex during generation of nerve impulses
D. Stabilizes neuronal membranes and decreases seizure activity by increasing the entrance of sodium ions across the cell membranes in the motor cortex during generation of nerve impulses

229. Which of the following does (do) NOT affect the dosage of phenytoin?

A. Phenytoin serum concentration
B. Number of seizures experienced
C. Adverse events experienced
D. Puncture sites available

230. Which of the following best explains the meaning of the sentence "Phenytoin has a narrow therapeutic window and monitoring of serum concentrations is necessary"?

A. There is a small difference in the serum concentrations known to produce seizures and the serum concentrations known to produce adverse experiences. Therefore, serum concentrations should be monitored.
B. There is no difference in the serum concentrations known to produce desirable effects and the serum concentrations known to produce undesirable effects. Therefore, serum concentrations should be monitored.
C. There is a small difference in the serum concentrations known to control migraines and the serum concentrations known to produce migraines. Therefore, serum concentrations should be monitored.
D. There is a small difference in the serum concentrations known to control seizures and the serum concentrations known to produce toxicities and adverse effects. Therefore, serum concentrations should be monitored.

231. Which of the following statements describe why phenytoin should NOT be administered at a rate greater than 50 mg per minute?

A. A higher rate takes longer to achieve adequate plasma concentrations.

B. A higher rate may lower blood pressure.

C. A higher rate increases arthritis pain.

D. A higher rate may cause a rash.

232. According to the passage, which of the following is NOT a common adverse reaction associated with phenytoin toxicity?

A. Blurred vision

B. Lethargy

C. Dysuria

D. Mental confusion

233. When is the therapeutic steady-state serum concentration generally achieved with an oral dosage of 300 mg daily of phenytoin?

A. Within 5 days

B. Within 24 hours

C. Within 6 days

D. Within 30 days

Passage 2

Hypercalcemia, increased serum calcium concentrations, occurs in approximately 15% of individuals with cancer. Occurrences of this condition have been reported in most types of malignancies. The most effective management of this life-threatening disease is successful treatment of the malignancy. Unfortunately, successful treatment of the cancer may not be possible. In these cases, treatment goals should include correcting intravascular depletion, enhancing renal excretion of calcium, and inhibiting bone resorption. First line treatment of acute hypercalcemia includes the administration of normal saline and furosemide. Since many patients suffering from acute hypercalcemia are dehydrated, the administration of normal saline is warranted. In addition to treating dehydration, normal saline helps to increase renal excretion of calcium. The optimal administration of normal saline is dependent on the severity of hypercalcemia, the degree of dehydration, and the clinical status of the patient. An infusion rate of 400 mL per hour of normal saline is typical. Furosemide, a diuretic, is useful in the treatment of hypercalcemia due to its ability to enhance urinary excretion and more importantly calcium excretion. Additionally, furosemide protects patients from becoming volume overloaded due to the administration of the normal saline. It is very important that patients be adequately hydrated prior to the administration of furosemide in order to get maximum benefits. Intravenous doses of

100 mg of furosemide every 2 hours may be used. Although normal saline and furosemide are the most commonly used agents to treat acute cancer hypercalcemia, only a modest decrease in calcium levels are achieved from this regimen. The use of normal saline and furosemide may be sufficient for the management of mild to moderate hypercalcemia, but it is commonly insufficient for treating severe hypercalcemia.

234. Hypercalcemia

  A. does not occur in any type of cancer.
  B. may occur in most types of cancer.
  C. may occur in bone cancer only.
  D. may occur in lung cancer only.

235. Which of the following is the most appropriate title for this passage?

  A. The Pathogenesis of Cancer-Related Hypercalcemia
  B. The Uses of Normal Saline and Furosemide
  C. Hypercalcemia—a Life-Threatening Disorder
  D. First Line Agents Used to Treat Acute Cancer-Related Hypercalcemia

236. In treating hypercalcemia with a diuretic, it is important to

  A. use the diuretic every hour.
  B. administer the diuretic by mouth.
  C. hydrate the patient before administrating the diuretic.
  D. give the diuretic before the normal saline.

237. Which of the following is the most effective method of treating cancer-related hypercalcemia?

  A. The use of normal saline
  B. The use of furosemide
  C. The use of dialysis
  D. Treatment of the malignancy

238. Which of the following is NOT a goal in the treatment of acute hypercalcemia?

  A. Administration of calcium carbonate
  B. Enhancing renal excretion of calcium
  C. Inhibiting bone resorption
  D. Correcting intravascular depletion

239. The use of normal saline and furosemide is NOT typically sufficient for which type of hypercalcemia?

  A. Mild cancer-related hypercalcemia
  B. Mild hypercalcemia
  C. Moderate hypercalcemia
  D. Severe hypercalcemia

Passage 3

Gastroesophageal reflux disease (GERD) is a common medical disorder seen by health care practitioners of all specialties. It is generally chronic in nature, and long-term therapy may be required. While the mortality associated with GERD is very low (1 death per 100,000 patients), the quality of life experienced by the patient can be greatly diminished.

GERD refers to any symptomatic clinical condition or histologic alteration that results from episodes of gastroesophageal reflux. Gastroesophageal reflux refers to the retrograde movement of gastric contents from the stomach into the esophagus. Many people experience some degree of reflux, especially after eating, which may be considered a benign physiologic process. When the esophagus is repeatedly exposed to refluxed material for prolonged periods of time, inflammation of the esophagus (i.e., reflux esophagitis) can occur. It is important to realize that gastroesophageal reflux must precede the development of GERD or reflux esophagitis. In severe cases, reflux may lead to a multitude of serious complications including esophageal strictures, esophageal ulcers, motility disorders, perforation, hemorrhage, aspiration, and Barrett's esophagus. While mild disease is often managed with life-style changes and antacids, more intensive therapeutic intervention with histamine (H$_2$) antagonists, sucralfate, prokinetic agents, or proton pump inhibitors is generally required for patients with more severe disease. Following discontinuation of therapy, relapse is common and long-term maintenance therapy may be required. Historically, surgical intervention has been reserved for patients in whom conventional treatment modalities fail. However, the recent development of laparoscopic antireflux surgical procedures has led to a reevaluation of the role of surgery in the long-term management of GERD. Some clinicians have suggested that laparoscopic antireflux surgery may be a cost-effective alternative to long-term maintenance therapy in young patients. However, long-term comparative trials evaluating the cost effectiveness of the various treatment modalities are warranted.

The pathogenesis of gastroesophageal reflux is related to the complex balance between defense mechanisms and aggressive factors. Understanding both the normal protective mechanisms and the aggressive factors that may contribute to or promote gastroesophageal reflux helps one to design rational therapeutic treatment regimens. Gastric acid, pepsin, bile acids, and pancreatic enzymes are considered aggressive factors and may promote esophageal damage upon reflux into the esophagus. Thus, the composition (potency) and volume of the refluxate are aggressive factors that may lead to esophageal injury. Conversely, normal protective mechanisms include anatomic factors, the lower esophageal sphincter pressure, esophageal clearing, mucosal resistance, and gastric emptying. Rational therapeutic regimens in the treatment of gastroesophageal reflux are designed to maximize normal defense mechanisms and/or attenuate the aggressive factors.

Excerpted with permission from *Pharmacotherapy, A Pathophysiological Approach*, Third Edition, by Joseph T. DiPiro, et al., page 675. Stamford, CT: Appleton & Lange, 1996.

240. Which of the following statements is FALSE?

A. GERD is a common medical disorder seen by healthcare practitioners of all specialties.
B. Gastroesophageal reflux must precede the development of reflux esophagitis.
C. The mortality associated with GERD is very high.
D. Mild GERD may be managed with life style changes and antacids.

241. One possible complication of reflux is

A. perforation.
B. mucosal resistance.
C. gastric emptying.
D. lower esophageal sphincter pressure.

242. In GERD patients, response to pharmacologic intervention is dependent on the

A. dosage regimen employed.
B. efficacy of the agent.
C. severity of the disease.
D. All of the above

243. Some clinicians have suggested that a cost-effective alternative therapy for GERD may be

A. histamine antagonists.
B. prokinetic agents.
C. laparoscopic antireflux surgery.
D. proton pump inhibitors.

244. Aggressive factors that may promote esophageal damage upon reflux into the esophagus are

A. gastric acid and pancreatic enzymes.
B. bile acids and esophageal clearing.
C. lower esophageal sphincter pressure and gastric emptying.
D. None of the above

Passage 4

Many people in the United States are diagnosed with diabetes mellitus. Non-insulin-dependent diabetes mellitus (NIDDM) is the most common type of diabetes and it is associated with a significant amount of morbidities and mortalities. NIDDM is classified as an endocrine disorder characterized by defects in insulin secretion as well as in insulin action. In NIDDM patients a defect also exists in insulin receptor binding. These defects lead to increased serum glucose concentrations or hyperglycemia.

Sulfonylureas are one of the most popular classes of agents used to treat NIDDM. One of the newest agents to treat NIDDM is acarbose, an oral alpha-glucosidase inhibitor. Acarbose interferes with the hydrolysis of dietary disaccharides and complex carbohydrates, thereby delaying absorption of glucose and other monosaccharides. Acarbose is available for oral administration only. To be most effective, it should be taken at the beginning of a meal. The recommended starting dose is 25 mg three times daily and doses as high as 200 mg three times a day have been safely used. The recommended starting dose is 25 mg three times daily and doses as high as 200 mg three times a day have been safely used. The most common adverse experiences associated with the use of acarbose are abdominal cramps, flatulence, diarrhea, and abdominal distension. Most of the adverse effects are due to the unabsorbed carbohydrates undergoing fermentation in the colon. Acarbose has also been associated with decreased intestinal absorption of iron, thereby possibly leading to anemia. The occurrence of hypoglycemia when using acarbose in combination with other agents used to lower serum glucose is great. Glucose should be administered to treat hypoglycemia in patients taking acarbose because sucrose may not be adequately hydrolyzed and absorbed. The effectiveness of this agent to lower serum glucose concentrations in patients with NIDDM has been clearly demonstrated in clinical trials. Acarbose provides another option for treating NIDDM.

245. Which of the following does NOT describe the term *non-insulin-dependent diabetes mellitus?*

   A. Endocrine in nature
   B. Hyperglycemia
   C. May be due to a defect in insulin receptor binding
   D. Results in iron deficiencies

246. Which of the following is the most common type of agent used to treat NIDDM?

   A. A sulfonylurea agent
   B. Glucose
   C. Sucrose
   D. Fructose

247. According to the passage, which of the following is the most common side effect associated with the use of acarbose?

   A. Hyperglycemia
   B. Anemia
   C. Gastrointestinal discomfort
   D. Rash

248. Which of the following is the best agent to treat hypoglycemia in patients taking acarbose?

   A. A sulfonylurea agent
   B. Glucose
   C. Sucrose
   D. Fructose

249. According to the passage, which of the following has NOT been associated with the use of acarbose?

   A. Low serum glucose concentrations
   B. Gastrointestinal discomfort
   C. Decreased iron absorption
   D. Obstruction of the urinary tract

250. Which of the following used in combination with acarbose increases the risk of experiencing hypoglycemia?

   A. A sulfonylurea agent
   B. Glucose
   C. Iron
   D. Increased caloric intake

251. Which of the following is the best title for this passage?

A. Diabetes in the United States
B. Agents Used to Treat Non-Insulin-Dependent Diabetes Mellitus
C. The Use of Acarbose in the Treatment of Non-Insulin-Dependent Diabetes Mellitus
D. Adverse Effects of Acarbose

Passage 5

Osteoporosis, the most common skeletal disorder associated with aging, is a significant cause of mortality and morbidity among the elderly. The two most common types of osteoporosis are type I (postmenopausal) osteoporosis and type II (senile) osteoporosis. Type I osteoporosis is due to a drastic decline in bone mass during the first five years of menopause and a slower rate of bone loss in subsequent years. Type II osteoporosis is characterized by a gradual, age-related loss of bone in females and males over the age of 65 years. By far, osteoporosis is most prevalent in the postmenopausal population. In addition to menopausal-associated hormonal changes, other risk factors for osteoporosis in women include low calcium intake, medical factors such as oophorectomy, and life-style factors such as inactivity and cigarette smoking. In osteoporosis, osteoclasts excavate areas in bone that the bone-forming cells, the osteoblasts, are unable to fully reconstitute. Often this defective bone loses compressive strength, thereby leading to an increased risk of fracture. Osteoporosis evolves as a silent disease with no obvious early warning signs. Many patients suffering from osteoporosis are not aware of their condition until a fracture occurs. This disease is responsible for at least 1.5 million fractures in Americans each year, with annual costs to the United States health care system of approximately $10 billion. Other consequences of osteoporosis include pain and spinal deformities such as dorsal kyphosis and dowager's or widow's hump. In addition, a decrease in appetite, fatigue, and weakness may be present. As the population continues to age, the cost of treating osteoporosis and its associated complications is predicted to double over the next 30 years.

252. Osteoporosis is most common in which population?

A. Postmenopausal women
B. Young males
C. Infants
D. Teenagers

253. Which of the following is NOT a risk factor for osteoporosis?

A. Age
B. Low calcium intake
C. Weight-bearing exercise
D. Cigarette smoking

254. Which of the following is a direct consequence of osteoporosis?

A. Height gain
B. Hypertension
C. Oophorectomy
D. Dowager's hump

255. What is the predicted U.S. cost of treating osteoporosis and its associated complications over the next 30 years?

A. $5 billion
B. $7 billion
C. $10 billion
D. $20 billion

256. Which cells are responsible for removing bone?

A. Osteoclasts
B. Osteoblasts
C. Osteomasts
D. Osteotrasts

257. Which cells are responsible for forming bone?

A. Osteoclasts
B. Osteoblasts
C. Osteomasts
D. Osteotrasts

Passage 6

Bronchial asthma is a common disease of children and adults. Although the clinical manifestations of asthma have been known since antiquity, it is a disease that still defies precise definition. The word *asthma* is of Greek origin and means "panting." More than 2000 years ago, Hippocrates used the word *asthma* to describe episodic shortness of breath; however, the first detailed clinical description of the asthmatic patient was made by Aretaeus in the second century. Since that time *asthma* has been used to describe any disorder with episodic shortness of breath or dyspnea; thus, the terms *cardiac asthma* and *bronchial asthma* have been used to delineate the etiologies of the dyspnea. These terms are now obsolete and *asthma* refers to a disorder of the respiratory system characterized by episodes of difficulty in breathing. An Expert Panel of the National Institutes of Health National Asthma Education Program (NAEP) has defined asthma as a lung disease characterized by (1) airway obstruction that is reversible (but not completely so in some patients) either spontaneously or with treatment; (2) airway inflammation; and (3) increased airway responsiveness to a variety of stimuli. This descriptive definition for asthma is attributed to our lack of knowledge of the precise pathogenic defect that results in the clinical syndrome we recognize as asthma. The current definition does allow for the important heterogeneity of the clinical presentation of asthma. New technologies have added substantially to our understanding of the interrelationships of immunology, biochemistry, and physiology to the clinical presentation of asthma, and further research may yet uncover a specific genetic defect associated with asthma. Until such time, asthma will continue to defy exact definition.

An estimated 10 million persons in the United States have asthma (about 5% of the population). The reported prevalence increased 29% from 1980 to 1987 to 40.1 per 1000 population. African-Americans have a 19% higher incidence of asthma than whites and are twice as likely to be hospitalized. The estimated cost of asthma in the United States in 1990 was $6.2 billion. The largest single direct medical expenditure was for inpatient hospital services (emergency care), reaching almost $1.5 billion, followed by prescription medications ($1.1 billion). The costs of medication increased 54% between 1985 and 1990. In total, 43% of the economic impact was associated with emergency room use, hospitalization, and death. Asthma accounted for 1% of all ambulatory care visits according to the National Ambulatory Medical Care Survey and results in more than 450,000 hospitalizations per year.

Excerpted with permission from *Pharmacotherapy, A Pathophysiological Approach*, Third Edition, by Joseph T. DiPiro, et al., page 553. Stamford, CT: Appleton & Lange, 1996.

258. According to the passage above, which of the following statements about the definition of asthma is true?

A. Asthma has been defined precisely since the second century.

B. Although asthma is a common disease of children and adults, it eludes a precise definition.

C. Two opposing views of the etiology of asthma, the cardiac and the bronchial, make it difficult to define the term precisely.

D. The NAEP's definition of asthma is widely regarded as exact but does not allow for the heterogeneity of the clinical presentation of asthma.

259. Which of the following statements is FALSE?

A. The cost of asthma in the United States in 1990 was $6.2 billion.

B. African-Americans have a 19% higher incidence of asthma than whites.

C. The cost of asthma medication decreased 54% between 1985 and 1990.

D. Prescription medications for asthma accounted for an expenditure of $1.1 billion in 1990.

260. The passage suggests that in the future researchers are likely to understand more about

A. new technologies to treat asthma.

B. wheezing and episodes of shortness of breath.

C. a specific genetic defect associated with asthma.

D. the interrelationship of immunology, biochemistry, and physiology.

261. The estimated number of persons in the United States who have asthma is

A. 100 million.

B. 2.5 million.

C. fewer than 2%.

D. 10 million.

262. In the 1990s, the term *asthma* refers to

A. panting.

B. dyspnea of cardiac or bronchial etiology.

C. Both A and B

D. a disorder of the respiratory system characterized by episodes of difficulty in breathing.

263. The passage contains which of the following?

A. A descriptive definition of asthma
B. Facts about the prevalence of asthma in the United States
C. An explanation of the worldwide increase in prevalence of asthma
D. Both A and B

Passage 7

Peptic ulcer disease affects approximately 10% of Americans each year. Peptic ulcer disease has been referred to as a chronic inflammatory condition of the stomach and duodenum and often requires lifelong therapy. Although this disease has a relatively low mortality rate, it results in substantial human suffering and high economic costs making treatment necessary. In the past, the pathogenesis of this disorder was believed to be related to diet and stress. However, new studies have suggested that peptic ulcer disease is commonly due to the presence of an organism, *Helicobacter pylori*. The recognition of gastritis due to *Helicobacter pylori* has revolutionized the therapeutic approach to treating peptic ulcer disease. Clinical trials demonstrate that the recurrence of ulcers can be drastically reduced by a single course of antimicrobial treatment that eradicates *Helicobacter pylori*, as compared to traditional therapy, which involves continuous suppression of gastric acid secretion. In light of this, the NIH Consensus Development Conference recommended that all patients with documented duodenal or gastric ulcers who are infected with *Helicobacter pylori* should receive antimicrobial therapy to cure the infection. Although *Helicobacter pylori* is difficult to eradicate and successful treatment requires concurrent administration of at least two antimicrobial drugs, many antibiotic regimens have been successfully used. Agents with antimicrobial activity such as amoxicillin, tetracycline, metronidazole, clarithromycin, and bismuth have been used to eradicate the organism. Peptic ulcer disease associated with *Helicobacter pylori* can now be cured with eradication of this organism.

264. According to the passage, approximately how many Americans are affected with peptic ulcer disease each year?

A. 2%
B. 5%
C. 7%
D. 10%

265. Which statement concerning peptic ulcer disease is FALSE?

A. It is an inflammatory condition of the gastrointestinal system.
B. It affects the stomach.
C. It affects the duodenum.
D. It affects the kidney.

266. Before the recent studies discussed in this passage, the pathogenesis of peptic ulcer disease was believed to be related to

A. dietary intake.
B. the bacterium *Escherichia coli.*
C. inflammatory bowel disease.
D. cancer.

267. Recent studies have suggested that peptic ulcer disease is commonly due to

A. viral load.
B. stress.
C. presence of the organism *Helicobacter pylori.*
D. ampicillin.

268. According to the passage, clinical trials demonstrate that the recurrence of ulcers can be reduced by

A. eating low sodium foods.
B. drinking more orange juice.
C. suppressing acid secretion.
D. eradicating *Helicobacter pylori.*

269. Which of the following is NOT an antimicrobial?

A. *Helicobacter pylori*
B. Amoxicillin
C. Tetracycline
D. Clarithromycin

270. Which of the following best expresses the main idea of the passage?

A. The treatment of gastric ulcer
B. The role of *Helicobacter pylori* in peptic ulcer disease
C. The use of antivirals in treating peptic ulcer disease
D. Treating gastritis by relieving stress

STOP

End of Reading Comprehension section. If you have any time left, you may go over your work in this section only.

PRACTICE PCAT 1 ANSWER KEY

Verbal Ability

1. A	11. B	21. C	31. A	41. D
2. B	12. D	22. C	32. B	42. B
3. D	13. C	23. C	33. A	43. D
4. C	14. C	24. D	34. C	44. C
5. A	15. B	25. B	35. D	45. B
6. B	16. B	26. C	36. A	46. C
7. D	17. D	27. A	37. B	47. B
8. A	18. A	28. B	38. C	48. C
9. A	19. C	29. C	39. A	49. B
10. C	20. A	30. A	40. B	50. D

Biology

51. A	61. D	71. D	81. A	91. A
52. C	62. B	72. A	82. A	92. C
53. A	63. C	73. B	83. B	93. C
54. B	64. A	74. A	84. B	94. A
55. D	65. C	75. B	85. B	95. B
56. A	66. B	76. D	86. C	96. A
57. B	67. C	77. A	87. C	97. C
58. A	68. C	78. B	88. A	98. B
59. B	69. A	79. D	89. B	99. A
60. C	70. B	80. C	90. D	100. C

Chemistry

101. A	113. D	125. D	137. B	149. B
102. B	114. B	126. D	138. A	150. C
103. B	115. B	127. C	139. A	151. B
104. C	116. B	128. B	140. C	152. C
105. A	117. C	129. D	141. B	153. B
106. C	118. A	130. C	142. C	154. B
107. A	119. B	131. D	143. B	155. A
108. A	120. B	132. B	144. A	156. C
109. C	121. A	133. C	145. B	157. C
110. C	122. A	134. B	146. C	158. D
111. A	123. A	135. B	147. A	159. B
112. D	124. B	136. C	148. C	160. C

Quantitative Ability

161. D	174. C	187. C
162. D	175. A	188. C
163. A	176. A	189. A
164. A	177. B	190. A
165. B	178. A	191. C
166. B	179. C	192. B
167. B	180. A	193. C
168. B	181. B	194. A
169. C	182. D	195. C
170. D	183. B	196. C
171. A	184. A	197. A
172. B	185. C	198. A
173. D	186. B	199. C

200. C	213. A
201. C	214. C
202. C	215. B
203. C	216. D
204. B	217. D
205. A	218. C
206. C	219. D
207. B	220. C
208. B	221. A
209. C	222. D
210. C	223. B
211. A	224. B
212. B	225. D

Reading Comprehension

226. A	235. D	244. A
227. C	236. C	245. D
228. C	237. D	246. A
229. D	238. A	247. C
230. D	239. D	248. B
231. B	240. C	249. D
232. C	241. A	250. A
233. D	242. D	251. C
234. B	243. C	252. A

253. C	262. D
254. D	263. D
255. D	264. D
256. A	265. D
257. B	266. A
258. B	267. C
259. C	268. D
260. C	269. A
261. D	270. B

EXPLANATORY ANSWERS FOR VERBAL ABILITY

1. Answer is **A**. To *retreat* means to retire, leave, or depart; the opposite is to *advance*, which means to move or cause to move forward.

2. Answer is **B**. To *abolish* means to end or eliminate; the opposite is to *establish*, which means to create.

3. Answer is **D**. *Brilliant* means bright, shining, radiant; the opposite is *dull*, which means lacking vividness or luster.

4. Answer is **C**. To *exaggerate* means to overstate, magnify; the opposite is to *diminish*, which means to make less or smaller.

5. Answer is **A**. To *preserve* means to keep, maintain, conserve, save; the opposite is to *discontinue*, which means to abandon, stop, or terminate.

6. Answer is **B**. *Relish* means satisfaction, delight, appreciation; the opposite is *disfavor*, which means disapproval, dislike, or disapprobation.

7. Answer is **D**. To *abandon* means to leave, quit, desert, forsake; the opposite is *retain*, which means to keep or hold.

8. Answer is **A**. *Subordinate* means inferior, lower; the opposite is *superior*, which means higher in rank or status.

9. Answer is **A**. *Summit* means top, peak, crown; the opposite is *base*, the lowest part.

10. Answer is **C**. *Desolate* means deserted, empty, lonely; the opposite is *crowded*.

11. Answer is **B**. *Uncivil* means rude, impolite, discourteous; the opposite is *polite*.

12. Answer is **D**. *Prosaic* means common, routine, lacking in imagination; the opposite is *imaginative*.

13. Answer is **C**. *Abrasive* means rough or irritating; the opposite is *silky*, which means soft and smooth.

14. Answer is **C**. *Iridescent* means shining with a rainbow of colors; the opposite is *colorless*.

15. Answer is **B**. To *distend* means to expand; the opposite is to *contract*.

16. Answer is **B**. To *imprecate* means to curse; the opposite is to *bless*.

17. Answer is **D**. To *reveal* is to make known or disclose; the opposite is to *hide*.

18. Answer is **A**. *Fundamental* means centrally important, primary, or basic; the opposite is *superficial*, which means unimportant, lacking depth, or affecting only the surface.

19. Answer is **C**. *Avid* means eager; the opposite is *averse*, which means disinclined or lacking the desire to do something.

20. Answer is **A**. *Drudgery* is dull, tiresome, or menial work; the opposite is *fun*.

21. Answer is **C**. *Animated* means full of life, movement, and activity; the opposite is *subdued*, or lacking in liveliness or intensity.

22. Answer is **C**. *Simultaneous* means existing or taking place at the same time; the oposite is *asynchronous*, which means not existing or occurring at the same time.

23. Answer is **C**. *Unintended* is the opposite of *planned*, which means intended.

24. Answer is **D**. *Bleak* means discouraging or not hopeful; the opposite is *encouraging*.

25. Answer is **B**. To *dwindle* means to decrease slowly or diminish; the opposite is to *increase*.

26. Answer is **C**. The analogy here is based on words that are synonyms, that is, that have the same or nearly the same meaning. To *fence* something in and to *enclose* it are the same. To *daub* means the same as to *smear*.

27. Answer is **A**. *Placate* and *pacify* have the same or nearly the same meaning, so you need to find the word that is synonymous with *confirm*. The answer is *ratify*.

28. Answer is **B**. This analogy is based on antonyms, words that are opposite in meaning. The first pair is simple: *melt* is clearly the opposite of *freeze*. But be careful in choosing your answer. You need a verb, so the correct choice is *work*.

29. Answer is **C**. In this example, you are looking for a word that means the opposite of *oblique* (indirect or deviating from a straight line), so the correct choice is *straight*. The analogy is one of antonyms.

30. Answer is **A**. This analogy involves causality. As a *virus* causes a *cold*, so a *deity* causes a *miracle*.

31. Answer is **A**. This analogy involves the relationship of part to whole. The *margin* of a wound is the part analogous to the *rim* of a volcano.

32. <u>Answer is</u> **B**. Here the analogy is based on the relationship of whole to part. A *book* is divided into parts, each of which is a *chapter*, and a *concerto* is divided into parts, each of which is a *movement*.

33. <u>Answer is</u> **A**. Here the relationship is that of whole to part. The *small intestine* contains a part called the *duodenum*, and the *hand* contains *fingers*. Since an echidna is a spiny anteater, that is clearly not the correct choice. The other alternatives must be rejected as well since neither completes an analogy based on a whole-to-part relationship.

34. <u>Answer is</u> **C**. This is a part to part analogy. Both the *raspberry* and *kiwi fruit* are part of the larger group of all fruits, and both *romaine* and *Boston lettuce* are part of the larger group of all kinds of lettuce.

35. <u>Answer is</u> **D**. In this example, the relationship is deceptively simple: purpose or use. We use a *needle to sew*, and we use a *hose to siphon*. Be careful not to choose the noun *lawn* erroneously; although we water the lawn with a hose, this word is not the correct choice in this case.

36. <u>Answer is</u> **A**. This analogy involves purpose or use. An *umbrella* shelters a *pedestrian* from rain; a *roof* shelters a *house*.

37. <u>Answer is</u> **B**. The correct answer is *egg* because this is an analogy of action to object. We *recycle* (action) *paper* (object), and *incubate* (action) an *egg* (object).

38. <u>Answer is</u> **C**. This is another analogy of action to object. Just as we *drink* (action) *juice* (object), we *mow* (action) the *lawn* (object). Obviously a noun is needed to complete this analogy.

39. <u>Answer is</u> **A**. Just as a *theory* is *refuted*, a *president* is impeached, so *impeach* is the correct choice. This analogy involves object to action.

40. <u>Answer is</u> **B**. In this analogy of place, all the examples are drawn from fiction. In Homer's epic poem *The Odyssey*, *Ithaca* was the home of the wanderer *Odysseus*, who longed to return there. In *The Wizard of Oz*, *Dorothy*, like Odysseus, often longed to go back to *Kansas*, her home.

41. <u>Answer is</u> **D**. This analogy expresses the relationship of part to whole: the *ear* is part of the *corn* plant, and the *boll* is part of the *cotton* plant.

42. <u>Answer is</u> **B**. *Debris* eventually becomes *compost* and can be used as fertilizer; *resin* eventually becomes *amber*. The analogy is one of sequence or time.

43. Answer is **D**. In this analogy of characteristic or description, the *cheetah* is *sleek*, whereas the *seal* is *rotund*.

44. Answer is **C**. A relationship of degree is implied here. The *flu* represents a much greater degree of severity than a *cold*. Likewise, a *depression* is a much greater economic problem than a recession.

45. Answer is **B**. Analogies may depend on grammar alone. In this grammatical analogy, you are asked to find the correct past tense of the verb *sweep*, which is *swept*.

46. Answer is **C**. This is also a grammatical analogy. This time you must find a verb that takes the preposition *out*, just as the verb *comment* takes the preposition *on*. The correct answer can only be *eke*.

47. Answer is **B**. In this analogy of association, the *pharmacist* is associated with a *pharmacy*, and the *diplomat* with an *embassy*.

48. Answer is **C**. An analogy may express the relationship between a worker and tool. In this example, a *painter* uses a *palette*, and a *cook* uses a *spatula*.

49. Answer is **B**. To understand this analogy of definition, it helps to know that an *ellipsis*, usually indicated by three successive dots . . . is an omission of words in a *sentence*. The correct answer is *pause*, a temporary cessation of utterance in a *speech*.

50. Answer is **D**. Since a *Panama* is one of many kinds of *hat*, and a *Mako* is one of many kinds of *shark*, the relationship expressed is part to whole.

EXPLANATORY ANSWERS FOR BIOLOGY

51. Answer is A. Monera is a taxonomic kingdom including bacteria, blue-green bacteria, and viruses. They are prokaryotic, not eukaryotic. Prokaryotic cells are small, have a simple internal structure, do not have their genetic material enclosed within a membrane nucleus, and lack organelles. Eukaryotic cells are characterized by the presence of a membrane-bound nucleus and other organelles.

52. Answer is C. Living organisms can be grouped into five major categories called kingdoms, making the only possible answer choice C. These five kingdoms are: Monera, Protista, Fungi, Plantae, and Animalia.

Figure 1 (Questions 53 and 54)

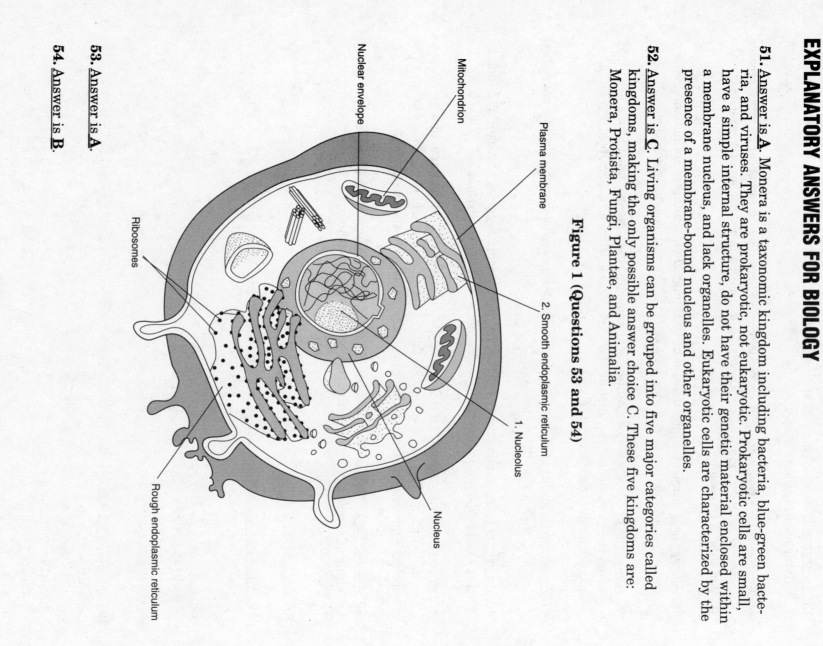

Nuclear envelope

Mitochondrion

Plasma membrane

2. Smooth endoplasmic reticulum

1. Nucleolus

Ribosomes

Rough endoplasmic reticulum

Nucleus

53. Answer is A.

54. Answer is B.

Figure 2 (Questions 55 and 56)

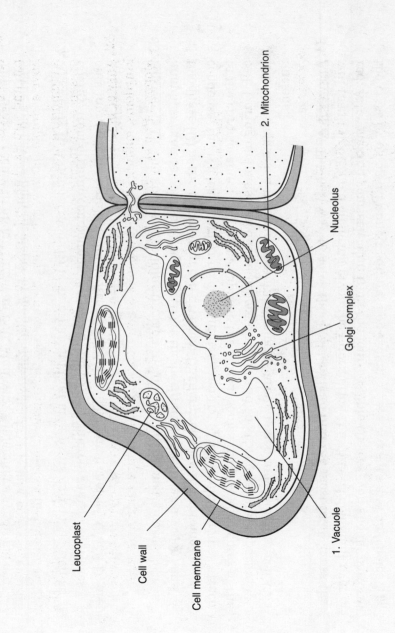

Leucoplast

Cell wall

Cell membrane

1. Vacuole

Golgi complex

Nucleolus

2. Mitochondrion

55. Answer is **D**.

56. Answer is **A**.

57. Answer is **B**. Cell locomotion is a function of flagella (A) and cilia (B). However, cells in the respiratory tract are mobile due to cilia.

58. Answer is **A**. Hypotonic situation (hypotonic solution) will favor water entering the cell, therefore causing the cell to swell (A), not shrivel. The cell will shrivel (B) in hypertonic solution. In isotonic solution, the cell will remain unchanged (D). Choice C is irrelevant.

59. Answer is **B**. Understanding the basic definition of the terms is the key to answering this question. A gene (B) is a unit of heredity containing information for a characteristic or factors that determine a given trait. Alleles (A) are defined as forms of a particular gene. Genotype (C) is basically the genetic composition (actual alleles) of an organism. Phenotype (D) is the physical (outward) properties of an organism.

60. Answer is **C**. The actual alleles carried by an individual are called genotype (C). See explanation for question 59.

61. Answer is D. Men with Klinefelter's syndrome have two X chromosomes. Since normal male chromosomes are XY, Klinefelter's syndrome is represented by XXY. This disease occurs in about 1 male in 500. Men with Klinefelter's syndrome are sterile and have a high incidence of mental deficiency.

62. Answer is B. A heterotroph (B) is an organism that obtains its carbon, as well as energy, from organic compounds. An autotroph (A) is a microorganism that uses only inorganic materials as its source of nutrients. The other choices, C and D, are irrelevant.

63. Answer is C. The stages of cellular division include prophase, metaphase, anaphase, and telophase. Anaphase (D) is the beginning of cellular division, and telophase (C) is the last step in cell division. During prophase the chromosomes condense, the nuclear membrane deteriorates, and the spindle microtubules attach to the chromosomes. During metaphase the chromosomes move to the center of the cell. During anaphase each kinetochore divides, and the chromosomes separate. During telophase a nuclear membrane reforms around each new daughter cell's nucleus.

64. Answer is A. The best way to solve this problem is to find the most likely cross that will result in 50% red offspring given the information that blue is dominant over red. After making your selection from the four possible choices, you should perform the cross by using a Punnett square. For example, let's cross Aa and aa (choice A):

	a	a
A	Aa	Aa
a	aa	aa

Aa = heterozygous blue;

aa = red.

The cross will result in 50% red and 50% blue.

To check the other choices, set up each of them in a Punnett square. Choice B will result in 100% heterozygous (Aa) blue offspring. Choice C will result in 75% blue offspring and 25% red. Choice D will result in 100% blue offspring. Only choice A results in 50% red and 50% blue.

65. <u>Answer is **C**</u>. Use the same method explained in question number 64. The cross of Aa and Aa (choice C) will result in 25% red offspring.

	A	a
A	AA	Aa
a	Aa	aa

AA (homozygous blue) and
Aa (heterozygous) = blue; aa = red.

This cross will result in 75% blue and 25% red.

66. <u>Answer is **B**</u>. For example, cones (A) provide daylight color vision and are responsible for visual acuity, while rods (B) respond to dim light for black-and-white vision. The iris (C) surrounds the pupil and regulates its diameter. The cornea (D) is the anterior portion of the outer layer of the eye.

67. <u>Answer is **C**</u>. Normal red blood cells (erythrocytes) have an average life span of 120 days.

68. <u>Answer is **C**</u>. The input region of the neuron is the dendrites (C), which pick up impulses. The signal conduction region of the neuron is the axon (A). The other choices are irrelevant.

69. <u>Answer is **A**</u>. See explanation for question 68.

70. <u>Answer is **B**</u>. Of the choices, the Golgi apparatus is the only one that modifies materials synthesized in the rough and smooth endoplasmic reticulum.

71. <u>Answer is **D**</u>. No explanation needed.

72. <u>Answer is **A**</u>. No explanation needed.

73. <u>Answer is **B**</u>. Since choices A and D are irrelevant to the question, a distinction in function needs to be made between choices B and C. Messenger RNA (mRNA) carries the code for the amino acid sequences of proteins from the genes of DNA out of the nucleus and into the cytoplasm. Each transfer RNA (B) carries an amino acid to a ribosome during protein synthesis, recognizes a codon of messenger RNA, and positions its amino acid for incorporation into the growing protein chain.

74. <u>Answer is **A**</u>. No explanation needed.

75. <u>Answer is **B**</u>. No explanation needed.

76. <u>Answer is **D**</u>. The principal autonomic and limbic functions of the hypothalamus are (1) cardiovascular (heart rate) regulation; (2) body temperature regulation; (3) regulation of water and electrolyte balance; (4) regulation of hunger and control of gastrointestinal activity; (5) regulation of sleeping and wakefulness; (6) regulation of sexual response; (7) regulation of emotions; and (8) control of endocrine functions. The respiratory center of the medulla oblongota controls the rate and depth of breathing.

77. <u>Answer is **A**</u>. The temporal lobe interprets some sensory experiences and stores memories of both auditory and visual experiences (A). The occipital lobe, not the temporal lobe, integrates eye movements by directing and focusing the eye.

78. <u>Answer is **B**</u>. Lobes of the cerebrum include the frontal lobe, parietal lobe, temporal lobe, occipital lobe, and insula.

79. <u>Answer is **D**</u>. Growth hormone (A), prolactin (B), antidiuretic hormone (C), thyroid-stimulating hormone, adrenocorticotropic hormone, follicle-stimulating hormone, luteinizing hormone, and oxytocin are secreted by the pituitary gland. Insulin (D) is secreted by the pancreas, not the pituitary gland.

80. <u>Answer is **C**</u>. The adrenal cortex secretes steroid hormones called corticosteroids (C). The other choices are either not steroid hormones or not secreted by the adrenal cortex.

81. <u>Answer is **A**</u>. The islet of Langerhans (pancreas) secretes insulin (A) and glucagon. Pepsinogen (C) is a proenzyme formed and secreted by the chief cells of the gastric mucosa, not the islet of Langerhans. Gastrin (B) is a hormone secreted by the mucosa of the pyloric area of the stomach.

82. <u>Answer is **A**</u>. Insulin promotes (A), not inhibits (C), cellular uptake of glucose and formation of glycogen and fat. Glucagon stimulates hydrolysis of glycogen and fat (B).

83. <u>Answer is **B**</u>. No explanation needed.

84. <u>Answer is **B**</u>. In order to answer this question, one must be familiar with the four chambers of the heart, the anatomy, and the circulation of blood flow. The heart has four valves (bicuspid, tricuspid, pulmonary, and aortic), thus ruling out choice C as the answer. Blood from the right atrium passes through the tricuspid valve (B) to fill the right ventricle. The bicuspid valve (A) is between the left atrium and left ventricle and therefore could not be the answer.

85. <u>Answer is **B**</u>. Contraction of the heart is called systole (A), and relaxation of the heart is called diastole (B). Choices C and D are irrelevant.

86. <u>Answer is **C**</u>. No explanation needed.

87. Answer is **C**. Functions of the skeletal system include support, protection, body movement, hemopoiesis (production of leukocytes, erythrocytes, and platelets) and mineral storage (calcium). Parietal cells in the gastric glands contribute to the production of hydrochloric acid (C).

88. Answer is **A**. Urea is the waste product of amino acid metabolism (A), not formation (B), that is formed in the liver and excreted in normal adult human urine. Choice C is irrelevant.

89. Answer is **B**. Aldosterone promotes sodium retention and potassium loss (B). Choice A is incorrect because it is the exact opposite of choice B.

90. Answer is **D**. No explanation needed.

91. Answer is **A**. The heart, brain, and pancreas are much smaller than the liver. In fact the liver is the largest internal organ of the body. The normal adult liver weighs approximately 3–4 pounds.

92. Answer is **C**. The liver (C) produces and secretes 250–1,500 ml of bile per day. The gallbladder (D) serves as a storage reservoir for bile. The pancreas (A) and the kidneys (B) are not associated with bile production.

93. Answer is **C**. No explanation needed.

94. Answer is **A**. No explanation needed.

95. Answer is **B**. No explanation needed.

96. Answer is **A**. No explanation needed.

97. Answer is **C**. No explanation needed.

98. Answer is **B**. No explanation needed.

99. Answer is **A**. No explanation needed.

100. Answer is **C**. No explanation needed.

EXPLANATORY ANSWERS FOR CHEMISTRY

101. Answer is **A**. Atoms of the same element having the same number of protons but different numbers of neutrons are called isotopes. Isomers are molecules having the same molecular formula but different structural formulas. Allotropes are different forms of the same element that have significantly different chemical and physical properties, for example, graphite and diamond. The term *diastereomer* is generally used in organic chemistry. Diastereomers are compounds that have two or more stereocenters and differ from each other at at least one of the stereocenters.

102. Answer is **B**. $KHCO_3$ may be called potassium hydrogen carbonate or potassium bicarbonate. The formula for sodium hydrogen carbonate is $NaHCO_3$. Potassium carbonic acid is incorrect nomenclature. The formula for sodium carbonate is $NaCO_3$.

103. Answer is **B**. Ions dissolved in water produce a solution that conducts electricity. Of the possible answers, only table salt, NaCl, produces ions when dissolved in water. Sugar, $C_6H_{12}O_6$, ethanol, C_2H_5OH, and oxygen, O_2, do not ionize in water but remain as molecules. Molecular substances dissolved in water do not conduct electricity.

104. Answer is **C**. This problem deals with finding the limiting reagent and then using it to calculate the number of grams of NO produced. To find the limiting reagent first find the number of moles of ammonia and oxygen. Next determine the smallest whole number ratio of moles of each reactant, SWNR, by dividing each number of moles by the smaller of the two numbers. Compare the ratio of moles which you HAVE with the ratio of moles needed in the balanced equation.

$$4NH_3(g) + 5O_2(g) \longrightarrow 4NO(g) + 6H_2O(g)$$

	NH_3	O_2
# moles	$\dfrac{42.5\text{ g}}{17\text{ g / mole}}$	$\dfrac{48.0\text{ g}}{32\text{ g / mole}}$
	2.5 moles	1.5 moles
SWNR	2.5/1.5	1.5/1.5
Have	1.7	1
Need	4	5

More oxygen is needed than ammonia, 5 to 4. However, more ammonia is present than oxygen, 1.7 to 1. Therefore oxygen is the limiting reagent.

grams O_2 $\longrightarrow$ moles O_2 $\longrightarrow$ moles NO $\longrightarrow$

48.0

$\dfrac{48.0}{32} = 1.5$ 1.5 moles $O_2 \times \dfrac{4 \text{ moles NO}}{5 \text{ moles } O_2}$

= 1.2 moles NO

grams NO

1.2 moles NO $\times \dfrac{30 \text{ g NO}}{1 \text{ mole NO}}$ = 36 g NO

105. <u>Answer is **A**</u>. The actual yield of the reaction, 32.0 g SO_2, is given. To calculate percent yield you must first calculate the theoretical yield which is the maximum possible yield of the reaction and then use the theoretical yield in the equation below to calculate percent yield.

$$\frac{\text{Actual yield}}{\text{Theoretical yield}} \times 100 = \% \text{ yield}$$

$$CS_2 + 3O_2 \longrightarrow CO_2 + 2SO_2$$

$$\text{g } CS_2 \longrightarrow \text{moles } CS_2 \longrightarrow \text{moles } SO_2 \longrightarrow$$

$$\frac{38.0 \text{ g}}{76 \text{ g / moles}} \qquad 0.50 \text{ mole } CS_2 \times \frac{2 \text{ moles } SO_2}{1 \text{ mole } CS_2}$$

38.0 gm

0.50 mole   1.00 mole SO_2

$$\text{g } SO_2$$

$$1.00 \text{ mole } SO_2 \times \frac{64 \text{ g } SO_2}{1 \text{ mole } SO_2} = 64 \text{ g } SO_2 \qquad \% \text{ yield} = \frac{32 \text{ g}}{64 \text{ g}} \times 100 = 50\%$$

106. <u>Answer is **C**</u>. Molarity is defined as moles of solute divided by liters of solution.

$$M = \frac{\text{moles of solute}}{\text{liters of solution}} = \frac{\text{g/molecular weight}}{\text{liters of solution}}$$

Sugar, $C_6H_{12}O_6$, has a molecular weight of 180 g/mole. Substituting 18.0 g, 180 g / mole, and 0.500 liter into the above equation gives 0.200 M as the molarity of the solution.

$$M = \frac{18.0 \text{ g} / 180 \text{ g} / \text{mole}}{0.500 \text{ liter}} = 0.200 \text{ M}$$

107. <u>Answer is **A**</u>. In a dilution problem, number of moles of solute before dilution = number of moles of solute after dilution. Therefore:

Molarity × volume (before dilution) = Molarity × volume (after dilution)

$$2.5 \frac{\text{moles}}{\text{L}} \times 0.250 \text{ L} = 5.0 \frac{\text{moles}}{\text{L}} \times \text{volume}$$

0.125 L = volume required

Dilute 125 mL of the 5.0 M solution with water to 250 mL to prepare the 2.5 M solution.

108. Answer is **A**. The density of a gas, O_2 (mol. wt. = 32 g/mole), can be determined by a rearrangement of the ideal gas law.

$$PV = \frac{\# g}{\text{mol. wt.}} RT$$

$$PV = nRT$$

$$\frac{P(\text{mol. wt.})}{RT} = \frac{\# g}{V} = D$$

$$PV = \frac{\# g}{\text{mol. wt.}} RT$$

$$\frac{1.0 \text{ atm}(32 \text{ g/mole})}{0.082 \dfrac{\text{L-atm}}{\text{mol-K}}(273+47)\text{K}}$$

$$= 1.2 \text{ g}/\text{L}$$

The densities of gases are reported as grams per liter because the same value as grams per milliliter would be very small. The volume of the gas is in liters because the value of R used is in liters.

109. Answer is **C**. The partial pressure of a gas in a mixture of gases is equal to the mole fraction of the gas times the total pressure of the mixture. First find the mole fraction x, of nitrogen, and then find the partial pressure of nitrogen.

$$P_{\text{total}} \cdot x_{\text{nitrogen}} = P_{\text{nitrogen}}$$

$$x_{\text{nitrogen}} = \frac{\# \text{moles N}_2}{\# \text{moles N}_2 + \# \text{moles O}_2}$$

$$x_{\text{nitrogen}} = \frac{84/28}{84/28 + 64/32} = 0.60$$

1.6 atm (0.60) = 0.96 atm = P_{nitrogen} = partial pressure of nitrogen

110. Answer is **C**. The heat capacity, C, of a substance equals the specific heat, s, times the mass of the material, m.

$$C = ms$$

$$C = 10 \text{ g}\left(\frac{0.385 \text{ J}}{\text{g} \cdot {}^{\circ}\text{C}}\right) = 3.85 \text{ J}/{}^{\circ}\text{C}$$

111. Answer is **A**. The wavelength times the frequency of light equals the speed of light, c. The wavelength is given in nanometers. Since the speed of light, c, is given in meters per second, convert the wavelength to meters. 1 m = 10^9 nm.

Wavelength × frequency = $c = 3.00 \times 10^8$ m/s

$$300 \text{ nm} \frac{(1\text{m})}{10^9 \text{nm}} = 3.00 \times 10^8 \text{ m/s}$$

Frequency = 1.0×10^{15} cps (cycles per second)

112. <u>Answer is **D**</u>. The electromagnetic spectrum consists of the energy coming from the sun. The spectrum may be characterized by different values of energy, wavelength, and frequency. Gamma rays have the highest energy, shortest wavelength, and highest frequency. These values progress to those of radio waves, which have the lowest energy, longest wavelength, and lowest frequency.

Electromagnetic Spectrum

Gamma rays, X-rays, ultraviolet light, visible light, infrared light, microwaves, radio waves

High energy	Low energy
Short wavelength	$\longrightarrow$ Long wavelength
High frequency	Low frequency

113. <u>Answer is **D**</u>. Atoms or ions of elements having the same numbers of electrons are said to be isoelectronic. Allotropes are different forms of the same element; for example diamond and graphite are allotropes of carbon. Isomers are compounds having the same molecular formulas but different structural formulas. Isotopes are elements having the same number of protons but different numbers of neutrons, for example hydrogen and deuterium.

$$^1_1H \qquad ^2_1D$$

114. <u>Answer is **B**</u>. A basic oxide is a compound that, when it reacts with water, produces a base. Another name for a basic oxide is a basic anhydride. The oxide K_2O reacts with water to produce KOH according to the following equation:

$$K_2O + H_2O \longrightarrow 2KOH$$

The other oxides, CO_2, SO_2, and P_2O_5, are all acid oxides or acid anhydrides.

$$CO_2 + H_2O \longrightarrow H_2CO_3$$
$$SO_2 + H_2O \longrightarrow H_2SO_3$$
$$P_2O_5 + 3H_2O \longrightarrow 2\ H_3PO_4$$

115. <u>Answer is **B**</u>. In order for hydrogen bonding to exist, the hydrogen must be bonded to nitrogen, oxygen, or fluorine: H - N, H - O, H - F. Hydrogen bonding is not possible between molecules of CH_4 because the hydrogen is bonded to carbon, C. Hydrogen bonding is possible, however, between molecules of H_2O, between molecules of CH_3OH, and between molecules of NH_3.

116. <u>Answer is **B**</u>. Vapor pressure is the pressure exerted by a gas in equilibrium with a liquid. The more gas above the surface of the liquid, the greater the vapor pressure. Boiling temperature is an indication of the attractive forces between molecules. The higher the boiling temperature of a pure liquid, the greater the attractive forces between

the molecules and the more energy that must be supplied in order for the molecules to separate in becoming a gas during boiling. The stronger the attractive forces between the molecules, the less liquid evaporates to become gas; conversely, the weaker the attractive forces between the molecules, the more liquid evaporates to become gas.

Boiling temperature and vapor pressure are inversely proportional; that is, the higher the boiling temperature of the liquid, the lower the vapor pressure of the gas at room temperature. Therefore, ethyl ether with the lowest boiling point, 34.6°C, of the answers given, has the highest vapor pressure.

117. Answer is C. Condensation is the conversion of a gas into a liquid. Sublimation is the conversion of a solid directly into a gas, for example the conversion of solid carbon dioxide, dry ice, into carbon dioxide vapor. Evaporation is the conversion of a liquid into a gas. Freezing is the conversion of a liquid into a solid.

118. Answer is A. Gases are usually most soluble in liquids at low temperature. As the temperature of a liquid increases, the gas molecules dissolved in it move faster and escape more readily from the surface of the liquid. Low pressure on the surface of a liquid will not keep a gas dissolved in the liquid, but rather will allow it to escape from the liquid. High agitation or extreme stirring of the liquid will cause the gas molecules to move faster than they would otherwise move and consequently will decrease the solubility of a gas in a liquid.

119. Answer is B. Weight measurements do not change as temperature changes. However, volume measurements do change as temperature increases or decreases. Therefore, any method of measuring concentration that includes a volume term, such as molarity, is temperature dependent.

120. Answer is B. When two equilibrium reactions are added to give a third reaction, the equilibrium constant for the third reaction is calculated by multiplying the two equilibrium constants for each original reaction, (K^1) (K^2). Add equations, multiply equilibrium constants.

121. Answer is A. In the given symbol, $^{35}_{21}X$, 35 is the atomic weight (number of protons plus number of neutrons), and 21 is the atomic number (number of protons) of element X. Subtracting 21 from 35 gives the number of neutrons, 14.

122. Answer is A. Nitrous acid, HNO_2, is a weak acid. The other acids—hydroiodic, HI; sulfuric H_2SO_4, and perchloric, $HClO_4$—are all strong acids. The common strong acids are the hydrohalic acids except for HF, for example, HCl, HBr, HI; nitric acid, HNO_3; sulfuric acid and perchloric acid. Most other common acids are weak acids.

123. Answer is A. Hydrofluoric acid, HF, is not a strong acid. Refer to the explanation given to question 122.

124. <u>Answer is **B**</u>. In determining the acidity of homologous compounds of members of the same family, as in HI, HBr, HCl, and HF, another concept besides electronegativity is invoked. HI is more acidic than HBr, which is more acidic than HCl, which is more acidic than HF. The larger the atom, I versus F, the more readily it can accommodate an extra electron and be stable. Therefore, I⁻ is more stable than F⁻ and consequently HI is more acidic than HF. Acidity increases as one progresses from top to bottom in a family, for example, HF < HCl < HBr < HI.

125. <u>Answer is **D**</u>. A small amount of acid or base may be added to a buffer solution; however, the pH of the solution remains approximately the same as before the acid or base was added. A buffer consists of a weak acid and its conjugate base or of a weak base and its conjugate acid. Sulfuric acid, H_2SO_4, is a strong acid and consequently is not a buffer either alone or with one of its salts. Acetic acid, written as either HAc or CH_3COOH, is a weak acid and in combination with an acetate salt is a buffer solution.

126. <u>Answer is **D**</u>. An alpha particle is the nucleus of the helium atom, ^4_2He.

   A beta particle is an electron, $^0_{-1}e$, while the gamma ray is high energy radiation.

   The symbol ^1_1H represents the proton, H^+; ^1_0n is a neutron.

   In each symbol the superscript (top number) represents the number of protons plus neutrons, that is, the atomic mass, while the subscript (bottom) number represents the number of protons, the number of positive charges, that is, the atomic number.

127. <u>Answer is **C**</u>. In the given reaction $^{90}_{38}Sr \longrightarrow ^{90}_{39}Y + ?$

   the total mass has remained the same, 90 for strontium, Sr, and 90 for yttrium, Y. The atomic number, however, has increased, from 38 to 39. The number of protons has increased by 1 because a neutron in the Sr nucleus has been converted into a proton and an electron. The proton has remained in the nucleus while the electron has been expelled from the nucleus. Therefore, the correct answer is the electron, $^0_{-1}e$.

128. <u>Answer is **B**</u>. The First Law of Thermodynamics considers the conversion of energy from one form to another form without subsequent formation or loss of any of the energy. The Second Law of Thermodynamics states that entropy, the measure of disorder, increases in spontaneous reactions and remains the same in equilibrium systems. The Third Law of Thermodynamics says that the entropy for a perfect crystal is zero at absolute zero temperature. The statement that the Gibbs Free Energy is a measure of the spontaneity of a reaction is true. Refer to the explanation given to question 129.

129. <u>Answer is **D**</u>. The Gibbs Free Energy measures energy changes which accompany a reaction. If the reaction releases usable energy, i.e. energy available to do work, the Gibbs Free Energy has a negative value and the reaction is spontaneous in the direction written. When the Gibbs Free Energy has a positive value, the reaction is not spontaneous in the direction written but is spontaneous in the opposite direction. When the Gibbs Free Energy equals zero, the reaction system is at equilibrium and no change occurs.

130. Answer is C. Color occurs in an object because the object absorbs some of the light and transmits or reflects some of the light which originates from the sun.

Absorbed Light	Color seen
violet	yellow
blue	orange
green	red
yellow	violet
orange	blue
red	green
(ROYGBV)	(GBVROY)

Reading both columns of colors from the bottom gives the acronym of the first letters of the colors, ROYGBV and GBVROY.

131. Answer is D. The following general formulas represent the general types of compounds indicated:

C_nH_{2n+2}	an alkane
C_nH_{2n}	an alkene or a cycloalkane
C_nH_{2n-2}	an alkyne or a cycloalkene
C_nH_n	benzene when $n = 6$

132. Answer is B. Refer to the explanation for question 131.

133. Answer is C. The formula C_2H_6O represents a compound capable of forming two structural isomers:

CH₃CH₂OH   CH₃OCH₃

ethyl alcohol   dimethyl ether

Each of the other molecular formulas given as answers represents a compound that is not capable of forming isomers.

134. Answer is B. The compound CH₃CH₂COOCH₃ is called methyl propanoate. An ester may be formed from a carboxylic acid and an alcohol. In this instance the acid is propanoic acid and the alcohol is methanol. The part of the molecule originating from the alcohol is named first, methyl. The part of the molecule derived from the acid is named by removing *-ic acid* from the name of the acid and adding the suffix *-ate.*

135. Answer is B. The formula C_2H_6 is the formula for the alkane ethane. Refer to the explanation given to question 131. The reaction of Br_2 with C_2H_6 has substituted one of the hydrogen atoms in ethane by a bromine atom. Whenever light or very high temperature is used in a reaction, the reaction usually occurs by a free radical mechanism. The reaction indicated is a free radical substitution reaction.

In a nucleophilic substitution reaction one nucleophile replaces another in a reaction. In the following example, $Br^{-1} + CH_3I \longrightarrow CH_3Br + I^{-1}$, the nucleophilic bromide ion replaces the weaker nucleophile, I^{-1}. There is no change in the total number of hydrogen atoms in a nucleophilic substitution reaction while there is such a change in a free radical substitution reaction.

In an electrophilic elimination reaction, a base reacts with a molecule to cause the loss of HZ from the molecule, where Z can be a leaving group. In the following example

$$CH_3 - \overset{\overset{\displaystyle CH_3}{|}}{\underset{\underset{\displaystyle Br}{|}}{C}} - CH_3 \ + \ NaOH \ (\text{in alcohol}) \ \longrightarrow \ CH_3 - \overset{\overset{\displaystyle CH_3}{|}}{C} = CH_2 + H_2O + NaBr$$

the hydroxide ion of sodium hydroxide, NaOH, removes the hydrogen bonded to one of the methyl carbon atoms to form water, H_2O. The sodium and bromide ions combine to form sodium bromide, NaBr. An alkene remains as the organic product.

Refer to the answer given to question 136 for an explanation of an electrophilic addition reaction.

136. <u>Answer is **C**</u>. The formula C_2H_4 is the formula for either an alkene or a cycloalkane. No cycloalkanes of fewer than three carbon atoms in the ring are common. Therefore, assume that C_2H_4 is an alkene, ethene. The electrophile bromine, Br_2, adds atoms to C_2H_4 to produce the dibromide $C_2H_4Br_2$, 1,2-dibromoethane,

$$CH_2 = CH_2 \ + \ Br_2 \ \longrightarrow \ \overset{\overset{\displaystyle Br}{|}}{CH_2} - \overset{\overset{\displaystyle Br}{|}}{CH_2}$$

137. <u>Answer is **B**</u>. Enantiomers are a form of stereoisomers, i.e. compounds which have the same groups within the molecules but differ from each other because of the arrangement of groups in the molecules. Enantiomers are two compounds having the same four different groups bonded to the stereocenter(s) in each compound, but, because of the different positions in which these groups are placed relative to each other, i.e. because of different configurations, they are nonsuperimposable mirror images. Enantiomers are identical in almost all their physical and chemical properties. The enantiomers of 1-chloro-1-iodoethane are shown below.

$$H - \overset{\overset{\displaystyle CH_3}{|}}{\underset{\underset{\displaystyle I}{|}}{C}} - Cl \qquad\qquad Cl - \overset{\overset{\displaystyle CH_3}{|}}{\underset{\underset{\displaystyle I}{|}}{C}} - H$$

Diastereomers are also a form of stereoisomers. Diastereomers are two compounds, each having at least two different stereocenters. The diastereomers have the arrangement of the four different groups at one of the stereocenters identical in both molecules but the arrangement of another four different groups at the other stereocenter different in both compounds. In other words, diastereomers with two stereocenters have the same configuration at one of the stereocenters but opposite configurations at the other stereocenter. Diastereomers are nonsuperimposable and have different physical and chemical properties. One pair of diastereomers of 2-bromo-3-chlorobutane are shown below.

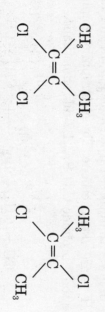

Geometric isomerism may occur in alkenes. It is not possible to freely rotate around a carbon-carbon double bond as it is around a carbon-carbon single bond. Therefore, when a carbon-carbon double bond is present in a compound, two different compounds, geometric isomers, may exist. In the example shown below:

the two chlorine atoms are on the same side of the double bond in one compound and on opposite sides of the double bond in the other compound. One could just as easily compare the position of the two methyl groups relative to the carbon-carbon double bond and arrive at the same conclusion. In order that geometric isomerism be present in alkenes, two identical groups cannot be bonded to the same carbon atom.

138. **Answer is A.** Pick the longest straight chain for the base name of the alkane, in this case octane. Next name each of the substituents, two methyl groups and one chloro group. Give each substituent the lowest possible number, and arrange the substituents in alphabetical order. The result is 5-chloro-3,4-dimethyloctane. The base names are listed below for the straight-chain alkanes with the general formula C_nH_{2n+2}. The names of compounds in other families can be derived from these names by using the proper suffix:

1 Carbon	methane
2 Carbons	ethane
3 Carbons	propane
4 Carbons	butane
5 Carbons	pentane
6 Carbons	hexane
7 Carbons	heptane
8 Carbons	octane
9 Carbons	nonane
10 Carbons	decane

139. <u>Answer is **A**</u>. The symbol R can be used to represent any akyl group. A generalized reaction is shown below for an acyl chloride reacting with a primary amine.

$$R - \overset{\overset{\displaystyle O}{\|}}{C} - Cl \quad + \quad NH_2 - R \quad \longrightarrow \quad R - \overset{\overset{\displaystyle O}{\|}}{C} - NH - R \quad + \quad HCl$$

acyl   primary   amide
chloride   amine

140. <u>Answer is **C**</u>. Complete hydrogenation of benzene, C_6H_6, adds six atoms of hydrogen or three molecules of hydrogen to one molecule of benzene.

141. <u>Answer is **B**</u>. Lipids have the following general structure where the R groups, which may or may not be the same, are large groups, usually a straight chain of twelve or more carbon atoms.

$$\begin{array}{l} CH_2OCR \overset{\displaystyle O}{\|} \\[2pt] CHOCR \overset{\displaystyle O}{\|} \\[2pt] CH_2OCR \overset{\displaystyle O}{\|} \end{array}$$

Lipids are triesters of the alcohol 1,2,3–trihydroxypropane.

142. <u>Answer is **C**</u>. The following generalized equation between an alcohol and a carboxylic acid produces an ester and water.

$$RCOH + HOR \longrightarrow RCOR + HOH$$
(with C=O on the RCOH and RCOR groups)

143. <u>Answer is **B**</u>. Proteins are polymers of alpha substituted amino acids which have the following generalized structure containing amide linkages.

$$x \; R-CH-C-O-H \longrightarrow -C-N-CH-C-N-CH-C-N-CH-$$

$$NH_2$$

alpha amino acid   protein

144. <u>Answer is **A**</u>. Carbohydrates contain mostly alcohol groups plus other functional groups, most frequently aldehydes or ketones. A formula for a carbohydrate is shown below.

```
      O
      =
      CH
      CHOH
      CHOH
      CHOH
      CHOH
      CH₂OH
```

145. <u>Answer is **B**</u>. It is not true that all bonds in benzene are equivalent in length. All of the C—C bonds are equivalent in length but the C—H bonds are a different length from the C—C bonds. Even though the C—C bonds in benzene may be represented by alternating single and double bonds, all of these C—C bonds are the same length because of delocation of pi electrons, that is, resonance. All of the other statements about benzene are correct.

146. <u>Answer is **C**</u>.

60 min = 1 hr   24 hr = 1 day   7 days = 1 wk

Convert each of these equalities into a fraction. Then multiply the appropriate fraction so that the only label remaining is min/wk, minutes per week, as shown below.

$$\frac{60 \text{ min}}{1 \text{ hr}} \times \frac{24 \text{ hr}}{1 \text{ day}} \times \frac{7 \text{ days}}{1 \text{ wk}} = 10,080 = \frac{1.01 \times 10^4 \text{ min}}{\text{wk}}$$

147. Answer is **A**. The compound is named 3-methylpentanoic acid. The carbonyl carbon is numbered 1, so the carbon atom to which the methyl group is attached is carbon 3. The acid is named by removing the -*e* from pentane and adding -*oic acid*. The formulas for the other answers are shown below.

$CH_3CH_2CH_2CHCOOH$
$\qquad\qquad\qquad | $
$\qquad\qquad\quad CH_3$

2-methylpentanoic acid

$CH_3CH_2CHCOOH$
$\qquad\qquad\quad | $
$\qquad\qquad CH_3$

2-methylbutanoic acid

CH_3CHCH_2COOH
$\qquad | $
$\quad CH_3$

3-methylbutanoic acid

148. Answer is **C**. Ordinarily, in the absence of other effects, compounds having the same molecular weight boil at approximately the same temperature. As molecular weight increases, boiling temperature increases. However, both of the alcohols 1-butanol and 2-butanol are capable of hydrogen bonding, which is possible when hydrogen is covalently bonded to nitrogen, oxygen, or fluorine. Both of the alcohols are capable of hydrogen bonding. Two molecules of 1-butanol can hydrogen bond to each other as can two molecules of 2-butanol.

When a liquid boils, heat is supplied to separate the molecules so that they can become gaseous. If the intermolecular forces between the molecules are weak, the boiling temperature is low. If the intermolecular forces between the molecules are strong, the boiling temperature is high. Since hydrogen bonding between molecules is a strong intermolecular force, the boiling temperatures of the alcohols will be higher than that of the ethyl ether, which is incapable of hydrogen bonding.

Of the two alcohols, 1-butanol will boil at the higher temperature. The alcohol 1-butanol is a straight chain compound, and, therefore, a molecule of this compound is able to fit closely with other molecules of 1-butanol, so that the intermolecular forces are relatively strong. The alcohol 2-butanol is a branched-chain compound; its molecules are not able to align themselves as closely, and the intermolecular forces are weaker. The correct decreasing order of boiling temperatures is 1-butanol > 2-butanol > ethyl ether.

149. Answer is **B**. Refer to the explanation for question 135.

150. Answer is **C**. Refer to the explanation for question 136.

151. Answer is **B**. Refer to the explanation for question 137.

152. Answer is **C**. An aldehyde is very easily oxidized and is converted to a carboxylic acid.

$$RCH \overset{O}{=} \xrightarrow{[O]} RCOH \overset{O}{=}$$

153. The answer is **B**. Dehydration means loss of water. In the example below, an alcohol is converted to an alkene by loss of water. The underlined OH group is lost from the carbon atom to which it is bonded and the underlined H atom is lost from a carbon atom adjacent to the carbon atom bonded to the OH group.

$$\begin{array}{c} CH_2 - CH - CH_3 \\ | \quad\quad | \\ \underline{H} \quad \underline{OH} \end{array} \quad \overset{heat}{\longrightarrow} \quad CH_2 = CH - CH_3 + H_2O$$

154. Answer is **B**. Density is defined as mass divided by volume. The density of the sample is its mass, 6.0 g, divided by the volume of water, which is the difference between the final volume and the initial volume, 20 mL − 16 mL, of the water displaced by the object.

$$\frac{6 \text{ g}}{4 \text{ mL}} = \frac{1.50 \text{ g}}{mL}$$

155. Answer is **A**. To convert temperatures from the Fahrenheit to Centigrade scale, use the following equation.

$$°C = \frac{5°C}{9°F}(10°F - 32°F) = -12.2°C = -12°C$$

156. Answer is **C**. In the given symbol, $_{21}^{35}X$, 35 is the atomic weight (number of protons plus number of neutrons), and 21 is the atomic number (number of protons) of element X. Subtracting 21 from 35 gives the number of neutrons, 14.

157. Answer is **C**. Molarity is defined as moles of solute divided by liters of solution.

$$M = \frac{\text{moles of solute}}{\text{liters of solution}} = \frac{\text{g/mol. wt.}}{\text{liters of solution}}$$

Sugar, $C_6H_{12}O_6$, has a molecular weight of 180 g/mole. Substitute 18 g, 180 g/mole, and 0.5 M into the above equation to obtain the volume of the solution.

$$M = \frac{18 \text{ g}/180 \text{ g}/\text{mole}}{x} = 0.5 \text{ M}$$

$$x = 0.2 \text{ L} = 200 \text{ ml}$$

158. Answer is **D**. Nuclear fission is the breakdown of a larger nucleus, usually by bombarding it with neutrons, to produce smaller atoms and more neutrons. A great deal of energy is released in this process, which is the basis for the atomic bomb. Radioactive decay is the spontaneous emission of nuclear particles, eg. alpha and beta particles, as well as gamma rays, by unstable nuclei. Carbon-14 dating is a method of determining the age of an object by comparing the amount of carbon-12 and the amount of radioactive carbon-14 present in the object. Nuclear fusion is the combination of small nucleii to produce a larger atom with the concomitant release of a large amount of energy. Nuclear fusion occurs on the sun. The hydrogen bomb is an example of nuclear fusion.

159. Answer is **B**. All radioactive decay occurs according to first order kinetics. The half life, $t_{1/2}$, i.e. the time needed for one-half of the sample to decay, is given by the following equation where k is the rate constant for the reaction

$$t_{1/2} = \frac{0.693}{k}$$

Since the concentration of the material decaying is not present in the above equation, the half life of any material which undergoes radioactive decay is independent of the initial concentration of the material.

160. Answer is **C**. Gamma rays are the most dangerous form of nuclear radiation to humans. They consist of short wavelength, high energy rays. Alpha particles are helium nuclei and are the least dangerous. Beta particles are electrons and are of intermediate danger.

EXPLANATORY ANSWERS FOR QUANTITATIVE ABILITY

161. Answer is **D**. Any number raised to zero power is 1, so $7^0 = 1$; $1 \cdot 5 = 5$.

162. Answer is **D**. $7 \div 20 = 0.35$. Convert to percent: $100 \cdot 0.35 = 35\%$.

163. Answer is **A**. The formula for calculating the circumference of a circle is $C = 2\pi r$; $\pi = 3.14$, $r = 3$. Therefore $C = 2(3.14)(3) = 18.84$.

164. Answer is **A**. At 300 mph the plane will fly 100 mi. in 20 min. Add 20 min. to 2:30 P.M. to arrive at the correct answer: 2:50 P.M.

165. Answer is **B**. $\frac{3}{9}$ can be reduced to $\frac{1}{3}$ by dividing the numerator and the denominator by 3; $1 \div 3 = 0.33$. Convert to percent: $100 \cdot 0.33 = 33\%$.

166. Answer is **B**. $\frac{8}{16}$ can be reduced to $\frac{1}{2}$ by dividing the numerator and the denominator by 8; $\frac{1}{2}$ is equivalent to 50%.

167. Answer is **B**. The truck must travel 50 mi. in 40 min. Set up a proportion:

$$\frac{50 \text{ mi.}}{40 \text{ min.}} = \frac{x \text{ mi.}}{60 \text{ min.}}$$

Cross multiply
and divide:

$$40x = 3,000$$

$$x = 75$$

50 mi. in 40 min. is equivalent to 75 mi. in 60 min. The required speed is 75 mph.

168. Answer is **B**. $10^4 = 10,000$; $9^3 = 9 \cdot 9 \cdot 9 = 729$; $10,000 + 729 = 10,729$.

169. Answer is **C**. $10^3 = 1,000$; $2^3 = 2 \cdot 2 \cdot 2 = 8$; $1,000 \cdot 8 = 8,000$.

170. Answer is **D**. $19 \div 20 = 0.95$. Convert to percent; $100 \cdot 0.95 = 95\%$.

171. Answer is **A**. The area of triangle ABE equals the area of triangle BED since they have the same altitude and base. Since the diagonal of a parallelogram (here BD) divides it equally, the area of triangle BAD is one-half that of the parallelogram, and the area of triangle ABE is one-half of that half, or 1/4. Therefore, the ratio of the two areas is 1 : 4.

172. Answer is **B**. $19\% = 0.19$; $0.19 \cdot 50 = 9.5$.

173. Answer is **D**. $6^3 = 6 \cdot 6 \cdot 6 = 216$; $4^2 = 4 \cdot 4 = 16$; $216 + 16 = 232$.

174. Answer is **C**. $0.50^2 = 0.50 \cdot 0.50 = 0.25$; $\dfrac{1}{4}$ is equivalent to 0.25; $0.25 + 0.25 = 0.50$.

175. Answer is **A**. Let x = number of minutes to fill $\dfrac{3}{5}$ of the basket. Set up a proportion, and solve for x:

$$\frac{\frac{2}{5}\ \text{basket}}{1\ \text{min.}} = \frac{\frac{3}{5}\ \text{basket}}{x\ \text{min.}}$$

$$x = 1\frac{1}{2} = 1.5\ \text{min.}$$

176. Answer is **A**. The plane travels 300 mi. in the first hour; 3,000 mi. (6 hr. • 500 mph), in the next 6 hr., and 100 mi. in the last hour. The total is 3,400 mi. in 8 hr.

177. Answer is **B**. Since $10^{-1} = \dfrac{1}{10}$, $\log \dfrac{1}{10} = -1$.

178. Answer is **A**. Since $0.0001 = 10^{-4}$, $\log 0.0001 = -4$.

179. Answer is **C**. Since $\log (ab) = \log a + \log b$, $\log (5 \times 3) = \log 5 + \log 3$.

180. Answer is **A**. 2.2 lb. = 1 kg; $160 \div 2.2 = 72.7$.

181. Answer is **B**. 2.2 lb. = 1 kg; $70 \cdot 2.2 = 154$.

182. Answer is **D**. Use the definition of slope and substitute the given values:

$$m = \frac{y_2 - y_1}{x_2 - x_1}$$

$$= \frac{6 - 3}{4 - 2} = \frac{3}{2}, \text{ or } 1.5$$

183. Answer is **B**. Since CD and DE are of equal length and BD is common to both the square and the triangle, the triangle is one-half the size of the square. Thus, the square has twice the area of the triangle: $16 \times 2 = 32$.

184. Answer is **A**. The probability of heads on a coin toss is $\dfrac{1}{2}$. Since there are four tosses, each with a probability of $\dfrac{1}{2}$ for heads, multiply by itself four times:

$$\frac{1}{2} \cdot \frac{1}{2} \cdot \frac{1}{2} \cdot \frac{1}{2} = \frac{1}{16}.$$

185. Answer is **C**. 1 in. = 2.54 cm; 120 ÷ 2.54 = 47 in.

186. Answer is **B**. 1 in. = 2.54 cm; 54 • 2.54 = 137 cm.

187. Answer is **C**. Since the sides of a square are equal, the square root of the area is the length of a side. In this case $\sqrt{144} = 12$. The perimeter is the sum of the sides: 12 + 12 + 12 + 12 = 48.

188. Answer is **C**. The reciprocal of 2 is $\frac{1}{2}$. Multiply the fractions:

$$\frac{1}{2} \cdot \frac{2}{5} = \frac{2}{10} \text{ or } \frac{1}{5}.$$

189. Answer is **A**. $\frac{2}{27} \cdot \frac{1}{3} = \frac{2}{81}$; $2 \div 81 = 0.025$.

190. Answer is **A**. If a line is parallel to the x-axis, its y-value will not change. The points along such a line could be (1,4), (2,4), (3,4), (4,4), and so forth. At each of these points, the value of $y = 4$.

191. Answer is **C**. $\frac{3}{4} \div \frac{1}{5} = \frac{3}{4} \cdot \frac{5}{1} = \frac{15}{4} = 3\frac{3}{4}$.

192. Answer is **B**. The mode of a list of numbers is the number that occurs most frequently. The number 6, which occurs four times, is the mode of the given data set.

193. Answer is **C**. $\sqrt[3]{64} = 4$: $4^3 = 4 \cdot 4 \cdot 4 = 64$.

194. Answer is **A**. $\sqrt[3]{8} = 2$: $2^3 = 2 \cdot 2 \cdot 2 = 8$.

195. Answer is **C**. Since the triangles are similar, the lengths of all sides are proportioned. The ratio between 3 and 6, which is 1:2, will also be the ratio between 18 and x, the value for DE. This can be set up as a proportion:

$$\frac{3}{6} = \frac{x}{18}$$

$$6x = 54$$

$$x = 9$$

196. Answer is **C**. 3 ÷ 10 = 0.30. Convert to percent: 0.30 × 100 = 30%.

197. Answer is **A**. $\sqrt[3]{1,000} = 10$: $10^3 = 10 \cdot 10 \cdot 10 = 1,000$.

198. Answer is **A**. $\sqrt{20} = \sqrt{4 \cdot 5} = 2\sqrt{5}$; $\sqrt{125} = \sqrt{25 \cdot 5} = 5\sqrt{5}$; $2\sqrt{5} + 5\sqrt{5} = 7\sqrt{5}$.

199. <u>Answer is **C**</u>. Solve for x as follows:

$$x^3 + 123 = 1{,}123$$
$$x^3 = 1{,}123 - 123$$
$$x^3 = 1{,}000$$

Take the cube root of each side: $x = 10$

200. <u>Answer is **C**</u>. Solve for x as follows:

$$2x^2 = 200$$
$$x^2 = 200 \div 2$$
$$x^2 = 100$$

Take the square root of each side: $x = 10, -10$

201. <u>Answer is **C**</u>. Solve for x as follows:

$$12x - 16 = 944$$
$$12x = 944 + 16$$
$$x = 960 \div 12$$
$$x = 80$$

202. <u>Answer is **C**</u>. Solve for x as follows:

$$3x = \frac{1}{2}$$

$$x = \frac{\frac{1}{2}}{3} = \frac{1}{2} \cdot \frac{1}{3} = \frac{1}{6}$$

203. <u>Answer is **C**</u>. Use the definition of slope and substitute the given values:

$$m = \frac{y_2 - y_1}{x_2 - x_1}$$

$$= \frac{3 - 2}{5 - 4} = 1$$

204. <u>Answer is **B**</u>. The square root of 0.36 is 0.6. Multiply: $0.6 \times 10^4 = 0.6 \times 10{,}000 = 6{,}000$.

205. <u>Answer is **A**</u>. Regardless of the number of previous tosses, or the results of those tosses, the probability of heads or tails on any one toss remains $\frac{1}{2}$.

206. <u>Answer is **C**</u>. Set up as a proportion and solve for x:

$$\frac{12 \text{ g}}{100 \text{ mL}} = \frac{x \text{ g}}{250 \text{ mL}}$$

Cross multiply and divide: $100x = 3,000$

$$x = 30 \text{ g}$$

207. <u>Answer is **B**</u>. 1 tbsp = 15 mL • 3 doses daily = 45 mL per day. To find a 7-day supply, multiply: 45 mL • 7 = 315 mL.

208. <u>Answer is **B**</u>. Convert 77% to a fraction: $77\% = \frac{77}{100}$. Set up as a proportion, and solve for x:

$$\frac{77 \text{ mcg of injection}}{100 \text{ mcg of tablets}} = \frac{x \text{ mcg of injection}}{200 \text{ mcg of tablets}}$$

Cross multiply and divide: $100x = 15,400$

$$x = 154 \text{ mcg}$$

209. <u>Answer is **C**</u>. $|-120| = 120$; $120 - 120 = 0$.

210. <u>Answer is **C**</u>. $\frac{1 \text{ lb.}}{16 \text{ oz.}} \cdot 128 \text{ oz.} = 8 \text{ lb.}$

211. <u>Answer is **A**</u>. $0.5 \cdot 10^3 = 0.05 \cdot 1,000 = 50$.

212. <u>Answer is **B**</u>. $4! = 4 \cdot 3 \cdot 2 \cdot 1 = 24$.

213. <u>Answer is **A**</u>. $6! = 6 \cdot 5 \cdot 4 \cdot 3 \cdot 2 \cdot 1 = 720$.

214. <u>Answer is **C**</u>. 50% of 100 = 50; 25% of 200 = 50.

215. <u>Answer is **B**</u>. The formula for the area of a circle is πr^2. The area of a semicircle is one-half the area of a circle. In the given figure, the radius of the semicircle is $\frac{1}{2}(2a)$, or a. Therefore, the area of the semicircle is $\frac{\pi a^2}{2}$.

The area of the rectangle is $2a \cdot a = 2a^2$.

Add the areas of the rectangle and the semicircle to get the total area: $2a^2 + \frac{\pi a^2}{2}$.

216. Answer is **D**. Solve for x as follows:

$$\sqrt[3]{x^3} = \sqrt[3]{729}$$

Take the cube root of each side: $x = 9$

217. Answer is **D**. Solve for x as follows:

$$3x - 4 = 20$$
$$3x = 24$$
$$x = 8$$

218. Answer is **C**. 2 divided by 3 = 0.67; 1 divided by 5 = 0.20; 0.67 + 0.20 = 0.87.

219. Answer is **D**. The area of a circle is πr^2; $\pi = 3.14$; $r = 4$. Therefore, area = $3.14(4)^2 = 50.24$.

220. Answer is **C**. Solve for x as follows:

$$x^2 + 50 = 131$$
$$x^2 = 81$$

Take the square root of each side: $x = 9, -9$

221. Answer is **A**. 5 divided by 8 = 0.625; 2 divided by 3 = 0.67; 0.625 + 0.67 = 1.29.

222. Answer is **D**. Convert 40% to a decimal by dividing by 100: 40% = 0.40; 0.40 • 160 = 64.

223. Answer is **B**. Convert 1% to a decimal by dividing by 100: 1% = 0.01; 0.01 • 50 = 0.5.

224. Answer is **B**. Convert 10% to a decimal by dividing by 100: 10% = 0.10; 0.10 • 220 = 22.

225. Answer is **D**. Convert 5% to a decimal by dividing by 100: 5% = 0.05; 0.05 • 200 = 10.

EXPLANATORY ANSWERS FOR READING COMPREHENSION

The numbers in the left margins of the reprinted passages indicate the statements in which the answer to the questions can be found.

Passage 1

226. __Although phenytoin may be used to treat cardiac arrhythmias, migraines, and trigeminal
227. neuralgia, the primary use of phenytoin is to treat seizure disorders.__ Phenytoin, one of the most
important agents used to manage seizures, works similarly to those of other hydantoin-
228. derivative anticonvulsants. __It decreases seizure activity by stabilizing neuronal membranes and by increasing efflux or decreasing influx of sodium ions across cell membranes
in the motor cortex during generation of nerve impulses.__ Phenytoin is commercially available
229. as oral suspension, tablets, and capsules. It is also available as an injection. __The dosage of
phenytoin varies according to the frequency of seizures, the type of seizures, and the
patient's tolerance for phenytoin.__ Therefore, it is extremely important to monitor the
230. patient for seizure activity as well as to monitor phenytoin serum concentrations. Phenytoin has a narrow therapeutic window and monitoring of serum concentrations is necessary.
Therapeutic serum concentrations of phenytoin are usually 10–20 mcg per mL (millimeter)
and depend on the assay method used. Serum concentrations above 20 mcg per mL often
232. result in toxicity. __Adverse reactions associated with dose related toxicities include blurred
vision, lethargy, rash, fever, slurred speech, nystagmus, and confusion.__ In some patients,
seizure control is not achieved when plasma concentrations are within the therapeutic
concentration range and therefore clinical response of the patient is more meaningful than
233. plasma concentrations. __Generally, therapeutic steady state serum concentrations are
achieved within 30 days of therapy with an oral dosage of 300 mg daily in adults.__ Follow-
231. ing an intravenous administration of 1000–1500 mg, at a rate not exceeding 50 mg per
minute, therapeutic concentrations can be attained within 2 hours. __Rapid administration
of intravenous phenytoin may result in adverse effects such as decreased blood pressure and
other cardiac complications.__ The use of phenytoin has been associated with osteomalacia,
thrombocytopenia, and gastrointestinal upset.

226. __Answer is A.__ Trigeminal neuralgia is treated with the phenytoin. Arthritis (B) is not
mentioned in the passage; osteomalacia (C) is mentioned as a possible adverse effect;
and nystagmus (D) is mentioned as an adverse reaction associated with toxicity.

227. __Answer is C.__ The first sentence clearly states that phenytoin is most commonly used to
treat seizure disorders. Cardiac arrythmias (A) and migraines (B) are mentioned as
other possible uses; arthritis (D) is not mentioned in the passage.

228. __Answer is C.__ Neither answer A nor answer B appears in the passage, and answer D
states the opposite of the correct answer.

229. Answer is **D**. Although phenytoin serum concentration (A), number of seizures (B), and adverse events (C) are listed as factors that affect the dosage of phenytoin, puncture sites available are not mentioned in the passage.

230. Answer is **D**. Answer A incorrectly implies that phenytoin produces seizures; answer B incorrectly states that there is no known difference between the serum concentrations known to produce desirable and undesirable effects; and answer C refers to migraines rather than to seizures.

231. Answer is **B**. A higher rate of administration may lower blood pressure. Answer A is irrelevant; answer C is inaccurate; and answer D refers to a condition (rash) that may be associated with phenytoin toxicity but not with the rapid administration of intravenous phenytoin.

232. Answer is **C**. Blurred vision (A), lethargy (B), and mental confusion (D) are mentioned in the passage as adverse reactions associated with drug-related toxicities. There is no reference to dysuria.

233. Answer is **D**. The passage states only that the therapeutic steady state serum concentration may be achieved within 30 days with an oral dosage of 300 mg daily of phenytoin. Therefore, 5 days (A), 24 hours (B), and 6 days (C) are all inaccurate.

Passage 2

Hypercalcemia, increased serum calcium concentrations, occurs in approximately 15% of individuals with cancer. Occurrences of this condition have been reported in most types of malignancies. The most effective management of treating this life-threatening disease is successful treatment of the malignancy. Unfortunately, successful treatment of the cancer may not be possible. In these cases, treatment goals should include correcting intravascular depletion, enhancing renal excretion of calcium, and inhibiting bone resorption. First line treatment of acute hypercalcemia includes the administration of normal saline and furosemide. Since many patients suffering from acute hypercalcemia are dehydrated, the administration of normal saline is warranted. In addition to treating dehydration, normal saline helps to increase renal excretion of calcium. The optimal administration of normal saline is dependent on the severity of hypercalcemia, the degree of dehydration, and the clinical status of the patient. An infusion rate of 400 mL per hour of normal saline is typical. Furosemide, a diuretic, is useful in the treatment of hypercalcemia due to its ability to enhance urinary excretion and more importantly calcium excretion. Additionally, furosemide protects patients from becoming volume overloaded due to the administration of the normal saline. It is very important that patients be adequately hydrated prior to the administration of furosemide in order to get maximum benefits. Intravenous doses of 100 mg of furosemide every 2 hours may be used. Although normal saline and furosemide are the most commonly used agents to treat acute cancer hypercalcemia, only

239. a modest decrease in calcium levels are achieved from this regimen. The use of normal saline and furosemide may be sufficient for the management of mild to moderate hypercalcemia, but it is commonly insufficient for treating severe hypercalcemia.

234. Answer is **B**. Hypercalcemia has been reported in most types of malignancies. Answer A is clearly incorrect, since it states the inverse of B; answers C and D are incorrect because they refer only to specific kinds of malignancies.

235. Answer is **D**. The passage is not concerned with the pathogenesis of cancer-related hypercalcemia (A); it does not cover all the uses of normal saline and furosemide (B); nor does it deal with the general characteristics or severity of cancer-related hypercalcemia (C). The focus is first line agents (normal saline and furosemide) used to manage acute cancer-related hypercalcemia.

236. Answer is **C**. To obtain maximum benefits from the administration of furosemide, it is important to hydrate the patient before administering the diuretic. Answers A, B, and D are not mentioned in the passage.

237. Answer is **D**. The passage states that cancer-related hypercalcemia is most effectively managed by successful treatment of the malignancy. Both normal saline (A) and furosemide (B) are agents used in first line treatment of cancer-related hypercalcemia when successful treatment of the cancer may not be possible. Dialysis (C) is not mentioned in the passage.

238. Answer is **A**. The passage states that treatment goals should include enhancing renal excretion of calcium (B), inhibiting bone resorption (C), and correcting intravascular depletion (D). However, administrating calcium carbonate (A) is not mentioned in the passage.

239. Answer is **D**. The last sentence of the passage clearly states that a normal saline-furosemide regimen alone is insufficient for treating severe hypercalcemia. However, it is usually effective in mild cancer-related hypercalcemia (A), mild hypercalcemia (B), and moderate hypercalcemia (C).

Passage 3

Gastroesophageal reflux disease (GERD) is a common medical disorder seen by health care practitioners of all specialties. It is generally chronic in nature, and long-term therapy may be required. While the mortality associated with GERD is very low (1 death per 100,000 patients), the quality of life experienced by the patient can be greatly diminished. GERD refers to any symptomatic clinical condition or histologic alteration that results from episodes of gastroesophageal reflux. Gastroesophageal reflux refers to the retrograde movement of gastric contents from the stomach into the esophagus. Many people experience some degree of reflux, especially after eating, which may be considered a benign physiologic process. When the esophagus is repeatedly exposed to refluxed material for prolonged periods of time, inflammation of the esophagus (i.e., reflux esophagitis) can occur. It is important to realize that gastroesophageal reflux must precede the development of GERD or

241. reflux esophagitis. In severe cases, reflux may lead to a multitude of serious complications including esophageal strictures, esophageal ulcers, motility disorders, perforation, hemorrhage, aspiration, and Barrett's esophagus. While mild disease is often managed with life-style changes and antacids, more intensive therapeutic intervention with histamine (H_2) antagonists, sucralfate, prokinetic agents, or proton pump inhibitors is generally required for

242. patients with more severe disease. In general, response to pharmacologic intervention is dependent on the efficacy of the agent, dosage regimen employed, duration of therapy, and severity of the disease. Following discontinuation of therapy, relapse is common and long-term maintenance therapy may be required. Historically, surgical intervention has been reserved for patients in whom conventional treatment modalities fail. However, the recent development of laparoscopic antireflux surgical procedures has led to a reevaluation of the

243. role of surgery in the long-term maintenance of GERD. Some clinicians have suggested that laparoscopic antireflux surgery may be a cost-effective alternative to long-term mainte-nance therapy in young patients. However, long-term comparative trials evaluating the cost effectiveness of the various treatment modalities are warranted.

The pathogenesis of gastroesophageal reflux is related to the complex balance between defense mechanisms and aggressive factors. Understanding both the normal protective mechanisms and the aggressive factors that may contribute to or promote gastroe-

244. sophageal reflux helps one to design rational therapeutic treatment regimens. Gastric acid, pepsin, bile acids, and pancreatic enzymes are considered aggressive factors and may promote esophageal damage upon reflux into the esophagus. Thus, the composition (potency) and volume of the refluxate are aggressive factors that may lead to esophageal injury. Conversely, normal protective mechanisms include anatomic factors, lower esophageal sphincter pressure, esophageal clearing, mucosal resistance, and gastric emptying. Rational therapeutic regimens in the treatment of gastroesophageal reflux are designed to maximize normal defense mechanisms and/or attenuate the aggressive factors.

240. Answer is **C**. Answers A, B, and D all consist of true statements taken directly from the passage. Answer C, however, is a false statement: the mortality associated with GERD is very low, not high.

241. Answer is **A**. One possible complication of reflux is perforation. Mucosal resistance (B), gastric emptying (C), and lower esophageal sphincter pressure (D) are all cited in the passage as normal protective mechanisms.

242. Answer is **D**. Dosage regimen employed (A), efficacy of the agent (B), and severity of the disease (C) all play a part in GERD patients' response to pharmacologic intervention.

243. Answer is **C**. The passage states that laparoscopic antireflux surgery has been suggested as a possible cost-effective alternative therapy.

244. Answer is A. Gastric acid and pancreatic enzymes are aggressive factors and may promote esophageal damage upon reflux into the esophagus. The factors in answer C are protective, and the factors in answer B are a combination of aggressive (bile acids) and protective (esophageal clearing).

Passage 4

Many people in the United States are diagnosed with diabetes mellitus. Non-insulin-dependent diabetes mellitus (NIDDM) is the most common type of diabetes and it is associated with a significant amount of morbidities and mortalities. NIDDM is classified as an endocrine disorder characterized by defects in insulin secretion as well as in insulin action. In NIDDM patients a defect also exists in insulin receptor binding. These defects lead to increased serum glucose concentrations or hyperglycemia. Sulfonylureas are one of the most popular classes of agents used to treat NIDDM. One of the newest agents to treat NIDDM is acarbose, an oral alpha-glucosidase inhibitor. Acarbose interferes with the hydrolysis of dietary disaccharides and complex carbohydrates, thereby delaying absorption of glucose and other monosaccharides. Acarbose is available for oral administration only. To be most effective, it should be taken at the beginning of a meal. The recommended starting dose is 25 mg three times daily and doses as high as 200 mg three times a day have been safely used. The most common adverse experiences associated with the use of acarbose are abdominal cramps, flatulence, diarrhea, and abdominal distension. Most of the adverse effects are due to the unabsorbed carbohydrates undergoing fermentation in the colon. Acarbose has also been associated with decreased intestinal absorption of iron, thereby possibly leading to anemia. The occurrence of hypoglycemia when using acarbose in combination with other agents used to lower serum glucose is great. Glucose should be administered to treat hypoglycemia in patients taking acarbose because sucrose may not be adequately hydrolyzed and absorbed. The effectiveness of this agent to lower serum glucose concentrations in patients with NIDDM has been clearly demonstrated in clinical trials. Acarbose provides another option for treating NIDDM.

245. Answer is D. Whereas "endocrine in nature" (A), "hyperglycemia" (B), and "may be due to a defect in insulin receptor binding" (C) are stated in, or may be inferred from, the passage, "results in iron deficiencies" is not listed as a characteristic of insulin-dependent diabetes. Rather, it is mentioned as a possible adverse effect of acarbose.

246. Answer is A. The passage states that a sulfonylurea agent is one of the most popular classes of agents used to treat NIDDM. Glucose (B), sucrose (C), and fructose (D) all represent types of sugar.

247. Answer is C. Hyperglycemia (A) is a characteristic of NIDDM; anemia (B) is a possible adverse effect of acarbose, but not one of the most common side effects; rash (D) is not mentioned in the passage. Gastrointestinal discomfort is stated to be the most common side effect of acarbose.

248. Answer is **B**. The passage states that glucose is the best choice for patients taking acarbose. A sulfurylurea agent (A) is the most popular class of agents used to treat NIDDM. Sucrose (C) is mentioned in the passage as a sugar that the patient may not be able to adequately hydrolyze and absorb, and fructose (D) is not mentioned at all.

249. Answer is **D**. Although low serum glucose concentration (A), gastrointestinal discomfort (B), and decreased iron absorption (C) are all described in the passage as possible adverse effects associated with the use of acarbose, obstruction of the urinary tract is not mentioned.

250. Answer is **A**. The passage states that sulfonylureas are one of the most popular classes of agents used to treat NIDDM and that using acarbose in combination with other agents may lead to hypoglycemia. Glucose (B), iron (C), and increased caloric intake (D) are not described as having this effect.

251. Answer is **C**. Since the passage does not cover the topic of diabetes in the United States, answer A cannot be the correct choice. Nor does the passage deal with all the various agents used to treat NIDDM, so answer B is ruled out. Answer D is too specific; the passage does deal with some adverse effects of acarbose, but it covers much more than that. The best title for the passage is The Use of Acarbose in the Treatment of Non-Insulin-Dependent Diabetes Mellitus.

Passage 5

252. Osteoporosis, the most common skeletal disorder associated with aging, is a significant cause of mortality and morbidity among the elderly. The two most common types of osteoporosis are type I (postmenopausal) osteoporosis and type II (senile) osteoporosis. Type I osteoporosis is due to a drastic decline in bone mass during the first five years of menopause and a slower rate of bone loss in subsequent years. Type II osteoporosis is characterized by a gradual, 252. age-related loss of bone in females and males over the age of 65 years. By far, osteoporosis 253. is most prevalent in the postmenopausal population. In addition to menopausal-associated hormonal changes, other risk factors for osteoporosis in women include low calcium intake, medical factors such as oophorectomy, and life-style factors such as inactivity and cigarette 256. smoking. In osteoporosis, osteoclasts excavate areas in bone that the bone forming cells, the 257. osteoblasts, are unable to fully reconstitute. Often this defective bone loses compressive strength, thereby leading to an increased risk of fracture. Osteoporosis evolves as a silent disease with no obvious early warning signs. Many patients suffering from osteoporosis are not aware of their condition until a fracture occurs. This disease is responsible for at least 1.5 million fractures in Americans each year, with annual costs to the United States health care 255. system of approximately $10 billion. Other consequences of osteoporosis include pain and spinal 254. deformities such as dorsal kyphosis and dowager's or widow's hump. In addition, a decrease in appetite, fatigue, and weakness may be present. As the population continues to age, the cost of treating osteoporosis and its associated complications are predicted to double over the next 255. 30 years.

252. Answer is <u>A</u>. Since the passage states that osteoporosis is associated with aging, infants (C) and teenagers (D) are clearly incorrect. Young males (B) is also incorrect; males with osteoporosis are described as over the age of 65. Postmenopausal women are the population in whom osteoporosis most commonly occurs.

253. Answer is <u>C</u>. Age (A), low calcium intake (B), and cigarette smoking (D) are all mentioned or implied as risk factors; however, weight-bearing exercises is not. In fact, answer C is the opposite of one of the stated risk ractors, inactivity.

254. Answer is <u>D</u>. The passage mentions dowager's hump as a consequence of osteoporosis. Height gain (A) is clearly not the best choice, since a decline in bone mass is more likely to lead to height loss. Oophorectomy (C) is mentioned in the passage as a risk factor for osteoporosis; hypertension (B) is irrelevant.

255. Answer is <u>D</u>. The passage states that the current cost of treating osteoporosis is approximately $10 billion. The last sentence in the passage states that the cost of treating osteoporosis and its associated complications is predicted to double over the next 30 years; thus $20 billion is the correct answer.

256. Answer is <u>A</u>. The passage states that osteoclasts excavate areas in bone. Osteoblasts (B) are also discussed in the passage, but they are the cells that form bone. The other two choices, osteomasts (C) and osteotrasts (D) are not mentioned in the passage and are therefore irrelevant.

257. Answer is <u>B</u>. Osteoblasts are responsible for forming bone. As stated in the explanation for question 256, osteoclasts remove bone. Again, osteomasts (C) and osteotrasts (D) are irrelevant.

Passage 6

258.   Bronchial asthma is a common disease of children and adults. Although the clinical manifestations of asthma have been known since antiquity, it is a disease that still defies precise definition. The word *asthma* is of Greek origin and means "panting." More than 2000 years ago, Hippocrates used the word *asthma* to describe episodic shortness of breath; however, the first detailed description of the asthmatic patient was made by Aretaeus in the second century. Since that time *asthma* has been used to describe any disorder with episodic shortness of breath or dyspnea; thus, the terms *cardiac asthma* and *bronchial asthma* have been used to delineate the etiologies of the dyspnea. These terms are now obsolete and asthma refers to a disorder of the respiratory system characterized by episodes of difficulty in breathing. An Expert Panel of the National Institutes of Health National Asthma Education Program (NAEP) has defined asthma as a lung disease characterized by (1) airway obstruction that is reversible (but not completely so in some patients) either spontaneously or with treatment; (2) airway inflammation; and (3) increased airway responsiveness to a variety of stimuli. This descriptive definition for asthma is attributed to our lack of knowledge of the precise pathogenic defect that results in the clinical syndrome we recognize as asthma. The current definition does allow for the important heterogeneity

260. of the clinical presentation of asthma. New technologies have added substantially to our understanding of the interrelationships of immunology, biochemistry, and physiology to

261. the clinical presentation of asthma, and further research may yet uncover a specific genetic defect associated with asthma. Until such time, asthma will continue to defy exact definition.

An estimated 10 million persons in the United States have asthma (about 5% of the population). The reported prevalence increased 29% from 1980 to 1987 to 40.1 per 1000 population. African-Americans have a 19% higher incidence of asthma than whites and are twice as likely to be hospitalized. The estimated cost of asthma in the United States in 1990 was $6.2 billion. The largest single direct medical expenditure was for inpatient hospital services (emergency care), reaching almost $1.5 billion, followed by prescription

259. medications ($1.1 billion). The costs of medication increased 54% between 1985 and 1990. In total, 43% of the economic impact was associated with emergency room use, hospitalization, and death. Asthma accounted for 1% of all ambulatory care visits according to the National Ambulatory Medical Care Survey and results in more than 450,000 hospitalizations per year.

258. Answer is **B**. Answer B sums up the main point of the first paragraph of the passage. Answer A is not true, since the passage states that the term *asthma* has been defined precisely. Answer C is incorrect since *cardiac asthma* and *bronchial asthma* are simply two terms that are no longer in use, although they were used for a long time to delineate the etiologies of the dyspnea associated with asthma. Answer D is incorrect because the statement that the NAEP's definition of asthma does *not* allow for the heterogeneity of the clinical presentation of the disease is false; in fact, the definition does allow for this.

259. Answer is **C**. Answers A, B, and D are true statements taken directly from the passage. In actuality, however, the cost of asthma medication *increased* (not decreased) 54% between 1985 and 1990.

260. Answer is **C**. Wheezing and episodes of shortness of breath (B) and the interrelationship of immunology, biochemistry, and physiology (D) are already understood, and answer A is irrelevant. Researchers hope to uncover a specific genetic defect in asthma.

261. Answer is **D**. The passage states that the estimated number of persons in the United States who have asthma is 10 million.

262. Answer is **D**. Answers A, B, and C are incorrect choices, since "panting" (A) and dyspnea of cardiac or bronchial etiology (B) are obsolete definitions. Answer D represents the current definition of asthma.

263. Answer is **D**. The passage does not go into the reasons for the worldwide increase in the prevalence of asthma. However, it does provide a descriptive definition of the disease (A) and also some facts about the prevalence of asthma in the United States (B).

Passage 7

264. Peptic ulcer disease affects approximately 10% of Americans each year. Peptic ulcer disease

265. has been referred to as a chronic inflammatory condition of the stomach and duodenum and often requires lifelong therapy. Although this disease has a relatively low mortality rate, it results in substantial human suffering and high economic costs making treatment

266. necessary. In the past, the pathogenesis of this disorder was believed to be related to diet

267. and stress. However, new studies have suggested that peptic ulcer disease is commonly due to the presence of an organism, *Helicobacter pylori*. The recognition of gastritis due to

268. *Helicobacter pylori* has revolutionized the therapeutic approach to treating peptic ulcer disease. Clinical trials demonstrate that the recurrence of ulcers can be drastically reduced by a single course of antimicrobial treatment that eradicates *Helicobacter pylori*, as compared to traditional therapy which involves continuous suppression of gastric acid secretion. In light of this, the NIH Consensus Development Conference recommended that all patients with documented duodenal or gastric ulcers who are infected with *Helicobacter pylori* should receive antimicrobial therapy to cure the infection. Although *Helicobacter pylori* is difficult to eradicate and successful treatment requires concurrent administration of at

269. least two antimicrobial drugs, many antibiotic regimens have been successfully used. Agents with antimicrobial activity such as amoxicillin, tetracycline, metronidazole, clarithromycin, and bismuth have been used to eradicate the organism. Peptic ulcer disease associated with *Helicobacter pylori* can now be cured with eradication of this organism.

264. Answer is **D**. The passage states that approximately 10% of Americans are affected with peptic ulcer disease each year.

265. Answer is **D**. Peptic ulcer disease is an inflammatory condition of the gastrointestinal system (A), and it affects the stomach (B) and duodenum (C). The statement that it affects the kidney is false.

266. Answer is **A**. The passage states that peptic ulcer disease was once believed to result from a combination of diet and stress. *Escherichia coli* (B) is a different organism from the one that actually causes peptic ulcers, and answers C and D are irrelevant.

267. Answer is **C**. The passage states that most peptic ulcers are caused by the presence of an organism called *Helicobacter pylori*. The answer viral load (A), stress (B), and ampicillin (D) are not supported by the passage.

268. Answer is **D**. The passage clearly states "Clinical trials demonstrate that the recurrence of ulcers can be drastically reduced by a single course of antimicrobial treatment that eradicates *Helicobacter pylori*, as compared to traditional therapy which involves continuous suppression of acid secretion." None of the other answers is supported by the passage.

269. Answer is **A**. While amoxicillin (B), tetracycline (C), and clarithromycin (D) are all mentioned in the passage as antimicrobials, *Helicobacter pylori* is identified as an organism. In fact, it is the organism associated with peptic ulcer disease.

270. Answer is **B**. The passage does not mention answer C, and both answer A and answer D are too general to express the main idea of the passage. "The roles of *Helicobacter pylori* in peptic ulcer disease" best expresses the main idea of the passage.

10

Practice PCAT 2

This second sample PCAT is not a copy of an actual PCAT, but it has also been designed to closely represent the types of questions that may be included in an actual exam. Proceed with this practice exam as if you were taking the actual PCAT, adhering to the time allowed for each section in the table below.

Please note: The order of the subjects can vary from test to test.

Section	Time Allowed*
Verbal Ability	30 minutes
Chemistry	50 minutes
Biology	45 minutes
Reading Comprehension	45 minutes
Quantitative Ability	45 minutes
Experimental Questions	45 minutes

*The times listed are an approximation of possible test section durations. Your actual test may vary slightly from these times.

PRACTICE PCAT 2 ANSWER SHEET

Verbal Ability

1 Ⓐ Ⓑ Ⓒ Ⓓ
2 Ⓐ Ⓑ Ⓒ Ⓓ
3 Ⓐ Ⓑ Ⓒ Ⓓ
4 Ⓐ Ⓑ Ⓒ Ⓓ
5 Ⓐ Ⓑ Ⓒ Ⓓ
6 Ⓐ Ⓑ Ⓒ Ⓓ
7 Ⓐ Ⓑ Ⓒ Ⓓ
8 Ⓐ Ⓑ Ⓒ Ⓓ
9 Ⓐ Ⓑ Ⓒ Ⓓ
10 Ⓐ Ⓑ Ⓒ Ⓓ

11 Ⓐ Ⓑ Ⓒ Ⓓ
12 Ⓐ Ⓑ Ⓒ Ⓓ
13 Ⓐ Ⓑ Ⓒ Ⓓ
14 Ⓐ Ⓑ Ⓒ Ⓓ
15 Ⓐ Ⓑ Ⓒ Ⓓ
16 Ⓐ Ⓑ Ⓒ Ⓓ
17 Ⓐ Ⓑ Ⓒ Ⓓ
18 Ⓐ Ⓑ Ⓒ Ⓓ
19 Ⓐ Ⓑ Ⓒ Ⓓ
20 Ⓐ Ⓑ Ⓒ Ⓓ

21 Ⓐ Ⓑ Ⓒ Ⓓ
22 Ⓐ Ⓑ Ⓒ Ⓓ
23 Ⓐ Ⓑ Ⓒ Ⓓ
24 Ⓐ Ⓑ Ⓒ Ⓓ
25 Ⓐ Ⓑ Ⓒ Ⓓ
26 Ⓐ Ⓑ Ⓒ Ⓓ
27 Ⓐ Ⓑ Ⓒ Ⓓ
28 Ⓐ Ⓑ Ⓒ Ⓓ
29 Ⓐ Ⓑ Ⓒ Ⓓ
30 Ⓐ Ⓑ Ⓒ Ⓓ

31 Ⓐ Ⓑ Ⓒ Ⓓ
32 Ⓐ Ⓑ Ⓒ Ⓓ
33 Ⓐ Ⓑ Ⓒ Ⓓ
34 Ⓐ Ⓑ Ⓒ Ⓓ
35 Ⓐ Ⓑ Ⓒ Ⓓ
36 Ⓐ Ⓑ Ⓒ Ⓓ
37 Ⓐ Ⓑ Ⓒ Ⓓ
38 Ⓐ Ⓑ Ⓒ Ⓓ
39 Ⓐ Ⓑ Ⓒ Ⓓ
40 Ⓐ Ⓑ Ⓒ Ⓓ

41 Ⓐ Ⓑ Ⓒ Ⓓ
42 Ⓐ Ⓑ Ⓒ Ⓓ
43 Ⓐ Ⓑ Ⓒ Ⓓ
44 Ⓐ Ⓑ Ⓒ Ⓓ
45 Ⓐ Ⓑ Ⓒ Ⓓ
46 Ⓐ Ⓑ Ⓒ Ⓓ
47 Ⓐ Ⓑ Ⓒ Ⓓ
48 Ⓐ Ⓑ Ⓒ Ⓓ
49 Ⓐ Ⓑ Ⓒ Ⓓ
50 Ⓐ Ⓑ Ⓒ Ⓓ

Chemistry

51 Ⓐ Ⓑ Ⓒ Ⓓ
52 Ⓐ Ⓑ Ⓒ Ⓓ
53 Ⓐ Ⓑ Ⓒ Ⓓ
54 Ⓐ Ⓑ Ⓒ Ⓓ
55 Ⓐ Ⓑ Ⓒ Ⓓ
56 Ⓐ Ⓑ Ⓒ Ⓓ
57 Ⓐ Ⓑ Ⓒ Ⓓ
58 Ⓐ Ⓑ Ⓒ Ⓓ
59 Ⓐ Ⓑ Ⓒ Ⓓ
60 Ⓐ Ⓑ Ⓒ Ⓓ
61 Ⓐ Ⓑ Ⓒ Ⓓ
62 Ⓐ Ⓑ Ⓒ Ⓓ

63 Ⓐ Ⓑ Ⓒ Ⓓ
64 Ⓐ Ⓑ Ⓒ Ⓓ
65 Ⓐ Ⓑ Ⓒ Ⓓ
66 Ⓐ Ⓑ Ⓒ Ⓓ
67 Ⓐ Ⓑ Ⓒ Ⓓ
68 Ⓐ Ⓑ Ⓒ Ⓓ
69 Ⓐ Ⓑ Ⓒ Ⓓ
70 Ⓐ Ⓑ Ⓒ Ⓓ
71 Ⓐ Ⓑ Ⓒ Ⓓ
72 Ⓐ Ⓑ Ⓒ Ⓓ
73 Ⓐ Ⓑ Ⓒ Ⓓ
74 Ⓐ Ⓑ Ⓒ Ⓓ

75 Ⓐ Ⓑ Ⓒ Ⓓ
76 Ⓐ Ⓑ Ⓒ Ⓓ
77 Ⓐ Ⓑ Ⓒ Ⓓ
78 Ⓐ Ⓑ Ⓒ Ⓓ
79 Ⓐ Ⓑ Ⓒ Ⓓ
80 Ⓐ Ⓑ Ⓒ Ⓓ
81 Ⓐ Ⓑ Ⓒ Ⓓ
82 Ⓐ Ⓑ Ⓒ Ⓓ
83 Ⓐ Ⓑ Ⓒ Ⓓ
84 Ⓐ Ⓑ Ⓒ Ⓓ
85 Ⓐ Ⓑ Ⓒ Ⓓ
86 Ⓐ Ⓑ Ⓒ Ⓓ

87 Ⓐ Ⓑ Ⓒ Ⓓ
88 Ⓐ Ⓑ Ⓒ Ⓓ
89 Ⓐ Ⓑ Ⓒ Ⓓ
90 Ⓐ Ⓑ Ⓒ Ⓓ
91 Ⓐ Ⓑ Ⓒ Ⓓ
92 Ⓐ Ⓑ Ⓒ Ⓓ
93 Ⓐ Ⓑ Ⓒ Ⓓ
94 Ⓐ Ⓑ Ⓒ Ⓓ
95 Ⓐ Ⓑ Ⓒ Ⓓ
96 Ⓐ Ⓑ Ⓒ Ⓓ
97 Ⓐ Ⓑ Ⓒ Ⓓ
98 Ⓐ Ⓑ Ⓒ Ⓓ

99 Ⓐ Ⓑ Ⓒ Ⓓ
100 Ⓐ Ⓑ Ⓒ Ⓓ
101 Ⓐ Ⓑ Ⓒ Ⓓ
102 Ⓐ Ⓑ Ⓒ Ⓓ
103 Ⓐ Ⓑ Ⓒ Ⓓ
104 Ⓐ Ⓑ Ⓒ Ⓓ
105 Ⓐ Ⓑ Ⓒ Ⓓ
106 Ⓐ Ⓑ Ⓒ Ⓓ
107 Ⓐ Ⓑ Ⓒ Ⓓ
108 Ⓐ Ⓑ Ⓒ Ⓓ
109 Ⓐ Ⓑ Ⓒ Ⓓ
110 Ⓐ Ⓑ Ⓒ Ⓓ

Biology

111 Ⓐ Ⓑ Ⓒ Ⓓ
112 Ⓐ Ⓑ Ⓒ Ⓓ
113 Ⓐ Ⓑ Ⓒ Ⓓ
114 Ⓐ Ⓑ Ⓒ Ⓓ
115 Ⓐ Ⓑ Ⓒ Ⓓ
116 Ⓐ Ⓑ Ⓒ Ⓓ
117 Ⓐ Ⓑ Ⓒ Ⓓ
118 Ⓐ Ⓑ Ⓒ Ⓓ
119 Ⓐ Ⓑ Ⓒ Ⓓ
120 Ⓐ Ⓑ Ⓒ Ⓓ

121 Ⓐ Ⓑ Ⓒ Ⓓ
122 Ⓐ Ⓑ Ⓒ Ⓓ
123 Ⓐ Ⓑ Ⓒ Ⓓ
124 Ⓐ Ⓑ Ⓒ Ⓓ
125 Ⓐ Ⓑ Ⓒ Ⓓ
126 Ⓐ Ⓑ Ⓒ Ⓓ
127 Ⓐ Ⓑ Ⓒ Ⓓ
128 Ⓐ Ⓑ Ⓒ Ⓓ
129 Ⓐ Ⓑ Ⓒ Ⓓ
130 Ⓐ Ⓑ Ⓒ Ⓓ

131 Ⓐ Ⓑ Ⓒ Ⓓ
132 Ⓐ Ⓑ Ⓒ Ⓓ
133 Ⓐ Ⓑ Ⓒ Ⓓ
134 Ⓐ Ⓑ Ⓒ Ⓓ
135 Ⓐ Ⓑ Ⓒ Ⓓ
136 Ⓐ Ⓑ Ⓒ Ⓓ
137 Ⓐ Ⓑ Ⓒ Ⓓ
138 Ⓐ Ⓑ Ⓒ Ⓓ
139 Ⓐ Ⓑ Ⓒ Ⓓ
140 Ⓐ Ⓑ Ⓒ Ⓓ

141 Ⓐ Ⓑ Ⓒ Ⓓ
142 Ⓐ Ⓑ Ⓒ Ⓓ
143 Ⓐ Ⓑ Ⓒ Ⓓ
144 Ⓐ Ⓑ Ⓒ Ⓓ
145 Ⓐ Ⓑ Ⓒ Ⓓ
146 Ⓐ Ⓑ Ⓒ Ⓓ
147 Ⓐ Ⓑ Ⓒ Ⓓ
148 Ⓐ Ⓑ Ⓒ Ⓓ
149 Ⓐ Ⓑ Ⓒ Ⓓ
150 Ⓐ Ⓑ Ⓒ Ⓓ

151 Ⓐ Ⓑ Ⓒ Ⓓ
152 Ⓐ Ⓑ Ⓒ Ⓓ
153 Ⓐ Ⓑ Ⓒ Ⓓ
154 Ⓐ Ⓑ Ⓒ Ⓓ
155 Ⓐ Ⓑ Ⓒ Ⓓ
156 Ⓐ Ⓑ Ⓒ Ⓓ
157 Ⓐ Ⓑ Ⓒ Ⓓ
158 Ⓐ Ⓑ Ⓒ Ⓓ
159 Ⓐ Ⓑ Ⓒ Ⓓ
160 Ⓐ Ⓑ Ⓒ Ⓓ

Reading Comprehension

161 Ⓐ Ⓑ Ⓒ Ⓓ	170 Ⓐ Ⓑ Ⓒ Ⓓ	179 Ⓐ Ⓑ Ⓒ Ⓓ	188 Ⓐ Ⓑ Ⓒ Ⓓ	197 Ⓐ Ⓑ Ⓒ Ⓓ
162 Ⓐ Ⓑ Ⓒ Ⓓ	171 Ⓐ Ⓑ Ⓒ Ⓓ	180 Ⓐ Ⓑ Ⓒ Ⓓ	189 Ⓐ Ⓑ Ⓒ Ⓓ	198 Ⓐ Ⓑ Ⓒ Ⓓ
163 Ⓐ Ⓑ Ⓒ Ⓓ	172 Ⓐ Ⓑ Ⓒ Ⓓ	181 Ⓐ Ⓑ Ⓒ Ⓓ	190 Ⓐ Ⓑ Ⓒ Ⓓ	199 Ⓐ Ⓑ Ⓒ Ⓓ
164 Ⓐ Ⓑ Ⓒ Ⓓ	173 Ⓐ Ⓑ Ⓒ Ⓓ	182 Ⓐ Ⓑ Ⓒ Ⓓ	191 Ⓐ Ⓑ Ⓒ Ⓓ	200 Ⓐ Ⓑ Ⓒ Ⓓ
165 Ⓐ Ⓑ Ⓒ Ⓓ	174 Ⓐ Ⓑ Ⓒ Ⓓ	183 Ⓐ Ⓑ Ⓒ Ⓓ	192 Ⓐ Ⓑ Ⓒ Ⓓ	201 Ⓐ Ⓑ Ⓒ Ⓓ
166 Ⓐ Ⓑ Ⓒ Ⓓ	175 Ⓐ Ⓑ Ⓒ Ⓓ	184 Ⓐ Ⓑ Ⓒ Ⓓ	193 Ⓐ Ⓑ Ⓒ Ⓓ	202 Ⓐ Ⓑ Ⓒ Ⓓ
167 Ⓐ Ⓑ Ⓒ Ⓓ	176 Ⓐ Ⓑ Ⓒ Ⓓ	185 Ⓐ Ⓑ Ⓒ Ⓓ	194 Ⓐ Ⓑ Ⓒ Ⓓ	203 Ⓐ Ⓑ Ⓒ Ⓓ
168 Ⓐ Ⓑ Ⓒ Ⓓ	177 Ⓐ Ⓑ Ⓒ Ⓓ	186 Ⓐ Ⓑ Ⓒ Ⓓ	195 Ⓐ Ⓑ Ⓒ Ⓓ	204 Ⓐ Ⓑ Ⓒ Ⓓ
169 Ⓐ Ⓑ Ⓒ Ⓓ	178 Ⓐ Ⓑ Ⓒ Ⓓ	187 Ⓐ Ⓑ Ⓒ Ⓓ	196 Ⓐ Ⓑ Ⓒ Ⓓ	205 Ⓐ Ⓑ Ⓒ Ⓓ

Quantitative Ability

206 Ⓐ Ⓑ Ⓒ Ⓓ	219 Ⓐ Ⓑ Ⓒ Ⓓ	232 Ⓐ Ⓑ Ⓒ Ⓓ	245 Ⓐ Ⓑ Ⓒ Ⓓ	258 Ⓐ Ⓑ Ⓒ Ⓓ
207 Ⓐ Ⓑ Ⓒ Ⓓ	220 Ⓐ Ⓑ Ⓒ Ⓓ	233 Ⓐ Ⓑ Ⓒ Ⓓ	246 Ⓐ Ⓑ Ⓒ Ⓓ	259 Ⓐ Ⓑ Ⓒ Ⓓ
208 Ⓐ Ⓑ Ⓒ Ⓓ	221 Ⓐ Ⓑ Ⓒ Ⓓ	234 Ⓐ Ⓑ Ⓒ Ⓓ	247 Ⓐ Ⓑ Ⓒ Ⓓ	260 Ⓐ Ⓑ Ⓒ Ⓓ
209 Ⓐ Ⓑ Ⓒ Ⓓ	222 Ⓐ Ⓑ Ⓒ Ⓓ	235 Ⓐ Ⓑ Ⓒ Ⓓ	248 Ⓐ Ⓑ Ⓒ Ⓓ	261 Ⓐ Ⓑ Ⓒ Ⓓ
210 Ⓐ Ⓑ Ⓒ Ⓓ	223 Ⓐ Ⓑ Ⓒ Ⓓ	236 Ⓐ Ⓑ Ⓒ Ⓓ	249 Ⓐ Ⓑ Ⓒ Ⓓ	262 Ⓐ Ⓑ Ⓒ Ⓓ
211 Ⓐ Ⓑ Ⓒ Ⓓ	224 Ⓐ Ⓑ Ⓒ Ⓓ	237 Ⓐ Ⓑ Ⓒ Ⓓ	250 Ⓐ Ⓑ Ⓒ Ⓓ	263 Ⓐ Ⓑ Ⓒ Ⓓ
212 Ⓐ Ⓑ Ⓒ Ⓓ	225 Ⓐ Ⓑ Ⓒ Ⓓ	238 Ⓐ Ⓑ Ⓒ Ⓓ	251 Ⓐ Ⓑ Ⓒ Ⓓ	264 Ⓐ Ⓑ Ⓒ Ⓓ
213 Ⓐ Ⓑ Ⓒ Ⓓ	226 Ⓐ Ⓑ Ⓒ Ⓓ	239 Ⓐ Ⓑ Ⓒ Ⓓ	252 Ⓐ Ⓑ Ⓒ Ⓓ	265 Ⓐ Ⓑ Ⓒ Ⓓ
214 Ⓐ Ⓑ Ⓒ Ⓓ	227 Ⓐ Ⓑ Ⓒ Ⓓ	240 Ⓐ Ⓑ Ⓒ Ⓓ	253 Ⓐ Ⓑ Ⓒ Ⓓ	266 Ⓐ Ⓑ Ⓒ Ⓓ
215 Ⓐ Ⓑ Ⓒ Ⓓ	228 Ⓐ Ⓑ Ⓒ Ⓓ	241 Ⓐ Ⓑ Ⓒ Ⓓ	254 Ⓐ Ⓑ Ⓒ Ⓓ	267 Ⓐ Ⓑ Ⓒ Ⓓ
216 Ⓐ Ⓑ Ⓒ Ⓓ	229 Ⓐ Ⓑ Ⓒ Ⓓ	242 Ⓐ Ⓑ Ⓒ Ⓓ	255 Ⓐ Ⓑ Ⓒ Ⓓ	268 Ⓐ Ⓑ Ⓒ Ⓓ
217 Ⓐ Ⓑ Ⓒ Ⓓ	230 Ⓐ Ⓑ Ⓒ Ⓓ	243 Ⓐ Ⓑ Ⓒ Ⓓ	256 Ⓐ Ⓑ Ⓒ Ⓓ	269 Ⓐ Ⓑ Ⓒ Ⓓ
218 Ⓐ Ⓑ Ⓒ Ⓓ	231 Ⓐ Ⓑ Ⓒ Ⓓ	244 Ⓐ Ⓑ Ⓒ Ⓓ	257 Ⓐ Ⓑ Ⓒ Ⓓ	270 Ⓐ Ⓑ Ⓒ Ⓓ

VERBAL ABILITY

50 Questions (#1–#50)

Directions: Choose the word that means the **opposite** or most nearly the opposite of the given word. You have 30 minutes to complete this section.

1. JOCULAR

A. Flaccid
B. Preponderance
C. Cantankerous
D. Fallacious

2. PAUCITY

A. Surfeit
B. Viscous
C. Capitulate
D. Laconic

3. INSIPID

A. Banal
B. Excite
C. Exonerate
D. Creative

4. RETICENT

A. Retiring
B. Requiring
C. Capitulate
D. Garrulous

5. NEFARIOUS

A. Trustworthy
B. Co-dependent
C. Radiate
D. Criminal

6. PROLIFERATION

A. Curtailment
B. Precision
C. Propagation
D. Unabated

7. SUBORDINATE

A. Enigmatic
B. Predecessor
C. Censorious
D. Superior

8. COMPLACENT

A. Laconic
B. Dissatisfied
C. Depressed
D. Assiduous

9. QUANDARY

A. Predicament
B. Resolution
C. Questioning
D. Superiority

10. COMMODIOUS

A. Bored
B. Inconvenient
C. Committed
D. Respectful

11. ICONOCLASTIC
A. Bombastic
B. Sedentary
C. Conventional
D. Terrestrial

12. LOUD
A. Raucous
B. Incoherent
C. Conscientious
D. Tranquil

13. PENURIOUS
A. Cynical
B. Lazy
C. Altruistic
D. Gregarious

14. UPBRAID
A. Unite
B. Verify
C. Welcome
D. Praise

15. ELUCIDATION
A. Elimination
B. Obscure
C. Paraphrase
D. Obligated

16. DETRIMENTAL
A. Pernicious
B. Beneficial
C. Harmful
D. Experimental

17. LETHARGIC
A. Dormant
B. Handicapped
C. Animated
D. Affable

18. LENIENT
A. Stern
B. Greedy
C. Easygoing
D. Gracious

19. EPILOGUE
A. Appendix
B. Library
C. Preface
D. Premise

20. FOLLY
A. Wisdom
B. Inanity
C. Dissolution
D. Creativity

21. REGULATE
A. Irrelevant
B. Tumultuous
C. Anecdote
D. Neglect

22. DIVERGENT
A. Schismatic
B. Similar
C. Unstoppable
D. Impudent

23. UNPRECEDENTED

A. Typical
B. Sinister
C. Esoteric
D. Soporific

24. TRUNCATE

A. Sever
B. Lengthen
C. Tacit
D. Infer

25. EPHEMERAL

A. Angelic
B. Eternal
C. Creative
D. Evanescent

<u>Directions:</u> Select the word that **best** completes the analogy.

---

26. SHALLOW: DEPTH:: APATHETIC:

A. Monopoly
B. Apology
C. Trying
D. Caring

27. SCISSORS: CUT:: SPICES:

A. Achieve
B. Season
C. Mesmerize
D. Decorate

28. GLUE: FASTEN:: ELEVATOR:

A. Launch
B. Service
C. Lift
D. Camp

29. ORACLE: FORESIGHT:: SAGE:

A. Wisdom
B. Talent
C. Wealth
D. Clarity

30. FLOWERS: FLORIST:: RINGS:

A. Tiara
B. Jeweler
C. Thorns
D. Roses

31. HOARD: SAVE:: REVERE:

A. Flirt
B. Sulk
C. Coyness
D. Admire

32. PLAYWRIGHT: ACTOR::
COMPOSER:

A. Melody
B. Trance
C. Musician
D. Memory

33. BUILDING: BLUEPRINT::
REPORT::

A. Outline
B. Canvas
C. Table
D. Artist

34. ANTISEPTIC: GERMS:: WATER:

A. Sterilized
B. Disinfectant
C. Thirst
D. Cook

35. SLUGGISH: ENERGY:: SATIATED:

A. Dissatisfied
B. Slothful
C. Wary
D. Hunger

36. LIBRARY: BOOK:: STABLE:

A. Horse
B. Automobile
C. Boat
D. Magazine

37. NEOPHYTE: EXPERIENCED::
INVALID:

A. Sickly
B. Healthy
C. Compliant
D. Wealthy

38. BUS: PASSENGERS:: FREIGHTER:

A. Requirement
B. Tires
C. Plane
D. Cargo

39. VERIFICATION: CONFIRM::
CONCILIATION:

A. Application
B. Appease
C. Reiteration
D. Affirm

40. EMBARGO: TRADE:: HELMET:

A. Injury
B. Respite
C. Football
D. Hearing

41. CONCEITED: HUMILITY::
IMPETUOUS:

A. Health
B. Perspective
C. Dedication
D. Patience

47. HUMIDITY: SWAMP:: ARIDITY:

A. Air-conditioning
B. Desert
C. Sea level
D. Beach

48. ANACONDA: SNAKE::
    BASKETBALL:

A. Serve
B. Sport
C. Shorts
D. Ball

49. BRUISE: SKIN:: STAIN:

A. Muscle
B. Bone
C. Fabric
D. Veneer

50. SPHYGMOMANOMETER: BLOOD
    PRESSURE:: THERMOMETER:

A. Temperature
B. Fahrenheit
C. Ampere
D. Air

42. RESOLUTE: DETERMINATION::
    SKEPTICAL:

A. Doubt
B. Mutiny
C. Hostility
D. Certainty

43. LEVEE: FLOOD:: IMMUNIZATION:

A. Avalanche
B. Hurricane
C. Catastrophe
D. Disease

44. METER: LENGTH:: POUND:

A. Inch
B. Yard
C. Heavy
D. Weight

45. ROSE: FLOWER:: ELM:

A. Street
B. Tree
C. Plant
D. Dew

46. POISON: TOXIC:: SUGAR:

A. Expensive
B. Cake
C. Sweet
D. Evil

STOP

**End of Verbal Ability section. If you have any time left, you may go over your
work in this section only.**

CHEMISTRY

60 Questions (#51–#110)

Directions: Choose the **best** answer to each of the following questions. You have 50 minutes to complete this section.

51. Convert –100°C to Kelvin.

A. –173
B. +173
C. –373
D. +373

52. Convert 5.86 milligrams to grams.

A. 5.86×10^{-2}
B. $5.86 \times 10^{+2}$
C. 5.86×10^{-3}
D. $5.86 \times 10^{+3}$

53. How many minutes are there in one day?

A. 1440
B. 2.50
C. 0.40
D. 1000

54. How many nanometers are present in 10 meters?

A. $1 \times 10^{+9}$
B. 1×10^{-8}
C. $1 \times 10^{+6}$
D. $1 \times 10^{+10}$

55. How many electrons are indicated in the following symbol for the iodide ion, $_{53}^{127}\text{I}^{-1}$?

A. 53
B. 127
C. 180
D. 54

56. How many protons are indicated in the following symbol for the lithium ion, $_{3}^{7}\text{Li}^{+1}$?

A. 3
B. 7
C. 10
D. 4

57. Which of the following is the correct formula for aluminum phosphide?

A. $\text{Al}_2(\text{HPO}_4)_3$
B. $\text{Al}(\text{H}_2\text{PO}_4)_3$
C. AlPO_4
D. AlP

58. Name the following compound, Na_2CO_3

A. Disodium carbonate
B. Disodium carbon trioxide
C. Sodium carbonate
D. Sodium carbon trioxide

59. Which of the following substances is NOT an allotrope of the others?

A. Graphite
B. Rust
C. Carbon
D. Diamond

60. Which of the following statements is a definition of an empirical formula?

A. A formula identifying the atoms present and their simplest whole number ratio.

B. A formula identifying the atoms present and the actual number of atoms.

C. A formula identifying the atoms present, the actual number of atoms, and showing how the atoms are bonded to each other.

D. None of the above

61. How many moles of carbon dioxide, CO_2, are present in 22 grams CO_2? (O = 16 amu, C = 12 amu)

A. 0.80
B. 0.50
C. 2.00
D. 1.30

62. What is the limiting reagent in the following reaction, given 8.0 grams oxygen, O_2, and 1.5 grams hydrogen, H_2 as the starting materials? (O = 16 amu, H = 1 amu)

$$O_2 + 2 H_2 \longrightarrow 2 H_2O$$

A. Oxygen
B. Hydrogen
C. Water
D. None of the above

63. What is the percentage yield of the following reaction if 1.0 gram of hydrogen, H_2, reacts with excess chlorine, Cl_2, to produce 18.3 grams of hydrogen chloride, HCl? (Cl = 35.5 amu, H = 1 amu)

$$H_2 + Cl_2 \longrightarrow 2 HCl$$

A. 100%
B. 75%
C. 50%
D. 25%

64. How many moles of copper, Cu, are present in 1.2×10^6 atoms of Cu? (Avogadro's Number = 6×10^{-23}, Cu = 63.5 amu)

A. $5.0 \times 10^{+17}$
B. $2.0 \times 10^{+4}$
C. 5.3×10^{-5}
D. 2.0×10^{-18}

65. What is the molar mass, in grams/mole, of an inorganic gaseous compound if 2.0 moles of this compound weigh 56 grams?

A. 28
B. 112
C. 0.04
D. 58

66. What is the percentage by weight of calcium, Ca, present in $Ca_3(PO_4)_2$? (Ca = 40 amu, P = 31 amu, O = 16 amu)

A. 38%
B. 18%
C. 49%
D. 56%

67. Which of the following reactions is a neutralization reaction?

A. $Mg + 2 HCl \longrightarrow MgCl_2 + H_2$

B. $2 HCl + CaCO_3 \longrightarrow CaCl_2 + H_2O + CO_2$

C. $BaCl_2 + Na_2SO_4 \longrightarrow BaSO_4 + 2 NaCl$

D. $2 KClO_3 \longrightarrow 2 KCl + 3O_2$

68. What is the oxidation number of phosphorus, P, in PO_4^{-3}?

A. −8

B. −3

C. +8

D. +5

69. What is the oxidation number of nitrogen, N, in NH_4^{+1}?

A. −3

B. +3

C. +1

D. −1

70. How many grams of sodium hydroxide, NaOH, is required to produce 800 milliliters of a 2.0 molar, 2.0 M, solution? (Na = 23 amu, O = 16 amu, H = 1 amu)

A. 8.0

B. 64

C. $1.6 \times 10^{+3}$

D. $6.4 \times 10^{+4}$

71. An autoclave has an initial pressure of 1.0 atmosphere and initial temperature of 27°C. The autoclave is heated until the final pressure inside the autoclave equals 5.0 atmospheres. What is the final temperature in degrees Celsius of the oven?

A. 1500

B. 1227

C. 135

D. 1000

72. How many grams of oxygen gas are present in a bulb of volume 2.0 liters, at 7°C and 1 atmosphere of pressure? (R = 0.082 liter-atm/mole-K, O = 16 amu)

A. 1.30

B. 112

C. 2.60

D. 55.8

73. In thermodynamics, a closed system is one that can

A. exchange energy and mass with the surroundings.

B. exchange energy but not mass with the surroundings.

C. exchange mass but not energy with the surroundings.

D. exchange neither energy nor mass with the surroundings.

Use the periodic table below in order to answer questions 74–86.

H																	He
Li	Be											B	C	N	O	F	Ne
Na	Mg											Al	Si	P	S	Cl	Ar
K	Ca	Sc	Ti	V	Cr	Mn	Fe	Co	Ni	Cu	Zn	Ga	Ge	As	Se	Br	Kr
Rb	Sr	Y	Zr	Nb	Mo	Tc	Ru	Rh	Pd	Ag	Cd	In	Sn	Sb	Te	I	Xe
Cs	Ba	La	Hf	Ta	W	Re	Os	Ir	Pt	Au	Hg	Tl	Pb	Bi	Po	At	Rn
Fr	Ra	Ac	Rf	Ha	Sg	Ns	Hs	Mt									

Ce	Pr	Nd	Pm	Sm	Eu	Gd	Tb	Dy	Ho	Er	Tm	Yb	Lu
Th	Pa	U	Np	Pu	Am	Cm	Bk	Cf	Es	Fm	Md	No	Lr

74. What is the electron configuration of the magnesium atom, Mg?

A. $1s^2 2s^2 2p^6 3s^2$
B. $1s^2 2s^2 2p^6$
C. $1s^2 2s^2 2p^6 3s^2 3p^4$
D. $1s^2 2s^2$

75. What is the electron configuration of the sodium ion, Na^{+1}?

A. $1s^2 2s^2 2p^6$
B. $1s^2 2s^2 2p^6 3s^1$
C. $1s^2 2s^2 2p^6 3s^2 3p^3$
D. $1s^2 2s^2$

76. What is the maximum number of electrons possible in the f orbitals of an atom?

A. 2
B. 6
C. 10
D. 14

77. Elements which place the last electron into an f orbital are called

A. transition elements.
B. actinide elements.
C. metalloids.
D. representative elements.

78. All the noble gases, except helium, He, have a completely filled

A. s subshell
B. p subshell
C. d subshell
D. f subshell

79. Indicate the correct order of the first ionization energy, IE, for the noble gases, with the highest IE being on the left, and the lowest IE being on the right.

A. He > Ne > Ar > Kr
B. Kr > Ar > Ne > He
C. Kr > Ne > Ar > He
D. He > Ar > Ne > Kr

80. Which of the following compounds is NOT ionic?

A. NaCl
B. ICl
C. CsF
D. LiBr

81. What is the outer electron configuration for the halogens, F, Cl, Br, I?

A. s^1
B. $s^2 p^5$
C. $s^2 p^6 d^5$
D. $s^2 p^6 d^{10} f^5$

82. Which of the following elements has the greatest electronegativity?

A. Cesium, Cs
B. Sodium, Na
C. Fluorine, F
D. Iodine, I

83. How many electrons are represented around the sulfur atom, S, in a Lewis dot structure?

   A. 2
   B. 4
   C. 6
   D. 8

84. Which of the following bonds is a nonpolar covalent bond?

   A. C - C
   B. Li - Cl
   C. H - F
   D. B - C

85. Indicate the correct order of boiling points for the following noble gases, with the lowest boiling point on the left, and the highest boiling point on the right.

   A. Kr < Ne < Ar < He
   B. Kr < Ar < Ne < He
   C. He < Ne < Ar < Kr
   D. He < Ar < Ne < Kr

86. Which of the following compounds has the highest boiling temperature?

   A. HCl
   B. H_2O
   C. HF
   D. NaCl

87. Which of the following substances is capable of hydrogen bonding to itself?

   A. CH_4
   B. HI
   C. NaH
   D. CH_3OH

88. What is the molecular geometry of BCl_3?

   A. Trigonal planar
   B. Trigonal pyramid
   C. Linear
   D. Tetrahedron

89. What is the geometry of the ammonium ion, NH_4^{+1}?

   A. Linear
   B. Bent
   C. Tetrahedral
   D. Trigonal planar

90. What is the geometry of the OF_2 molecule?

   A. Linear
   B. Bent
   C. Tetrahedral
   D. Trigonal planar

91. What is the approximate value of the bond angle for the O = C = O bond in carbon dioxide, CO_2?

   A. 90
   B. 105
   C. 120
   D. 180

92. What is the hybridization state of oxygen, O, in water, H_2O?

   A. sp
   B. sp^2
   C. sp^3
   D. sp^3d^2

93. What is the hybridization state of the carbon, C, atom in $H_2C = CH_2$?

A. sp
B. sp^2
C. sp^3
D. sp^3d^2

94. Which of the following molecules is NOT polar?

A. CCl_4
B. HCl
C. $CHCl_3$
D. CH_3Cl

95. What is the pH of a solution in which the hydrogen ion concentration equals 1×10^{-5} M (moles/liter)?

A. 5
B. 9
C. 6
D. 7

96. Some substances can function as both a Brönsted acid and Brönsted base. Which of the following substances can function as both acid and base?

A. H_3O^{+1}
B. H_2O
C. OH^{-1}
D. NO_3^{-1}

97. Which of the following acid-base reactions will produce a basic solution?

A. Strong acid and strong base
B. Weak acid and strong base
C. Strong acid and weak base
D. Weak acid and weak base

98. A solution of the following salt, sodium acetate, CH_3COONa, in water will be

A. acidic
B. basic
C. nearly neutral
D. independent of pH

99. Which of the following solutions is a buffer solution?

A. Hydrochloric acid and sodium chloride, $HCl + NaCl$
B. Acetic acid and sodium acetate, $CH_3COOH + CH_3COONa$
C. Nitric acid and sodium nitrate, $HNO_3 + NaNO_3$
D. Sulfuric acid and sodium sulfate, $H_2SO_4 + Na_2SO_4$

100. How many sigma bonds are present in the ethylene molecule shown below?

$$
\begin{array}{c c}
H & H \\
| & | \\
C & = C \\
| & | \\
H & H \\
\end{array}
$$

A. 1
B. 2
C. 4
D. 5

101. According to the kinetic molecular theory, in which of the following states of matter do atoms or molecules have the greatest freedom of motion?

A. Solid
B. Gas
C. Liquid
D. All states have the same freedom of motion.

102. The conversion of a solid directly to a gas, without passing through the liquid state, is known as

A. condensation.
B. vaporization.
C. sublimation.
D. freezing.

103. According to Henry's law, the solubility of a gas in a liquid increases with

A. an increase in temperature of the solution.
B. a decrease in pressure on the surface of the liquid.
C. an increase in pressure on the surface of the liquid.
D. stirring of the solution.

104. In order to measure the rate of the general reaction shown below

$$A \rightarrow B + C$$

one could measure the

A. increase in A
B. decrease in C
C. increase in B
D. decrease in B

105. A chemical reaction may have several steps through which the reactants proceed in order to form the products. The individual step which determines the rate of the overall reaction is called the rate determining step. The rate determining step would be which of the following in the sequence of steps?

A. Fastest
B. Slowest
C. First
D. Last

106. A catalyst is added to a reaction and is regenerated at the end of the reaction. During the reaction the catalyst

A. speeds up the reaction by raising the activation energy.
B. slows down the reaction by lowering the activation energy.
C. speeds up or slows down the reaction by lowering or raising the activation energy respectively.
D. has no effect on the rate of the reaction.

107. In the thermodynamic reaction

$$\Delta G = \Delta H - T \Delta S$$

ΔG represents the change in free energy in a reaction, ΔH the change in enthalpy, and ΔS the change in entropy. The reaction is spontaneous when ΔG is

A. +
B. –
C. 0
D. The sign of ΔG has no significance.

108. Which of the following reactions shows an increase in entropy?

A. $2 \, KClO_3 \, (s) \longrightarrow 2 \, KCl \, (s) + 3 \, O_2 \, (g)$
B. $H_2O \, (g) \longrightarrow H_2O \, (l)$
C. $2 \, H_2 \, (g) + O_2 \, (g) \longrightarrow 2 \, H_2O \, (l)$
D. $PCl_3 \, (l) + Cl_2 \, (g) \longrightarrow PCl_5 \, (s)$

109. A change in which of the following factors causes a change in the equilibrium constant of the reversible reaction shown?

$$A + B \longleftrightarrow C + D \qquad K = \frac{[C][D]}{[A][B]}$$

A. Temperature
B. Volume
C. Concentration
D. Catalyst

110. Which of the following types of radiation is the most dangerous?

A. Alpha particles
B. Beta particles
C. Gamma rays
D. All the above types of radiation are equally dangerous.

STOP

End of Chemistry section. If you have any time left, you may go over your work in this section only.

BIOLOGY

50 Questions (#111–#160)

Directions: Choose the **best** answer to each of the following questions. You will have 50 minutes to complete this section.

111. What is the name of the Kingdom that mushrooms belong to:

A. Animalia
B. Plantae
C. Protista
D. Fungi

112. Which of the Kingdoms have cells that do not have a true nucleus?

A. Monera
B. Protista
C. Fungi
D. Plantae

113. Which statement is <u>not true</u> concerning the plasma membrane?

A. It controls exchange of materials between the inside and outside of the cell.
B. It is the outermost layer of animal cells.
C. It regulates cell's chemical composition.
D. It is the power plant of the cell.

114. Plastids that contain green pigment chlorophyll and are involved in photosynthesis are characteristic of:

A. vacuole
B. chloroplast
C. rough endoplasmic reticulum
D. microtubules

Use Figure 1 to answer questions 115–118.

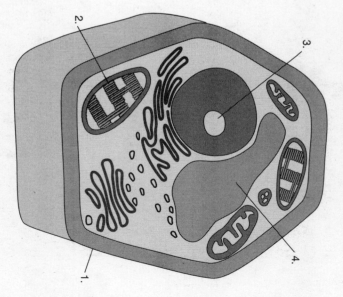

Figure 1.

115. In Figure 1, number 1 is pointing to what part of the plant cell?

A. Cell Wall
B. Nucleus
C. Vacuole
D. Mitochondrion

116. In Figure 1, number 2 is pointing to what part of the plant cell?

A. Cell Wall
B. Nucleus
C. Vacuole
D. Mitochondrion

117. In Figure 1, number 3 is pointing to what part of the plant cell?

A. Cell Wall
B. Nucleus
C. Vacuole
D. Mitochondrion

118. In Figure 1, number 4 is pointing to what part of the plant cell?

A. Cell Wall
B. Nucleus
C. Vacuole
D. Mitochondrion

119. Solutions that cause blood cells to shrink are called:

A. hypertonic
B. isotonic
C. mestonic
D. hypotonic

120. Solutions that cause blood cells to swell are called:

A. hypertonic
B. isotonic
C. mestonic
D. hypotonic

121. Which of the following represent the proper sequence for the stages of mitosis?

A. Prophase, Metaphase, Anaphase, Telophase
B. Prophase, Anaphase, Telophase, Metaphase
C. Anaphase, Telophase, Prophase, Metaphase
D. Anaphase, Prophase, Telophase, Metaphase

122. This process involves the synthesis of polypeptide chains at the ribosome in response to information contained in mRNA molecules.

A. Transcription
B. Translation
C. Transduction
D. Transmetric

123. This process occurs when double strands of a DNA segment separate and RNA nucleotides pair with DNA nucleotides.

A. Transcription
B. Translation
C. Transduction
D. Transmetric

124. An endocrine gland:

A. lacks a duct
B. depends on the blood for transport of its secretions
C. releases its hormone into the surrounding interstitial fluid
D. all of the above

125. Oxytocin is responsible for:

A. preventing milk release from the mammary glands

B. causing contraction of the uterus

C. preventing goiter

D. maintaining normal thyroid and calcium levels

126. Thyroid hormones:

A. are transported in the blood bound to thyroxin-binding globulin

B. are made from the amino acid tyrosine

C. require iodine for their production

D. all of the above

127. Calcitonin:

A. is produced by the pancreas

B. levels increase when blood calcium levels decrease

C. causes blood calcium levels to decrease

D. insufficiency results in weak bones and tetany

128. Parathyroid hormone secretion increases in response to:

A. a decrease in blood calcium

B. increased production of parathyroid-stimulating hormone from the anterior pituitary

C. increase secretion of parathyroid-releasing hormone from the hypothalamus

D. all of the above

129. The adrenal medulla:

A. is formed from a modified portion of the sympathetic nervous system

B. has epinephrine as its major secretory product

C. increases its secretions during exercise

D. all of the above

130. Which type of blood is the universal donor?

A. O

B. B

C. A

D. AB

131. Which type of blood is the universal recipient?

A. O

B. B

C. A

D. AB

132. The valve between the right atrium and right ventricle is:

A. Bicuspid (mitral) valve

B. Tricuspid valve

C. Atrioventricular valve

D. Chamber valve

133. Given these blood vessels below:

1. aorta
2. inferior vena cava
3. pulmonary trunk
4. pulmonary vein

Choose the arrangement that lists the vessels in the order a red blood cell would encounter them in going from the systemic veins back to the systemic arteries.

A. 1, 3, 4, 2
B. 2, 3, 4, 1
C. 2, 4, 3, 1
D. 3, 2, 1, 4

134. Oxygen is mostly transported in the blood:

A. in white blood cells
B. bound to albumin
C. bound to gamma globulins
D. bound to the heme portion of hemoglobin

135. Which of these structures function to increase the mucosal surface of the small intestine?

A. The length of the small intestine
B. Villi
C. Microvilli
D. all of the above

136. Which of the following statements are true concerning vitamins?

A. They function as coenzymes.
B. Most can be synthesized by the body.
C. They are normally broken down before they can be used by the body.
D. A, D, E, and K are water-soluble vitamins.

137. Functions of the kidney involve:

A. maintaining blood volume
B. disposing nitrogenous wastes
C. maintaining electrolyte balance
D. all of the above

138. In the reaction versus substrate concentration graph, below, the curve plateaus because:

A. a noncompetitive inhibitor is present
B. a competitive inhibitor is present
C. the active site is saturated with substrate
D. all the substrate has been converted to product

139. In a heterozygous monohybrid cross, the dominant trait would be expressed _____ of the time.

A. 0 percent
B. 25 percent
C. 75 percent
D. 100 percent

140. Which of the following is the specialized absorptive structure in the intestine?

A. Alveoli
B. Villi
C. Bowman's capsule
D. Nephron

141. Which of the following is an instinct in many species?

A. Caring for offspring
B. Operating a car
C. Playing baseball
D. all of the above

142. The process that allows higher plants to be autotrophic is:

A. protein synthesis
B. digestion
C. fermentation
D. photosynthesis

143. The process that leads to the production of ethyl alcohol or lactic acid is:

A. lactation
B. digestion
C. fermentation
D. respiration

144. In minks, the gene for brown fur (B) is dominant to the gene for silver fur (b). Which set of genotypes represents a cross that could produce offspring with silver fur from parents that both have brown fur?

A. Bb × Bb
B. BB × Bb
C. BB × bb
D. Bb × bb

145. HIV (human immunodeficiency virus) infects mostly:

A. red blood cells
B. D-killer cells
C. T-helper cells
D. none of the above

146. Carbohydrate digestion begins in the _____ with the action of the enzyme _____.

A. mouth, amylase
B. stomach, pepsin
C. small intestine, cholecystokinin
D. large intestine, water

147. Which of the crosses would most likely give offspring of 50% dominant and 50% recessive?

A. BB × Bb
B. Bb × bb
C. BB × bb
D. BB × BB

148. The chromosome number is reduced from diploid to haploid in cell division is

- **A.** meiosis.
- **B.** mitosis.
- **C.** hapnosis.
- **D.** triosis.

149. Responsible for transmitting genetic information from the DNA molecule in the nucleus to the cytoplasm is

- **A.** transmitting RNA.
- **B.** transfer RNA.
- **C.** receiving RNA.
- **D.** messenger RNA.

150. _____ carries amino acids to the messenger RNA-ribosome complex during protein synthesis.

- **A.** Transmitting RNA
- **B.** Transfer RNA
- **C.** Receiving RNA
- **D.** Ribosomal RNA

151. A major function of white blood cells is to fight:

- **A.** pain
- **B.** infections
- **C.** glucose intolerance
- **D.** none of the above

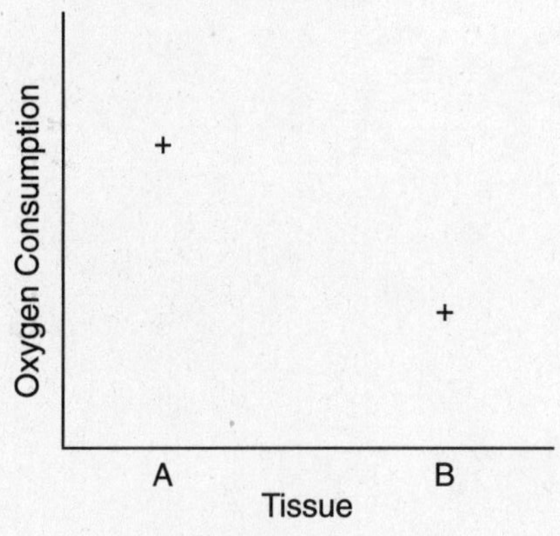

152. In Figure 2, the oxygen consumption of tissues A and B were determined with the following results:

- **A.** tissue A has either a greater number of mitochondria, larger mitochondria, or more enzymatic activity.
- **B.** tissue A has a lesser number of mitochondria, smaller mitochondria, or less enzymatic activity.
- **C.** tissue A has a lesser number of mitochondria, medium-sized mitochondria, or less enzymatic activity.
- **D.** tissue A has to have a smaller nucleus.

Use Figure 3 to answer questions 153 and 154.

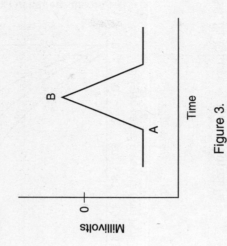

Figure 3.

153. In Figure 3, the ascending portion of the action potential observed in the cell in the graph is caused by:

- **A.** potassium efflux out of the cell
- **B.** potassium influx into the cell
- **C.** sodium efflux out of the cell
- **D.** sodium influx into the cell

Figure 2.

154. In Figure 3, the descending portion of an action potential after the initial spike potential is caused by:

A. potassium efflux out of the cell
B. potassium influx into the cell
C. sodium efflux out of the cell
D. sodium influx into the cell

155. Hormones are distributed throughout the body by means of the

A. gallbladder
B. blood
C. pancreas
D. stomach

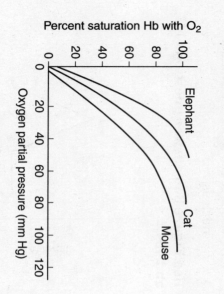

Percent saturation Hb with O₂

Figure 4.

156. In Figure 4, for an animal's hemoglobin to unload more readily it must

A. have a high metabolic rate and high oxygen requirements.
B. have a low metabolic rate and low oxygen requirements.
C. have an intermediate oxygen requirement.
D. not require oxygen.

157. Acetylcholine is:

A. a hormone in the endocrine system
B. an androgen in the reproductive system
C. a neurotransmitter in the nervous system
D. an angiotensin antagonist in the circulatory system

158. Transmission across a synapse is slower than impulse conduction along a neuron because:

A. there is more surface area in a synapse than a neuron
B. synaptic vesicles clog the neural pathways and the signal takes longer
C. it involves a series of events
D. partial depolarization requires more time to accomplish

159. Neurological drugs alter synaptic function in which ways?

A. Interferes with synthesis of the appropriate transmitter.
B. Blocks uptake of the transmitter into synaptic vesicles.
C. Prevents the release of transmitter from the vesicles into the cleft
D. all of the above

160. Which statement is NOT characteristic of red blood cells?

A. Red blood cells carry oxygen from the lungs to the tissues.

B. Mature red blood cells lack a nucleus.

C. The normal life span of a red blood cell is about 30 days.

D. Hemoglobin is present in red blood cells.

STOP

End of Biology section. If you have any time left, you may go over your work in this section only.

READING COMPREHENSION

45 Questions (#161–#205)

Directions: Read each of the following passages, and choose the **best** answer to each of the questions that follows each passage. You have 45 minutes to complete this section.

Passage 1:

As many as 50 million Americans have high blood pressure, defined as a systolic blood pressure ≥140 mm Hg and a diastolic blood pressure ≥90 mm Hg. Although blood pressure generally increases with age, the onset of hypertension most often occurs in the third, fourth, or fifth decade of life. The prevalence of hypertension in the elderly population (age ≥65 years) is approximately 63% in whites and 76% in blacks. In younger generations (35 to 45 years of age), the prevalence is markedly different with 44% among black men, 37% among black women, 26% among white men, and 17% among white women.

A specific cause of sustained hypertension cannot be found in the vast majority of individuals with high blood pressure. Genetic factors have been suggested to play a role in essential hypertension due to the fact that high blood pressure may be hereditary. Evidence that a single gene may account for specific subtypes of hypertension has also been suggested. Genetic traits include high angiotensin levels, increased aldosterone and other adrenal steroids, and high sodium-lithium counter-transport. More direct approaches for preventing or treating hypertension could be achieved by identifying individuals with these traits. Factors such as sodium excretion and transport rates, blood pressure response to plasma volume expansion, electrolyte homeostasis, and glomerular filtration rate help explain the predisposition for a person to develop hypertension.

Anti-hypertensive drug therapy should be individualized according to various patient characteristics and fundamental pathophysiologic circumstances. Dietary intake has been shown to be similar in all races but blacks ingest less potassium and calcium than whites. Supplemental potassium and calcium has shown to cause a modest reduction in blood pressure in some studies. Therefore, it would seem reasonable to ascertain the affects of increasing the amount of potassium and calcium in the diet as part of the non-pharmacologic regulation of hypertension. The initial treatment for hypertension is lifestyle changes unless target-organ damage is present. These changes include sodium restriction, weight reduction, increased physical activity, and ethanol reduction or abstinence. In terms of target-organ damage, diuretics and beta-blockers are first-line therapy. Control of blood pressure and prevention of cardiovascular morbidity and mortality are the goals of antihypertensive therapy. By maintaining arterial blood pressure below 140 mm Hg systolic and 90 mm Hg diastolic and by controlling other risk factors such as smoking, hyperlipidemia, and diabetes, morbidity and mortality may be averted.

161. The onset of hypertension most often occurs in which decades?

A. Third and fifth.
B. Third, fourth, and fifth.
C. Fourth, fifth, and sixth.
D. Fifth, sixth, and seventh.

162. According to the passage, initial treatment for hypertension is lifestyle changes which include:

A. smoking cessation, weight reduction, decreased physical activity, and ethanol restriction.
B. sodium restriction, weight reduction, increased physical activity, and ethanol reduction or abstinence.
C. ethanol reduction or abstinence, sodium restriction, reduced mental activity or stress, and gaining weight.
D. weight reduction, increase sodium intake, ethanol reduction, and increase stress.

163. Genetic factors have been suggested to play a role in essential hypertension based on the fact that:

A. parents can get it from their children.
B. if ancestors have high angiotensin levels they have a higher rate of morbidity.
C. geneticists know which gene causes hypertension.
D. high blood pressure may be hereditary.

164. Anti-hypertensive therapy should be individualized according to:

A. patients characteristics and fundamental pathophysiologic circumstances.
B. number of offspring and dietary habits stemming from care of those offspring.
C. features found in their family tree.
D. the climate of the state where the patient lives.

165. How many Americans currently suffer from high blood pressure?

A. As many as 60 billion.
B. As many as 50 billion.
C. As many as 50 million.
D. As many as 40 million.

Passage 2:

Non-adherence to medication therapy results in numerous adverse effects such as increased hospitalizations and even death. Additionally, it costs the U.S. healthcare system billions of dollars each year. It is important to assess patients adherence to medications.

Improper medication adherence encompasses an assortment of behaviors. These include not having a prescription filled, forgetting or intentionally not taking a medication, consuming an incorrect amount of a medication, taking a medication at the wrong time, ceasing therapy too soon, or continuing therapy after advised to discontinue. All forms of improper medication taking behavior may jeopardize health outcomes.

Measuring medication taking behavior is often difficult. The ideal method of measurement should be simultaneously unobtrusive (to avoid patient sensitization and maximize cooperation), objective (to produce discrete and reproducible data for each subject), and practical (to maximize portability and minimize cost). Refill records, pill counts, electronic medication dispensers/caps, patient surveys (interviews), blood-drug level monitoring, and urine assay for drug metabolites can be used as clues to identify improper medication use.

Before altering therapy based on the assumption that a patient is taking a medication as prescribed, practitioners should ascertain patient's medication taking behavior. This becomes especially important when modifying dosages of medications. Due to the advantages and disadvantages of each measurement, it is important for practitioners to use a combination of methods to assess a patient's medication usage behavior and relate these findings to the patient's clinical presentation.

166. The ideal method of medication compliance measurement should be:

A. simultaneously functional, easy, and reliable.

B. simultaneously fun, personalized, and fancy-free.

C. simultaneously practical, objective, and unobtrusive.

D. simultaneously advantageous, creative, and unpretentious.

167. According to the passage, current techniques for assessing a patients medication usage include:

A. blood-drug level monitoring, pill counts, refill records, and half-life tables.

B. refill records, patient interviews, electronic medication dispensers, and nucleic acid levels.

C. pill counts, electronic medication dispensers, patient interviews, patient examinations, and refill records.

D. blood-level drug monitoring, refill records, electronic medication dispensers, and urine assays for drug metabolites.

168. Improper medication adherence encompasses:

  A. taking a medication too soon, not taking enough of the drug, and forgetting to take the medication.

  B. not having the prescription filled, continuing to take the medication after therapy has been discontinued, forgetting or intentionally not taking the medication, and consuming the wrong amount of medication.

  C. not having the prescription filled, taking the medication before therapy has been continued, forgetting or intentionally not taking the medication, and consuming too much medication.

  D. all of the above

169. Before altering therapy based on the assumption that the medication is being taken as prescribed, practitioners should:

  A. assess the patients behavior concerning taking their medication.

  B. check the patients blood glucose levels and ask about their dietary intake.

  C. discern the patients refill rate and whether they were on schedule.

  D. decide if the patient is in the maintenance phase of compliance.

170. It is important to assess patients adherence to compliance because:

  A. if they are not compliant then their medication will not work

  B. it can result in adverse reactions such as increased hospitalizations and perhaps death.

  C. it costs the U.S. government trillions in lawsuits each year.

  D. maintenance of adherence contributes to an increase in suicides.

Passage 3:

Alzheimer's disease, first described by Alois Alzheimer in 1907, is a type of progressive dementia for which no cause is known or no cure exists. People with Alzheimer's disease eventually lose their identity, memories, and all associated analytical, cognitive, and physical functions.

Several trials have been conducted to discover and evaluate drugs that may help Alzheimer's patients. One such trial of the drug memantine raised ethical and policy issues. Decline in cognitive and behavioral functioning was slower in trial participants with moderately severe disease receiving memantine than in those receiving placebo.

The benefits produced by this and other potential therapies for later-stage Alzheimer's must be carefully evaluated. There are many questions that need to be answered. Do patients receiving the investigational drug exhibit less personal distress or improved well-being during their last months? Does the drug improve patients' quality of life? Is the drug cost-effective?

These are hard questions with controversial moral dimensions. But they must be addressed if research is to offer meaningful help to patients and families coping with the effects of this awful disease. Currently, all treatments for Alzheimer's are palliative.

171. According to the passage, treatments for Alzheimer's disease are:

A. a partial frontal lobotomy to ensure new brain growth.
B. memory aids and cognitive functioning treatment.
C. the new drug, memantine.
D. palliative.

172. The benefits produced by this new drug therapy:

A. are numerous and more are being discovered everyday.
B. should be carefully evaluated.
C. can affect both the patient and their family.
D. can increase correspondingly to the drug dose.

173. The most important concern of the new drug memantine is:

A. the patients get addicted to the medication and their behavioral function is altered.
B. the drug is not strong enough to halt the progress of the disease for those with late stage Alzheimer's.
C. decline in cognitive function and behavioral function was slower in those receiving the drug than those receiving a placebo.
D. the cost of the drug exceeds its beneficial efficacy for the patients involved.

174. People with Alzheimer's disease:

A. look older than their age.
B. cannot wear certain colors.
C. have a hard time remembering who they are or where their place of residence is located.
D. are younger and more intelligent.

175. According to the passage, which statement is incorrect:

A. Alzheimer's disease was first described by Alois Alzheimer.
B. a cure exists for Alzheimer's.
C. many trials have been conducted to discover and evaluate drugs that may help Alzheimer's patients.
D. the memantine trial raised ethical and policy issues.

Passage 4:

Imagine picking up a 10-kilogram piece of steak with your tongue. That's more or less what a chameleon can do with its so-called ballistic tongue. Its secret is suction, researchers reveal in the November issue of the *Journal of Experimental Biology*.

Scientists have determined that other lizards catch prey by using mainly surface tension—the stickiness created when a wet tongue contacts dry prey. But chameleons consume creatures much too large for surface tension alone to handle. So evolutionary biologists at the University of Antwerp in Belgium and Northern Arizona University in Flagstaff decided to find out what else is going on. Dissecting tongues from several chameleon species, they found that two muscles form a pouch at the tip. Slow-motion film of chameleons capturing crickets, grasshoppers, and other lizards revealed that these muscles retract just before the tongue makes contact with the target.

The team suspected that the tongue pouch was behaving like a suction cup. So they anesthetized chameleons, inserted a glass tube into the pouch, and measured the force required to remove the tube as the pouch muscles were electrically stimulated. It took 10 times greater force to remove a sealed tube than a hollow (nonsuctionable) tube. The team also cut the nerve that controls the pouch muscles and found that although the animals could still extend their tongues, they couldn't latch onto prey.

Scientists seem to believe that these vacuum-generating tongues may be unique. A better understanding of this unusual mechanism should help scientists understand how it evolved.

Reprinted with permission from *Science*, Vol 290, October 2000. Page 79.

176. The **main** topic of this summary is:

A. evolutionary biology is making advances.

B. chameleons have weak tongues.

C. understanding how the chameleon tongue works.

D. chameleons eat prey with tongue.

177. The chameleon tongue works by

A. instantly killing and then latching onto its prey.

B. stabbing its prey.

C. using tongue muscles to create a suction cup and latching onto prey.

D. slapping its prey and immobilizing it with the force of its tongue.

178. The tongue experiment was conducted and accomplished by what means?

A. Examining the tongue in action many times.

B. Genetically creating a lab chameleon and watching it eat.

C. Dissecting the tongue and measuring it with a ruler.

D. Measuring the force created by the pouch muscles using a glass tube.

179. What size prey can a chameleon attain with its tongue?

A. 22 pounds

B. 100 pounds

C. 1000 pounds

D. 1000 tons

180. When the experimental team cut the nerve which controls the pouch muscles,

A. the tongue was useless but the chameleon could still swallow.

B. the animals could still latch onto prey but couldn't extend their tongue.

C. the nerve never healed normally and the animal expired.

D. the animals could extend their tongue but could not latch onto prey.

Passage 5:

A dreaded disease is striking California's coast live oaks with the ferocity of an oak-tree Ebola virus, causing the trees to sprout sores, hemorrhage sap, and become infested with beetles and various fungi. The trees die within a few weeks of their first symptoms. Pathologists at the University of California, Davis, announced that his team had found the cause of the disease dubbed "Sudden Oak Death." The tree-slayer is a new member of the genus Phytophthora, whose name means "plant destroyer." Its kin include pathogens responsible for the Irish potato famine and die-offs in Australian eucalyptus forests and European oak groves. "We don't know if (the new species) was just recently introduced, or if it has always been here and something else has changed that has allowed it to go crazy," one pathologist says.

The first trees to succumb to the plague 5 years ago were tan oaks, which often grow in the under-story of redwood forests. Last year the disease began hitting large numbers of coast live oaks, the signature species in scenic coastal woodlands. Alarmingly, the pathogen has begun to blight another species, the black oak.

Knowing the culprit doesn't make the outlook much brighter. Fungicides can save individual oaks, says one pathologist, but we can't go to Mount Tamalpais and spray 10,000 trees." And prevention is largely limited to warning people not to carry oak firewood to uninfected areas. The Sierra Nevada hosts black oaks, and pathologists fear the deadly spores could strike groves in beloved Yosemite Valley.

Reprinted with permission from *Science*, Vol 289, August 2000. Page 859.

181. "Sudden Oak Death" causes trees to

A. grow multiple trunks and become infested with mold.

B. sprout sores, hemorrhage sap, and become infested with beetles and various fungi.

C. lose all leaves, branches and wilt.

D. hemorrhage at the tips, spout new branches, and become infested with termites.

182. This plague began

A. 5 years ago.
B. 10 years ago.
C. 15 years ago.
D. 2 years ago.

183. The cause of this disease is

A. Phytohemagglutinin.
B. Phytosterol.
C. Phytophthora.
D. Phytoalexin.

184. The first trees to succumb were

A. tan oaks.
B. coast live oaks.
C. black oaks.
D. European oak.

185. The greatest fear of this plague is that it will strike

A. Redwood Forests.
B. Yosemite Valley.
C. Australian Eucalyptus Forests.
D. Coastal Woodlands.

Passage 6:

We humans sense old age through feeling those creaky joints or observing those graying hairs but, according to Apfeld and Kenyon reporting in a recent issue of *Nature*, the nematode worm senses its age by smelling and tasting the environment. These investigators show that worms with defective olfactory organs (that would normally detect odor molecules in the environment) live longer than their comrades with a keener sense of smell. By comparing these worms with other mutant nematodes that live an unusually long time, the researchers found clues to how a reduced ability to "smell the roses" might lengthen life-span.

The worm's olfactory sense organs—amphids on the head and plasmids on the tail—are composed of a cluster of nerve cells, the ends of which are modified into cilia. The cilia are encircled by a sheath and a socket cell that form a pore in the worm's skin through which the tips of the cilia protrude. Odor molecules and soluble compounds bind to G protein-coupled receptors (similar to the olfactory and taste receptors of mammals) located at the tip of each cilium. Worms with a poor sense of smell—because their olfactory organs have defective or absent cilia, blocked pores, or damaged sheaths—live much longer, yet are otherwise normal (for example, their feeding and reproductive behaviors are unchanged). Mutations in TAX-4—a channel regulated by cyclic GMP that sits under the G-protein-coupled receptor and transduces the sensory signals into electrical impulses—also imbue the worm with a longer life.

But mutations in the worms olfactory machinery are not the only defects that extend its life-span. In an earlier study, Kenyon's group found that defects in the reproductive system could prolong life by decreasing the activity of DAF-2 (a receptor for an insulin-like molecule) and increasing the activity of DAF-16 (a transcription factor). By looking at worms defective in both sensory perception and reproduction, Apfeld and Kenyon worked out a putative pathway through which smell might influence a worm's longevity.

An environmental signal, perhaps produced by bacteria (the worm's favorite food), binds to G protein-coupled olfactory receptors on sensory cilia activating TAX-4, which then incites electrical activity in the sensory neurons. This activity triggers secretory vesicles in the neurons to release insulin-like molecules, which bind to DAF-2 and activate the insulin-like signaling pathway. This then switches on genes that will ensure the worm dies at the usual age of 2 weeks. A reduced ability to sense olfactory cues would result in a decrease in DAF-2 activation and an increase in life-span.

This chain of events is not proven, but insulin-like molecules that might bind to DAF-2 have been identified in the nematode. Such a pathway would also make physiological sense. After all, if food is scarce it may behoove the worm to live longer to ensure that it has the chance to produce its full quota of offspring. A scarcity of food also promotes longevity in rodents and primates. But so far it seems that in these more complicated creatures a poor sense of smell is not a harbinger of a ripe old age.

Reprinted with permission from *Science*, Vol 287, January 2000. Page 54.

186. A worm usually lives to the 'old age' of

- **A.** 3 weeks.
- **B.** 5 weeks.
- **C.** 1 week.
- **D.** 2 weeks.

187. TAX-4 is

- **A.** a channel regulated by cyclic GMP which sits beneath the G protein-coupled receptor and transduces the sensory signals into electrical impulses.
- **B.** a cyclic regulated AMP which lies above the G protein-coupled receptor and transduces the neurological signals into electrical impulses.
- **C.** a liability which the nematode has to deal with four times the amount of cyclic GMP next to the G protein-coupled receptor.
- **D.** a receptor for an insulin-like molecule which activate the insulin-like pathway.

188. A nematode worm detects its age by

- **A.** a biological stopwatch which notes sunrise and sunset.
- **B.** burrowing through the soil at speeds up to 0.01 mph.
- **C.** whether it has had the chance to produce its full quota of offspring.
- **D.** smelling and tasting the environment.

189. The worm's olfactory sense organs are composed of

- **A.** a cluster of nervous tissue surrounded by a sheath which protects it.
- **B.** socket cells that are embedded in the head and tail of the worm.
- **C.** a cluster of nerve cells which the ends are modified into cilia.
- **D.** their individual mouths and noses which are covered with cilia.

190. What other traits in the worm extend its lifespan?

- **A.** Defects in the circulatory system.
- **B.** Mutations in the excretory system.
- **C.** Alterations in the lymphatic system.
- **D.** Aberrations in the reproductive system.

191. DAF-2 is

- **A.** a receptor for an insulin-like molecule.
- **B.** a transcription factor.
- **C.** a transduction factor.
- **D.** a binding site for a glucose molecule.

192. A logical pathway by which smell might influence a worm's longevity was achieved by studying

A. worms flawed in both circulatory and sensory perception.

B. worms defective in both reproduction and sensory perception.

C. worms deficient in only the reproductive system.

D. worms impaired in the nervous and circulatory system.

193. Secretory vesicles in the neurons are stimulated by what to release insulin-like molecules?

A. TAX-4 excites electrical activity.

B. DAF-2 activates the insulin-like pathway.

C. DAF-16 regulates the electrical activity.

D. TAX-2 initiates the secretory vesicles.

194. A scarcity of food is known to promote longevity in

A. nematodes.

B. nematodes and rodents.

C. nonprimates and nematodes.

D. rodents and primates.

195. The reduced ability to sense olfactory cues results in

A. a decrease in life-span and an increase in DAF-2 activation.

B. a decrease in DAF-2 activation and an increase in lifespan.

C. a decrease in TAX-4 which incites electrical activity.

D. a decrease in DAF-16 which creates more gene activity.

Passage 7:

Presidents of the United States are not like you and me. A new personality assessment presented this week at the American Psychological Association conference in Washington, D.C., shows that, compared to the public they serve, presidents are more likely to be extroverted, assertive, and disagreeable. They're also less modest and straightforward.

Says who? Historians who have written book-length biographies of Oval Office occupants. Psychologist Steve Rubenzer of the Mental Health and Mental Retardation Authority of Harris County in Houston, Texas, and colleagues asked the biographers to fill out three standard personality inventories on their subjects, basing answers on the presidents' behavior during the 5 years preceding their reigns. The researchers compared the presidents' scores to population norms and compared the profiles of successful commanders-in-chief with those history hasn't smiled upon.

"Great" presidents, such as Jefferson and Lincoln, they find, "are attentive to their emotions, willing to question traditional values ... imaginative, and more interested in art and beauty than less successful Chief Executives." They're also more assertive, stubborn, and "tender-minded", which is a measure of concern for the less fortunate. Rubenzer hasn't analyzed the current presidential contenders yet—he prefers to have at least three "unbiased" historians fill out the forms for each president or presidential wanna-be.

Reprinted with permission from *Science*, Vol 289, August 2000. Page 859.

196. This personality assessment was presented at a conference of which group?

A. The American Pharmacists Association
B. The Annual Physicians Association
C. The American Psychological Association
D. The Association of Practicing Psychiatrists

197. This book was written by

A. historians.
B. presidents.
C. psychologists.
D. historiographers.

198. According to the passage, "great" presidents include those such as

A. Kennedy and Roosevelt.
B. Jefferson and Lincoln.
C. Bush and Wilson.
D. Adams and Carter.

199. In this article, use of the word "tender-minded" meant

A. less stubborn.
B. more concerned for the less-fortunate.
C. more apathetic toward the environment.
D. less concerned for the more-fortunate.

200. Presidents are more likely to be

A. disagreeable, extroverted, and assertive.
B. agreeable, apathetic, and introverted.
C. unwilling to question traditional values.
D. less interested in art and beauty.

Passage 8:

Drug interactions, a common type of drug-related problem, are categorized as pharmacokinetic, pharmacodynamic, or a combination of both. Pharmacokinetic drug interactions include changes in absorption, distribution, excretion, and metabolism; whereas, pharmacodynamic drug interactions may lead to antagonist or synergistic effects. Not all drug interactions are undesirable, in fact, many drug interactions are used to produce desirable effects. Patients who take drugs with narrow therapeutic indices and drugs that interfere with the pharmacokinetic properties of other drugs are at increased risk of experiencing a drug interaction. Also, patients who take multiple medications per day or take multiple doses of medications per day are at increased risk. Because renal transplant patients take immunosuppressive agents that have narrow therapeutic indices and are subjected to multiple medications per day they are vulnerable to experiencing adverse drug events. To prevent adverse drug interactions, an alternative therapy should be considered when possible or the dose or schedule of the drugs should be adjusted to reduce the occurrence of an adverse experience. Additionally, adequate monitoring to prevent and detect adverse effects is an essential part of patient care.

A common pharmacokinetic interaction involves drugs that interfere with the absorption of other medications. Drugs that bind and decrease the gastrointestinal absorption of another drug, such as cholestyramine decreasing the absorption of tacrolimus, typically can be prevented by administering the agents two to three hours apart from each other. Prokinetic agents interfere with the rate of absorption. Since many transplant patients take prokinetic agents, such as metochlopromide, this may increase the bioavailability of other medications. This is of significant importance since immunosuppressive agents have narrow therapeutic indices and toxicity may result from this interaction. If the prokinetic agent cannot be avoided, careful monitoring (e.g., serum drug levels, clinical presentation of patient) and adjustments should be made to prevent immunosuppressant toxicity.

201. Prokinetic agents

A. interfere with the rate of metabolism.

B. affect all interactions in the gastrointestinal tract.

C. interfere with the rate of absorption.

D. should be monitored and adjusted.

202. Pharmokinetic drug interactions include

A. changes in allocation, circulation, and dispersion.

B. changes in absorption, distribution, excretion, and metabolism.

C. reactions which affect composition of other medications.

D. cumulative and additive effects.

203. Patients that are at increased risk of experiencing a drug interaction include

A. patients who take multiple medications per day or multiple doses of medications per day.

B. patients who take drugs with narrow therapeutic indices.

C. patients who take drugs that interfere with the pharmacokinetic properties of other drugs.

D. all of the above.

204. To prevent adverse drug reactions

A. consult neighbors regularly.

B. consider an alternate therapy or alter the dose or schedule of the drugs.

C. time medication regimens with meals.

D. increase water intake.

205. If the prokinetic agent cannot be avoided, to prevent immunosuppressant toxicity

A. carefully arrange the patients medication consumption schedule.

B. monitor compliance to see if the prokinetic factor is really necessary.

C. monitor serum levels and the clinical presentation of the patient and make appropriate adjustments.

D. educate the patient on the types of adverse drug reactions which may occur.

STOP

End of Reading Comprehension section. If you have any time left, you may go over your work in this section only.

QUANTITATIVE ABILITY
65 Questions (#206–#270)

Directions: Choose the **best** answer to each of the following questions. You will have 45 minutes to complete this section.

206. If a square plot of land 210 feet on one side contains one acre, approximately how many square feet are in the one acre of land?

A. 44,100
B. 28,400
C. 2,860
D. 840

207. For the expression $6x - 12 = 60$, $x =$

A. 18
B. 12
C. 9
D. 8

208. To solve the equation $x^2 + 50 = 66$, the value of x is

A. 4
B. 7
C. 8
D. 12

209. One tablespoonful contains 15mL of volume. If a patient takes one tablespoonful three times a day, how many days supply will be provided by a 12 ounce bottle? (One ounce = 30mL)

A. 6
B. 8
C. 12
D. 16

210. Sixty-six percent (66%) can be expressed as

A. $\dfrac{1}{2}$
B. $\dfrac{2}{3}$
C. $\dfrac{8}{15}$
D. $\dfrac{15}{25}$

211. Solve for x in the equation $2x^2 = 800$.

A. 100
B. 80
C. 40
D. 20

212. $0.025\,(10^4) =$

A. 0.25
B. 2.5
C. 25
D. 250

213. $0.3^3 + \dfrac{1}{2} =$

A. 9.5
B. 5.27
C. 0.527
D. 0.0527

214. 0.5 is _____ of 50

  A. 0.1%
  B. 1%
  C. 2.5%
  D. 10%

215. $10^2 + 9^2 =$

  A. 90^4
  B. 19^4
  C. 1.81×10^2
  D. 1^4

216. $10^0 \times 10 =$

  A. 0.1
  B. 1
  C. 10
  D. 100

217. 10^5 minus $10^3 =$

  A. 9.9×10^4
  B. 10^2
  C. 10^{-2}
  D. 9.9×10^2

218. $\dfrac{11}{33} =$

  A. 66%
  B. 50%
  C. 33%
  D. 24%

219. $\dfrac{2}{5} \div 4 =$

  A. $\dfrac{2}{9}$
  B. $\dfrac{5}{8}$
  C. $\dfrac{2}{10}$
  D. $\dfrac{1}{10}$

220. $\dfrac{2}{3} + \dfrac{4}{5} =$

  A. $\dfrac{8}{15}$
  B. $\dfrac{6}{15}$
  C. $1\dfrac{3}{7}$
  D. $1\dfrac{7}{15}$

221. 25% of 100 = 10% of

  A. 2500
  B. 250
  C. 150
  D. 12.5

222. $\dfrac{3}{5} =$

  A. 15%
  B. 30%
  C. 60%
  D. 75%

223. $\dfrac{3}{5} + 6 =$

A. $\dfrac{63}{5}$

B. $\dfrac{33}{5}$

C. $\dfrac{18}{5}$

D. $\dfrac{9}{5}$

224. $\dfrac{4}{5} \div 3 =$

A. 0.5

B. 0.44

C. 0.27

D. 0.15

225. $5^3 + 4^4 =$

A. 31

B. 63

C. 381

D. 32,000

226. 5! =

A. 120

B. 25

C. 6

D. 2.24

227. A truck travels at a steady speed of 100 kilometers per hour from 12 noon until 6 P.M. How many miles will be driven?

A. 968

B. 600

C. 372

D. 106

228. A line contains the points (2,2) and (4,6). What is the slope of this line?

A. 0.5

B. 1

C. 2

D. 4

229. A teenager is 152.4 centimeters (cm) tall. This can also be expressed as _____ feet.

A. 4.5

B. 5

C. 5.5

D. 6

230. A box is labeled as containing lemons that weigh 4 ounces each. How many lemons will be needed if a shopper wants 6 pounds of lemons?

A. 96

B. 32

C. 24

D. 16

231. A person weighing 220 pounds would weigh _____ kilograms.

A. 70

B. 100

C. 242

D. 484

232. A man is tossing a coin. The first three tosses have been heads. What are the chances that heads will occur on the fourth toss?

A. 50%
B. 25%
C. 12.5%
D. 6.25%

233. A worker can put 10 oranges a minute into a basket. How long will it take to put 2400 oranges into baskets?

A. 2 hours
B. 3 hours
C. 4 hours
D. 6 hours

234. An airplane is due to land at 4 P.M. If the plane is 1500 miles away at 10 A.M., how fast must it fly to arrive on time?

A. 600 mph
B. 500 mph
C. 300 mph
D. 250 mph

235. Calculate the expression $3\sqrt{1,000}$

A. 333
B. 111
C. 100
D. 10

236. Calculate the value of x in the expression $4x = \dfrac{1}{2}$

A. $\dfrac{1}{42}$

B. $\dfrac{1}{24}$

C. $\dfrac{1}{16}$

D. $\dfrac{1}{8}$

237. A newborn child weighs 8.8 pounds. This is _____ kilograms.

A. 3
B. 4
C. 6.6
D. 19.36

238. Determine 80% of $\sqrt{16}$.

A. 6.4
B. 5.4
C. 3.2
D. 1.6

239. Determine the value of $\sqrt{49} \times 10^3$.

A. 7
B. 70
C. 700
D. 7000

240. Digoxin Injection is supplied in ampules of 500 micrograms per 2 ml. What quantity must a nurse administer to provide a dose of 0.25 milligrams?

A. 0.2 mL
B. 0.5 mL
C. 1.0 mL
D. 2.0 ml

241. Express the value of $\frac{2}{3} + \frac{1}{4}$ as a decimal.

A. 3.33
B. 0.92
C. 0.60
D. 0.46

242. For the figure shown below; $ED = 4$ and $BD = 5$. What is the length of BE?

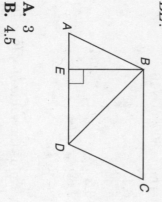

A. 3
B. 4.5
C. 5.5
D. 6

243. If a drug product contains 2.5% active ingredient, then 30 grams of the drug product will contain _____ of the active ingredient.

A. 900 mg
B. 750 mg
C. 550 mg
D. 25 mg

244. If a coin is tossed 3 times, what is the probability that the result will be three tails?

A. $\frac{1}{2}$
B. $\frac{1}{3}$
C. $\frac{1}{4}$
D. $\frac{1}{8}$

245. If one acre is approximately 4900 square yards, what is the perimeter of four contiguous acres that form a perfect square?

A. 420 feet
B. 840 feet
C. 1260 feet
D. 1680 feet

246. If a prescription calls for 30 capsules that contain 15 mg of codeine per capsule, what will be the total amount of codeine used to fill the prescription?

A. 450 mcg
B. 450 grams
C. 0.45 mg
D. 0.45 grams

247. In the equation $x^2 + 50 = 66$, the value of x is

A. −4
B. 27
C. 8
D. 12

248. In the equation $x^2 + 5 = 54$, the value of x is

A. 24
B. 7
C. 13
D. 6

249. Morphine Sulfate is available in 15 mg tablets. How many tablets would provide the 0.3 grams needed for a prescription?

A. 2
B. 20
C. 40
D. 200

250. One acre is approximately 4900 square yards. This is equivalent to _____ square feet.

A. 14,700
B. 29,400
C. 44,100
D. 62,400

251. One teaspoonful contains 5 mL of volume. How many mL will be needed for a 10-day supply if a patient takes one teaspoonful four times a day?

A. 240
B. 200
C. 120
D. 100

252. Sixteen fluid ounces equal one _____.

A. cup
B. pint
C. quart
D. gallon

253. Solve for x in the equation $3x^2 = 300$.

A. 100
B. 33.33
C. 10
D. 1.5

254. Sixty percent (60%) can be expressed as

A. $\dfrac{1}{2}$
B. $\dfrac{2}{3}$
C. $\dfrac{8}{15}$
D. $\dfrac{15}{25}$

255. The value of $\log(6 \times 4)$ can also be expressed as

A. $\log 2.4$
B. $\log 240$
C. $\log 6 \times \log 4$
D. $\log 6 + \log 4$

256. Forty percent (40%) can be expressed as

A. $\dfrac{2}{5}$

B. $\dfrac{1}{10}$

C. $\dfrac{1}{20}$

D. $\dfrac{1}{2}$

257. The circumference of a circle with a diameter of 6 centimeters would be

A. 18.84 cm

B. 16.88 cm

C. 12.44 cm

D. 9.14 cm

258. Two inches can also be expressed as _____ centimeters.

A. 0.78

B. 5.08

C. 25.48

D. 39.37

259. What is the value of $\sqrt{45} + \sqrt{80}$?

A. $4\sqrt{125}$

B. $5\sqrt{35}$

C. $4\sqrt{9}$

D. $7\sqrt{5}$

260. What is the slope of the line shown in the graph below?

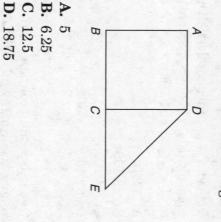

A. 1

B. 2

C. 4

D. 10

261. For the figure shown below, the area of the square is 25. If $AB = BC = CE$, what is the area of the triangle?

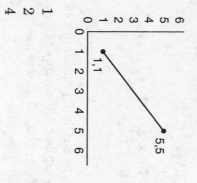

A. 5

B. 6.25

C. 12.5

D. 18.75

262. What is the average of the following values?   10, 12, 9, 10, 11, 9, 9, 10, 8, 12

A. 2

B. 9.5

C. 10

D. 12

263. What is 22% of 50?

A. 4.4

B. 11

C. 28

D. 44

264. What is the value of x in the expression: $x^3 + 27 = 54$?

A. 3
B. 9
C. 11
D. 14

265. What is the value of $|-100| + 50 = ?$

A. 150
B. 50
C. 0
D. −50

266. What is the area of the circle shown below?

$\pi = 3.14;\ d = 8$

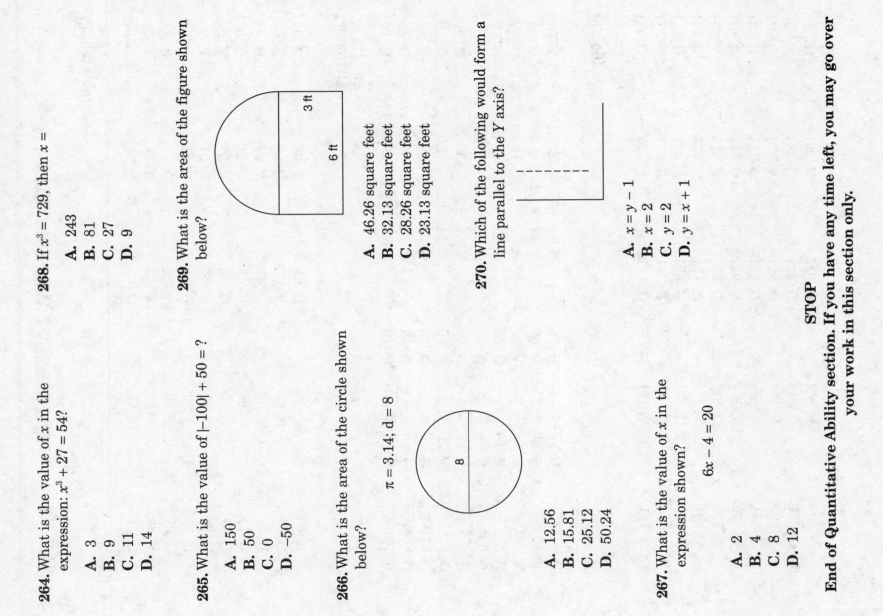

8

A. 12.56
B. 15.81
C. 25.12
D. 50.24

267. What is the value of x in the expression shown?

$6x - 4 = 20$

A. 2
B. 4
C. 8
D. 12

268. If $x^3 = 729$, then $x =$

A. 243
B. 81
C. 27
D. 9

269. What is the area of the figure shown below?

6 ft

3 ft

A. 46.26 square feet
B. 32.13 square feet
C. 28.26 square feet
D. 23.13 square feet

270. Which of the following would form a line parallel to the Y axis?

A. $x = y - 1$
B. $x = 2$
C. $y = 2$
D. $y = x + 1$

STOP

End of Quantitative Ability section. If you have any time left, you may go over your work in this section only.

PRACTICE PCAT 2 ANSWER KEY

Verbal Ability

1. C	11. C	21. D	31. D	41. D
2. A	12. D	22. B	32. C	42. A
3. B	13. C	23. A	33. A	43. D
4. D	14. D	24. B	34. C	44. D
5. A	15. B	25. B	35. D	45. B
6. A	16. B	26. D	36. A	46. C
7. D	17. C	27. B	37. B	47. B
8. B	18. A	28. C	38. D	48. B
9. B	19. C	29. A	39. B	49. C
10. B	20. A	30. B	40. A	50. A

Chemistry

51. B	61. B	71. B	81. B	91. D	101. B
52. C	62. A	72. C	82. C	92. C	102. C
53. A	63. C	73. B	83. C	93. B	103. C
54. D	64. D	74. A	84. A	94. A	104. C
55. D	65. A	75. A	85. C	95. A	105. B
56. A	66. A	76. D	86. D	96. B	106. C
57. D	67. B	77. B	87. D	97. B	107. B
58. C	68. D	78. B	88. A	98. B	108. B
59. B	69. A	79. A	89. C	99. B	109. A
60. A	70. B	80. B	90. B	100. D	110. C

Biology

111. D	121. A	131. D	141. A	151. B
112. A	122. B	132. B	142. D	152. A
113. D	123. A	133. B	143. C	153. D
114. B	124. D	134. D	144. A	154. A
115. A	125. B	135. D	145. C	155. B
116. D	126. D	136. A	146. A	156. A
117. B	127. C	137. D	147. B	157. C
118. C	128. A	138. C	148. A	158. C
119. A	129. D	139. C	149. D	159. D
120. D	130. A	140. B	150. B	160. C

Reading Comprehension

161. B	170. B	179. A	188. D	197. A
162. B	171. D	180. D	189. C	198. B
163. D	172. B	181. B	190. D	199. B
164. A	173. C	182. A	191. A	200. A
165. C	174. C	183. C	192. B	201. C
166. C	175. B	184. A	193. A	202. B
167. D	176. C	185. B	194. D	203. D
168. D	177. C	186. D	195. B	204. B
169. A	178. D	187. A	196. C	205. C

Quantitative Ability

206. A	219. D	232. A	245. D	258. B
207. B	220. D	233. C	246. D	259. D
208. A	221. B	234. D	247. A	260. A
209. B	222. C	235. D	248. B	261. C
210. B	223. B	236. D	249. B	262. C
211. D	224. C	237. B	250. C	263. B
212. D	225. C	238. C	251. B	264. A
213. C	226. A	239. D	252. B	265. A
214. B	227. C	240. C	253. C	266. D
215. C	228. C	241. B	254. D	267. B
216. C	229. B	242. A	255. D	268. D
217. A	230. C	243. B	256. A	269. B
218. C	231. B	244. D	257. A	270. B

EXPLANATORY ANSWERS FOR VERBAL ABILITY

1. Answer is **C**. *Jocular* means jolly or playful; the opposite is *cantankerous*, which means cranky or disagreeable.

2. Answer is **A**. *Paucity* means deficit or poverty; the opposite is *surfeit*, which means abundance or surplus.

3. Answer is **B**. *Insipid* means bland or boring; the opposite is *excite*, which means interesting or poignant.

4. Answer is **D**. *Reticent* means quiet or latent; the opposite is *garrulous*, which means talkative or verbose.

5. Answer is **A**. *Nefarious* means corrupt or criminal; the opposite is *trustworthy*, which means dependable or honest.

6. Answer is **A**. *Proliferation* means increase or expansion; the opposite is *curtailment*, which means cessation or reduction.

7. Answer is **D**. *Subordinate* means inferior or apprentice; the opposite is *superior*, which means sovereign or commanding.

8. Answer is **B**. *Complacent* means content; the opposite is *dissatisfied*, which means displeased.

9. Answer is **B**. *Quandary* means dilemma, doubt, or problem; the opposite is *resolution*, which means settlement or agreement.

10. Answer is **B**. *Commodious* means favorable or timely; the opposite is *inconvenient*, which means inappropriate or untimely.

11. Answer is **C**. *Iconoclastic* means radical or unorthodox; the opposite is *conventional*, which means classic or characteristic.

12. Answer is **D**. *Loud* means noisy; the opposite is *tranquil*, which means quiet or sedate.

13. Answer is **C**. *Penurious* means greedy or miserly; the opposite is *altruistic*, which means to be generous or kind.

14. Answer is **D**. *Upbraid* means to admonish or scold; the opposite is *praise*, which means to compliment or commend.

15. Answer is **B**. *Elucidation* means clarify or translate; the opposite is *obscure*, which means concealed or blurry.

16. Answer is **B**. *Detrimental* means unwanted or harmful; the opposite is *beneficial* which means advantageous or desirable.

17. Answer is **C**. *Lethargic* means drowsy or passive; the opposite is *animated* which means energetic or perky.

18. Answer is **A**. *Lenient* means easygoing or liberal; the opposite is *stern* which means firm or rigorous.

19. Answer is **C**. *Epilogue* means conclusion or postscript; the opposite is *preface* which means beginning or prelude.

20. Answer is **A**. *Folly* means foolishness or nonsense; the opposite is *wisdom* which means knowledge or prudence.

21. Answer is **D**. *Regulate* means monitor or control; the opposite is *neglect* which means unattended or free.

22. Answer is **B**. *Divergent* means varied or diverse; the opposite is *similar* which means consistent or congruent.

23. Answer is **A**. *Unprecedented* means unusual or revolutionary; the opposite is *typical* which means average or common.

24. Answer is **B**. *Truncate* means cut or shorten; the opposite is *lengthen* which means extend or elongate.

25. Answer is **B**. *Ephemeral* means fading or elusive; the opposite is *eternal* which means unchanging or ceaseless.

26. Answer is **D**. This is an analogy of a "lack of" or "without" relationship where one word means lack of or without the other. Shallow is lack of depth and apathetic is lack of caring.

27. Answer is **B**. This is an analogy of "used to" or "serves to" relationship. Scissors are used to cut and spices are used to season.

28. Answer is **C**. This is an analogy of "used to" or "serves to" relationship. Glue is used to fasten and an elevator is used to lift.

29. Answer is **A**. This is an analogy of characteristics or description. An oracle by definition has foresight and a sage has wisdom.

30. Answer is **B**. This is an analogy of characteristic or description. A florist sells flowers and a jeweler sells rings.

31. Answer is **D**. This analogy is based on synonyms in a degree relationship. To revere someone is to admire them to a greater degree, whereas, to hoard is to save to a greater degree.

32. Answer is **C**. This is an analogy of characteristic or description. A playwright provides the material that an actor performs and a composer provides the material that a musician performs.

33. Answer is **A**. This is an analogy of characteristic or description in which the blueprint is the plan of the building and the outline is the plan of a report.

34. Answer is **C**. This is an analogy of characteristic or description. An antiseptic helps to eliminate germs, water helps to eliminate thirst.

35. Answer is **D**. This is an analogy of a "lack of" or "without" relationship. Sluggish means lack of energy and satiated means lack of hunger.

36. Answer is **A**. This is an analogy of characteristic or description. A book can be located in a library and a horse can be found in a stable.

37. Answer is **B**. This is an analogy of a "lack of" or "without" relationship. A neophyte is without experience and an invalid is not healthy.

38. Answer is **D**. This is an analogy of characteristic or description. A bus carries passengers and freighter carries cargo.

39. Answer is **B**. This is an analogy of synonyms. To verify is to confirm and conciliation is to appease.

40. Answer is **A**. This is an analogy of characteristic or description. An embargo prevents trade and a helmet prevents injury.

41. Answer is **D**. This is an analogy of a "lack of" or "without" relationship. A person who is conceited has no humility and one who is impetuous lacks patience.

42. Answer is **A**. This is an analogy of synonyms. To be resolute means full of determination and to be skeptical means full of doubt.

43. Answer is **D**. This is an analogy of characteristic or description. A levee prevents a flood and immunization prevents disease.

44. Answer is **D**. This is an analogy of "used to" or "serves to" relationship. A meter is used to measure length and a pound is used to measure weight.

45. Answer is **B**. This is an analogy of characteristic or description. A rose is a type of flower and an elm is a type of tree.

46. Answer is **C**. This is an analogy of characteristic or description. A poison is toxic and sugar is sweet.

47. Answer is **B**. This may also be considered an analogy of description or characteristic. A swamp is associated with humidity and a desert is associated with aridity (which means dry).

48. Answer is **B**. This is a part to whole analogy. An anaconda is a type of snake and basketball is a type of sport. To help clarify this kind of analogy, think of the group of all snakes and the group of all sports as "wholes," of which the anaconda and basketball are merely parts.

49. Answer is **C**. This is an analogy of characteristics or description. A bruise is a mark on the skin and a stain is a mark on fabric.

50. Answer is **A**. This is an analogy of purpose or use. A sphygmomanometer is used to measure blood pressure, and a thermometer is used to measure temperature.

EXPLANATORY ANSWERS FOR CHEMISTRY

51. Answer is B. To convert between °C and Kelvin, the following formula is used.

$$K = 273 + °C$$

The value, −273°C, or 0K is absolute zero, the temperature at which all molecular movement is believed to stop.

$$K = 273 + (-100) = +173$$

52. Answer is C. One gram contains 1000 milligrams, $1\,g = 10^{+3}\,mg$. In using dimensional analysis to solve this problem, any equality can be converted into two fractions:

$$\frac{1\,g}{10^{+3}\,mg} \quad \text{and} \quad \frac{10^{+3}\,mg}{1\,g}$$

Multiply 5.86 mg by the appropriate fraction of the two fractions above, so that the milligrams cancel and only the gram unit remains.

$$5.86\,mg \times \frac{1\,g}{10^{+3}\,mg} = 5.86\,mg \times 10^{-3}\,g$$

Don't forget that in moving an exponential term from the denominator to the numerator, *i.e.* dividing, the sign of the exponential term changes.

53. Answer is A. Using dimensional analysis as explained in question 52 above and knowing that

$$60 \text{ minutes} = 1 \text{ hour} \quad \text{and} \quad 24 \text{ hours} = 1 \text{ day}$$

multiply one day by the two appropriate fractions formed from the two equalities above.

$$1\,day \times \frac{24\,hrs}{1\,day} \times \frac{60\,min}{1\,hour} = 1440\,min$$

54. Answer is D. Using dimensional analysis as explained in question 52 and knowing that

$$1\,m = 10^{+9}\,nm$$

multiply ten meters by the appropriate fraction formed from the equality above.

$$10\,m \times \frac{10^{+9}\,nm}{1\,m} = 10 \times 10^{+9}\,nm = 1 \times 10^{10}\,nm$$

55. <u>Answer is **D**</u>. In the symbol for the iodide ion

$$^{127}_{53}\text{I}^{-1}$$

the bottom number, 53, is the number of protons, the atomic number, and the top number, 127, is the number of protons plus neutrons, the atomic mass. In a neutral atom, the number of protons equals the number of electrons. This ion has a −1 charge, indicating that it has one more electron than it has protons. Therefore the number of electrons is 53 + 1 = 54.

56. <u>Answer is **A**</u>. As explained in question 55 above, in the symbol for the lithium ion

$$^{7}_{3}\text{Li}^{+1}$$

the bottom number, 3, is the number of protons. One could obtain the number of neutrons, 4, by subtracting the number of protons, 3, from the number of protons plus neutrons, 7.

57. <u>Answer is **D**</u>. In naming binary compounds, *i.e.* compounds derived from two elements, one a metal and the other a nonmetal, the name of the first element is that of the metal present, while the name of the second element, the nonmetal, has its ending removed and replaced by -ide. For example, AlP is called aluminum phosphide. The name of the first element is aluminum. The ending -orus is removed from phosphorus, the second element, and replaced by -ide. The other formulas given as possible answers to this problem represent salt derivatives of phosphoric acid, H_3PO_4. Each of these compounds, derivatives of an acid ending in -ic, is named by removing the -ic acid and replacing it with -ate as its ending. In addition, the name of each formula indicates the number of hydrogen atoms remaining. For example, if one H^+ is removed from the neutral molecule H_3PO_4, the resulting anion will have a charge of −1 and be $H_2PO_4^{-1}$, dihydrogen phosphate. With two H^+ removed, the anion is HPO_4^{-2}, hydrogen phosphate. With three H^+ removed, the anion is PO_4^{-3}, phosphate.

Therefore, the name of **A**, $Al_2(HPO_4)_3$, is aluminum hydrogen phosphate, of **B**, $Al(H_2PO_4)_3$, is aluminum dihydrogen phosphate, and of **C**, $AlPO_4$, is aluminum phosphate.

58. <u>Answer is **C**</u>. When the formula of a compound contains both a metal and nonmetal or ion containing a nonmetal, the number of atoms of each element is not indicated. Sodium carbonate is the correct name for Na_2CO_3. Answers **A**, **B**, and **D** are nonsense answers.

59. <u>Answer is **B**</u>. Allotropes are different forms of the same element. Each allotrope has vastly different properties from the others. Answers **A**, graphite, and **D**, diamond, are both made of carbon, answer **C**. Rust is an iron oxide.

60. <u>Answer is **A**</u>. Each of the following types of formulas show the atoms present. In addition, an empirical formula shows the simplest whole number ratio of these atoms, for example, HO. Answer **B**, a molecular formula, shows the actual number of atoms present, for example, H_2O_2. Answer **C**, a structural formula, shows the actual number of atoms present, as well as how the atoms are bonded to each other, for example H - O - O - H.

61. <u>Answer is **B**</u>. Moles may be defined as grams/molar mass.

$$\text{Moles} = \frac{\text{Grams}}{\text{MolarMass}}$$

The molar mass of carbon dioxide, CO_2, is

$$1\ C = 1(12) = 12$$
$$2\ O = 2(16) = \underline{32}$$
$$44\ \text{grams / mole}$$

Dividing 22 grams by 44 grams/mole gives 0.50 mole.

62. <u>Answer is **A**</u>. In a stoichiometric problem dealing with the limiting reagent it is necessary to remember that the numbers in front of the formulas in a chemical equation represent either molecules or moles. From the balanced equation

$$O_2 + 2\ H_2 \longrightarrow 2\ H_2O$$

it can be seen that 1 mole of O_2 needs to react with 2 moles of H_2 to produce 2 moles of H_2O. Grams of oxygen and of hydrogen are given in this problem, so it is necessary to convert the grams to moles in order to see which reagent is present in excess and to determine that the other reagent is the limiting reagent. The number of moles of O_2 is 8 grams/ 32 grams per mole or 0.25 mole. The number of moles of H_2 is 1.5 grams/2 grams per mole or 0.75 mole. The number of moles of O_2, 0.25, would require 0.50 mole of H_2 for complete reaction of both reactants, according to the balanced equation. There are 0.75 mole of H_2 and therefore, there are 0.25 mole of H_2 in excess, 0.75 – 0.50. Oxygen is then the limiting reagent, determining how much product, H_2O, can theoretically be produced.

63. <u>Answer is **C**</u>. Percentage yield is defined as $100 \times$ actual yield/theoretical yield. Theoretical yield is the number of grams calculated as being possible to produce in a reaction. Actual yield is the number of grams actually isolated in a reaction.

$$H_2 + Cl_2 \longrightarrow 2\ HCl$$

From the balanced equation above it can be seen that 1 mole of hydrogen reacts with 1 mole of chlorine to produce 2 moles of hydrogen chloride. In the problem, grams of hydrogen are given and they react with excess chlorine. Therefore hydrogen is the limiting reagent and is used to calculate the theoretical yield. Theoretical yield may be calculated as follows:

$$\text{grams } H_2 \longrightarrow \text{moles } H_2 \longrightarrow \text{moles } Cl_2 \longrightarrow \text{grams HCl}$$

Refer to explanation to question 61 for definition of moles.

Grams H_2
1.0

Moles H_2

$$\frac{1.0 \text{ gram}}{2 \text{ grams per mole}} = 0.5 \text{ moles } H_2$$

Moles Cl_2

$$0.5 \text{ moles } H_2 \times \frac{2 \text{ moles HCl}}{1 \text{ mole } H_2} = 1.0 \text{ mole HCl}$$

Grams HCl

$$1.0 \text{ mole HCl} \times \frac{36.5 \text{ grams HCl}}{1 \text{ mole HCl}} = 36.5 \text{ grams HCl(theoretical yield)}$$

$$\text{Percentage yield} = \frac{\text{Actual Yield}}{\text{Theoretical Yield}} \times 100 = \frac{18.3 \text{ grams HCl}}{36.5 \text{ grams HCl}} \times 100$$

$$= 50\%$$

64. Answer is D. There are 6×10^{23} atoms, Avogadro's number, present in one mole of any element. To calculate the number of moles in 1.2×10^6 atoms of copper, divide the number of atoms by the number of atoms in one mole.

$$\frac{1.2 \times 10^6 \text{ atoms Cu}}{6 \times 10^{23} \text{ atoms / mole}} = 0.2 \times 10^{-17} = 2.0 \times 10^{-18} \text{ mole}$$

65. Answer is A. The number of moles of a substance equals the number of grams divided by the molar mass of the substance. Molar mass has the units of grams/mole. Divide the mass, 56 grams, by the number of moles, 2 moles, to obtain the molar mass, 28 grams/mole.

66. Answer is A. To calculate the percentage by weight, divide the weight of the part by the weight of the whole, *i.e.*, divide the weight of Ca by the molar mass of $Ca_3(PO_4)_2$, and multiply by 100 to convert to percentage.

67. Answer is B. A neutralization reaction is one in which an acid and a base react to produce a salt and water. In equation **B**, the acid, HCl, reacts with the base, $CaCO_3$, to produce the salt, $CaCl_2$, and initially H_2CO_3, carbonic acid.

$$2HCl + CaCO_3 \longrightarrow CaCl_2 + H_2CO_3$$

However, carbonic acid is unstable and decomposes to carbon dioxide, CO_2, and water, H_2O.

$$H_2CO_3 \longrightarrow CO_2 + H_2O$$

Equation **A** is a single displacement reaction, displacement of the H in HCl by Mg.

$$Mg + 2HCl \longrightarrow MgCl_2 + H_2$$

Equation **C** is a double displacement reaction, in which the positive and negative ions change partners. The Ba replaces the Na and the Na replaces the Ba.

$$BaCl_2 + Na_2SO_4 \longrightarrow BaSO_4 + 2NaCl$$

Equation **D** is a decomposition reaction, in which $KClO_3$ decomposes to KCl and O_2.

$$2KClO_3 \longrightarrow 2KCl + 3O_2$$

68. Answer is D. In order to determine the oxidation number of an element in a formula, it is necessary to assign oxidation numbers to all the other elements in the formula. For example, in PO_4^{-3}, oxygen has an oxidation number of –2. There are four atoms of oxygen in the formula, so the total oxidation value of oxygen is $4(-2) =$ –8. Since the ion has a charge of –3, the oxidation number of phosphorus should be such that when it is combined with –8, a charge of –3 remains. Therefore, the oxidation number of phosphorus is $-3 = -8 + ?$. The value of $+5 = ?$. Oxygen is assigned an oxidation number of –2, except when it is present in a peroxide, eg. H_2O_2, when the oxidation number is –1.

69. Answer is A. The oxidation number assigned to hydrogen is +1. There are 4 atoms of hydrogen in NH_4^{+1}, so the total oxidation value for hydrogen is $4(+1) = +4$. Since the ion has a charge of +1, the nitrogen must have an oxidation value of –3. Hydrogen is assigned an oxidation number of +1, except when it is present in a hydride, eg. NaH, when the oxidation number is –1.

$$\frac{\text{Part}}{\text{Whole}} \times 100 = \frac{3\,Ca}{3\,Ca + 2\,P + 8\,O} \times 100 =$$

$$\frac{3(40)}{3(40) + 2(31) + 8(16)} \times 100 = 38\%$$

70. <u>Answer is **B**</u>. Molarity is defined as moles of solute divided by liters of solution.

$$M = \frac{\text{moles solute}}{\text{liters solution}} = \frac{\text{grams / molar mass}}{\text{liters solution}}$$

Substituting the given values for sodium hydroxide, NaOH, (molar mass = 40 grams/mole) into the above formula gives

$$2.0\ M = \frac{x/40\ \text{gm per mole}}{0.8\ \text{liter}}$$

Solving for $\times$ gives a value of 64 grams.

71. <u>Answer is **B**</u>. Since volume is constant in an autoclave, the equation

$$\frac{P_1V_1}{T_1} = \frac{P_2V_2}{T_2} \quad \text{reduces to} \quad \frac{P_1}{T_1} = \frac{P_2}{T_2}$$

Temperature in the gas equations is always in Kelvin. Refer to explanation to question 51. Substituting the values given in the problem into the above equation gives

$$\frac{1\ \text{atm}}{27 + 273} = \frac{5.0\ \text{atm}}{x} \qquad x = 1500\ K$$

$$1500 - 273 = 1227°C$$

72. <u>Answer is **C**</u>. The ideal gas law, $PV = nRT$, is used to solve this problem. Pressure is used in atmospheres, volume in liters, and temperature in Kelvin. Moles of gas is represented by n. The molar mass of oxygen gas is 32 grams/mole since oxygen is a diatomic molecule, O_2. Substituting the given data into the above formula gives

$$1\ \text{atm}\ (2.0\ \text{liters}) = \frac{x}{32\ \text{grams / mole}} \frac{(0.082\ \text{l-atm})}{\text{K-mole}} (273 + 7)\ K$$

$$x = 2.60\ \text{grams}$$

73. <u>Answer is **B**</u>. By definition, a closed system is one that can exchange energy but not mass with the surroundings. An open system allows the exchange of the mass and energy of the system with that of the surroundings, answer **A**. An isolated system does not allow the exchange of either the mass or energy of the system with that of the surroundings, answer **D**. Answer **C** is a nonsense answer.

74. <u>Answer is **A**</u>. The correct electron configuration for magnesium, Mg, is $1s^2 2s^2 2p^6 3s^2$. Magnesium is the 12th element in counting the elements from left to right across each row. Therefore, the atomic number, the number of protons, is 12 and the number of electrons is 12 for the neutral atom. The letters s, p, d, and f indicate the type of orbital. The number in front of the symbols, as in 1s, indicates the number of the orbit, in this case 1. The superscript, as in $1s^2$, indicates the number of electrons present in the orbital, in this case 2. The electron configuration of Mg, $1s^22s^22p^63s^2$, shows the 12 electrons in the neutral atom.

75. Answer is **A**. The correct electron configuration for the sodium ion is $1s^22s^22p^6$. Sodium, Na, is element 11 and the neutral atom would have 11 electrons in its electron configuration. However, Na^{+1} is the ion which has lost one electron. The sodium ion has 10 electrons as shown in the configuration above.

76. Answer is **D**. There are seven f orbitals, each capable of containing two electrons. Therefore the maximum number of electrons possible in the f orbitals of an atom is 14. In the periodic table the 4f orbitals begin in the row across with the element Ce and end with the element Lu. The 5f orbitals begin in the row across with the element Th and end with the element Lr. There are fourteen elements in each row.

77. Answer is **B**. Elements which place the last electron in an f orbital are called either lanthanides or actinides. The row beginning with Ce and ending with Lu follows the element lanthanum, La, and hence is known as the lanthanides. The row beginning with Th and ending with Lr follows the element actinium, Ac, and hence is known as the actinides. The representative elements are those in the columns down which begin with the elements hydrogen, H; beryllium, Be; boron, B; carbon, C; nitrogen, N; oxygen, O; fluorine, F; and helium, He. The transition elements constitute the four rows across in the middle of the periodic table, from Sc to Zn, from Y to Cd, from La to Hg, and from Ac to Mt. The metalloids are elements which can act as either metals or nonmetals. The metalloids consist of the following elements, B, Si, Ge, As, Sb, Te, Po, At. All the elements to the left of the metalloids are metals; all the elements to the right of the metalloids are nonmetals.

78. Answer is **B**. The electron configuration of helium, He, ends with $1s^2$. The electron configuration of neon, Ne, ends with $2p^6$; that of argon, Ar, ends with $3p^6$; that of krypton, Kr, ends with $4p^6$; that of xenon, Xe, ends with $5p^6$; and that of radon, Rn, ends in $6p^6$.

79. Answer is **A**. The first ionization energy may be defined as the amount of energy that must be added to cause a neutral atom to lose an electron.

$$Atom + Energy \longrightarrow Atom^{+1} + Electron^{-1}$$

The first electron lost from an atom is usually one of those in the outermost shell. In a small atom the distance between the negatively charged outermost shell electron and the positively charged proton in the nucleus is small and the attractive force between the electron and the proton is large. The smaller an atom is, the more energy is needed to lose an electron from the outermost shell. Conversely, the larger an atom, the less energy is required to lose an electron from the outermost shell. The size of elements in a column down, a family, increases from top, He, to bottom, Rn, or krypton, Kr, in the case given. Hence, more energy is needed to remove an electron from a small atom than from a large atom.

80. **Answer is B.** Compounds formed from elements located close together in the periodic table are generally covalently bonded, for example ICl. Compounds formed from elements located far apart in the periodic table are generally ionically bonded. The element hydrogen, H, is an exception to this general rule. Sometimes hydrogen is covalently bonded, as in CH_4, other times hydrogen is ionically bonded as in hydrochloric acid, HCl.

81. **Answer is B.** The electron configuration for the first member of the halogen family, fluorine, F, is

$1s^2 2s^2 2p^5$

The OUTER electron configuration for F, for the electrons in the second or outermost shell, is $2s^2 2p^5$. Each of the other halogens has a similar outer electron configuration:

Cl	$3s^2 3p^5$
Br	$4s^2 4p^5$
I	$5s^2 5p^5$

Therefore, the outer electron configuration for the halogens is $s^2 p^5$. Elements in the same family, column down, have similar electron configurations. The similar electron configurations give the elements similar chemical and physical properties.

82. **Answer is C.** Electronegativity is a measure of the ability of an atom to draw covalently bonded electrons towards itself. For example, in the molecule hydrogen fluoride, H - F, the fluorine has a greater electronegativity than does hydrogen, and, consequently, the shared electrons comprising the bond between the hydrogen and the fluorine, are closer to fluorine than to hydrogen. Elements with the highest electronegativity are in the upper right corner of the periodic table, while elements with the lowest electronegativity are in the lower left corner. Of the elements given in the problem, F has the highest electronegativity and Cs has the lowest electronegativity.

83. **Answer is C.** A Lewis dot formula shows the electrons in the outermost shell. The electron configuration of sulfur, S, is

$1s^2 2s^2 2p^6 3s^2 3p^4$

The electrons in the outermost, the third, shell are $3s^2 3p^4$. The total number of electrons represented around sulfur is six, $2 + 4$, in the outermost shell. All of the members of the sulfur or oxygen family would have six electrons represented in a Lewis dot formula. In the halogen family, F, Cl, Br, I, seven electrons would be represented in a Lewis dot formula.

84. **Answer is A.** A nonpolar covalent bond is a bond in which electrons are equally shared between the two atoms forming the bond, *i.e.* both atoms have the same electronegativity. Atoms have identical electronegativities only when they are the same element. Therefore, the C - C bond is nonpolar. The bond between lithium and chlorine, Li - Cl, is ionic, answer **B**. The bond between hydrogen and fluorine, H - F, answer **C**, is polar. The electrons comprising the bond between the two atoms, are unequally shared, with fluorine, which has the higher electronegativity, having more electron density around itself than does hydrogen. The bond between boron and carbon, B - C, answer **D** is slightly polar, with the electrons being drawn slightly more towards carbon than towards boron, B. Electronegativity increases from left to right across the rows of the periodic table and decreases from top to bottom in the columns or families. The closer elements are to each other, the more likely their electronegativities are to be close in value. The following statement is an important relationship. Generally, as the size of the atom decreases, electronegativity increases.

85. **Answer is C.** The boiling temperature of a substance is a measure of the strength of the attractive forces between particles of the substance. When a substance is boiled, it is converted from a liquid to a gas. In the absence of other effects, boiling point is determined by molar mass. The higher the molar mass, the stronger the attractive forces between the particles. The higher the molar mass of a substance, the higher the boiling temperature. The molar mass of He is less than that of Ne, which is less than that of Ar, which is less than that of Kr.

86. **Answer is D.** Ionic compounds boil at higher temperatures than do covalent compounds, because positive and negative ions are strongly attracted to each other and much energy (high boiling point) is needed to separate them. Sodium chloride, NaCl, is the only ionic compound indicated in the problem. Three covalent compounds are included, hydrogen chloride, HCl, answer **A**, water, H_2O, answer **B**, and hydrogen fluoride, HF, answer **C**. The more polar the compound, the stronger the attractive forces between the molecules. Both water and hydrogen fluoride exhibit hydrogen bonding, a strong intermolecular force. The amount of hydrogen bonding between water molecules is greater than that between hydrogen fluoride molecules, and, consequently, the boiling temperature of water is greater than that of hydrogen fluoride. Hydrogen chloride does not exhibit hydrogen bonding, *i.e.* the intermolecular forces between the molecules of hydrogen chloride are not as strong as those between water molecules and between hydrogen fluoride molecules.

Consequently the boiling temperature of hydrogen chloride is less than that of hydrogen fluoride.

87. **Answer is D**. In order for hydrogen bonding to occur, hydrogen must be bonded to a nitrogen, oxygen, or fluorine atom, N - H, O - H, or F - H. The hydrogen atom in these bonds can then be strongly attracted to another nitrogen, oxygen, or fluorine atom. This strong attractive force is called the hydrogen bond. The only molecule indicated in the problem which fulfills these conditions is CH_3OH.

88. **Answer is A**. The shape of a molecule is believed to be determined by the number of electron pairs around the central atom. In the molecule BCl_3, the central B atom is bonded to three Cl atoms by three bonds which are made up of three electron pairs. Three electron pairs around the central atom equates to a trigonal planar shape. Two electron pairs around the central atom gives a linear shape. Four electron pairs around the central atom gives a tetrahedral shape.

89. **Answer is C**. The ammonium ion, NH_4^{+1}, has four bonds, four electron pairs, around the central atom and therefore the ion has a tetrahedral shape. On the other hand, the ammonia molecule, NH_3, has three bonding pairs of electrons and one nonbonding pair of electrons around the central nitrogen, N, atom. Ammonia has a trigonal pyramid shape.

90. **Answer is B**. The OF_2 molecule has two bonding electron pairs and two nonbonding electron pairs around the central oxygen, O, atom. The molecule has a bent shape.

91. **Answer is D**. Carbon dioxide, CO_2, a linear molecule, has a bond angle of $180°$. A trigonal planar molecule, for example aluminum chloride, $AlCl_3$, has bond angles of $120°$. A bent molecule, for example, water, H_2O, has a bond angle of approximately $105°$. A tetrahedral molecule, for example, carbon tetrachloride, CCl_4, has bond angles of approximately $90°$.

92. **Answer is C**. For the bent molecule, H_2O, the trigonal pyramidal molecule, NH_3, and the tetrahedral molecule, CH_4, the hybridization of the central atom, O, N, and C, respectively, is sp^3. For the linear molecule, CO_2, the hybridization of the central atom, C, is sp. For the trigonal planar molecule, BF_3, the hybridization of the central atom, B, is sp^2.

93. **Answer is B**. Each carbon atom in $H_2C = CH_2$ is bonded to three other atoms, bonded by two single bonds to two hydrogen atoms and bonded by a double bond to the other carbon atom. To determine the shape of the molecule, the double bond is considered to be one pair of electrons. Therefore, each carbon is assumed to have three electron pairs around itself and the shape of the molecule around each carbon atom is trigonal planar with a $120°$ bond angle. The hybridization of the trigonal planar carbon atom is sp^2.

94. Answer is **A**. In order to determine the polarity of a molecule, both the shape of the molecule and the polarity of each bond in the molecule must be considered. The CCl_4 molecule is tetrahedral and at each corner of the tetrahedron there is a chlorine, Cl, atom. Chlorine is more polar than carbon and, consequently, each bond is polar. However, since the molecule is symmetrical and the polarity is equal at each corner of the tetrahedron, overall the molecule is nonpolar. The H - Cl molecule, answer **B**, is linear, with chlorine being more polar than hydrogen. Hence, the H - Cl molecule is polar. Both $CHCl_3$, answer **C**, and CH_3Cl, answer **D**, have a tetrahedron shape. In the case of $CHCl_3$, three corners of the tetrahedron are occupied by chlorine atoms and one corner by the hydrogen atom. The polarity is not equal in all directions and the molecule is polar. The same explanation holds for CH_3Cl, where three corners of the tetrahedron are occupied by the three hydrogen atoms and one corner by the chlorine atom. The polarity is not equal in all directions and the molecule is polar.

95. Answer is **A**. The value of the pH measures the acidity or basicity of a solution and is defined as $pH = -\log[H^{+1}]$. Substituting $[H^{+1}] = 1 \times 10^{-5}$ into the pH equation gives a pH = 5.

96. Answer is **B**. A Brönsted acid is a substance that donates a proton. A Brönsted base is a substance that accepts a proton. A few examples of Brönsted acids include HCl(aq), hydrochloric acid; H_2SO_4, sulfuric acid; and CH_3COOH or HAc, acetic acid. Each of these acids contains the hydrogen atom, which can be donated as a proton. A few examples of Brönsted bases include OH^{-1}, hydroxide ion; : NH_3, ammonia; and HCO_3^{-1}, bicarbonate ion. Brönsted bases can be any substance with either a nonbonded pair of electrons, as in : NH_3, or a negative charge. A sample equation is shown below. The H_2SO_4 is the reactant acid, the NaOH is the reactant base. The H_2O is the product acid or the conjugate acid of OH^{-1} and the SO_4^{-2} is the product base or the conjugate base of H_2SO_4. Since H_2SO_4 is a strong acid, its, conjugate, SO_4^{-2}, is a weak base. Since OH^{-1} is a strong base, its conjugate, H_2O is a weak acid.

$$H_2SO_4 + 2 NaOH <-> Na_2SO_4 + 2 H_2O$$

The Brönsted acid-base definitions allow many different substances to be classified as bases.

97. Answer is **B**. A strong acid or base is one that totally ionizes, while a weak acid or base ionizes only partially. A strong base and a weak acid react together as shown in the example below.

$$NaOH + HAc --> NaAc + H_2O$$

Sodium hydroxide, the strong base, and acetic acid, the weak acid, react to produce a salt, sodium acetate, NaAc, plus water. Because the acetate ion, Ac^{-1}, is the conjugate base of a weak acid, acetic acid, HAc, it is a strong base, and capable of further reaction with water to produce hydroxide ions, OH^{-1}, as shown below.

$$NaAc + H_2O \longrightarrow NaOH + HAc$$

Because hydroxide ion is produced, the solution is basic.

A weak base, ammonia, NH_3, and a strong acid, hydrochloric acid, HCl, answer **C**, react, as shown below, to produce the salt ammonium chloride, NH_4Cl.

$$NH_3 + HCl \longrightarrow NH_4Cl$$

Because NH_4^{+1} is the conjugate acid of the weak base NH_3, it is a strong acid, and capable of further reaction with water to produce hydronium ion, H_3O^{+1}, as shown below.

$$NH_4^{+1} + H_2O \longrightarrow NH_3 + H_3O^{+1}$$

Because hydronium ion is produced, the solution is acidic.

When a strong base and a strong acid, answer **A**, react together, a salt and water are produced as shown below.

$$NaOH + HCl \longrightarrow NaCl + H_2O$$

Because the sodium ion, Na^{+1}, is the conjugate acid of the strong base, NaOH, it is a weak acid, and doesn't react further with water. Because the chloride ion, Cl^{-1}, is the conjugate base of the strong acid, HCl, it is a weak base, and doesn't react further with water. The solution is neutral.

When a weak acid and a weak base react, answer **D**, as shown below, to produce the salt, both the NH_4^{+1} and the Ac^{-1} ions react with H_2O. Whether the resulting solution is acidic, basic, or neutral depends upon the relative abilities of the two ions to react with water.

$$NH_3 + HAc \longrightarrow NH_4Ac$$

98. **Answer is B**. The acetate ion, CH_3COO^{-1} or Ac^{-1}, reacts with water to produce hydroxide ion and consequently the solution is basic.

$$Ac^{-1} + H_2O \longrightarrow HAc + OH^{-1}$$

99. **Answer is B**. A buffer solution is one in which the pH remains constant even when small amounts of acid or base are added to the solution. A buffer solution consists of a weak acid and its salt, or a weak base and its salt. Acetic acid, CH_3COOH, is the

only weak acid present, along with its salt sodium acetate, CH_3COONa. The other acids, HCl, HNO_3, H_2SO_4, are all strong acids.

100. Answer is **D**. Molecular orbital, MO, theory includes both sigma and pi bonds. Sigma bonds have a symmetrical concentration of electron density along the bond between the two bonded atoms. Pi bonds have electron density both above and below the plane of the bond. Single bonds in molecules are sigma bonds. The double bond, $C = C$, in the ethylene molecule consists of one sigma bond and one pi bond. A triple bond, for example, consists of one sigma and two pi bonds.

101. Answer is **B**. According to the Kinetic Molecular Theory of Matter, the molecules in a solid are close together, the molecules of a liquid are farther apart, and the molecules of a gas are farthest apart. The farther apart molecules are, the more freely they can move.

102. Answer is **C**. Sublimation is the direct conversion of a solid to a gas. For example, dry ice, solid carbon dioxide, is converted from solid to gas, without becoming liquid, at room temperature and pressure. Condensation, answer **A**, is the conversion of a gas to a liquid. Vaporization, answer **B**, is the conversion of a liquid to a gas. Freezing, answer **D**, is the conversion of a liquid to a solid.

103. Answer is **C**. An increase of pressure on the surface of a liquid, atmospheric pressure, decreases the opportunity for gas molecules in solution to leave the surface of the liquid. An increase in pressure on the surface of the liquid increases the solubility of the gas. All the other options, an increase in temperature of the solution, answer **A**, a decrease in pressure on the surface of the liquid, answer **B**, and stirring of the solution, answer **D**, decrease the solubility of the gas in the liquid.

104. Answer is **C**. As a chemical reaction proceeds, the concentration of the reactants decreases, while the concentration of the products increases. In studying the kinetics of a reaction, a decrease in reactants, A, or an increase in products, B or C, can be followed to determine the rate of the reaction.

105. Answer is **B**. The rate determining step in a sequence of reactions leading from reactants to products is always the slowest step.

106. Answer is **C**. A catalyst is a substance that is added to a reaction in order to alter the rate of the reaction. The catalyst can increase the rate of the reaction by lowering the activation energy of the reaction, or can decrease the rate of the reaction by raising the activation energy of the reaction. A catalyst changes the mechanism of a reaction and subsequently changes the activation energy of the reaction. A catalyst can be recovered unchanged at the end of the reaction.

107. Answer is **B**. The change in free energy, ΔG, represents the energy which can be used to do work in a reaction. The change in free energy may be used to determine whether a reaction will take place as written or not.

If $\Delta G < 0$, the reaction occurs spontaneously in the direction written
If $\Delta G > 0$, the reaction does not occur spontaneously in the direction written, but
    does occur spontaneously in the opposite direction
If $\Delta G = 0$, the reaction is at equilibrium and no change occurs.

108. Answer is **A**. Entropy is a measure of the amount of disorder in a reaction system. More freedom of movement, or disorder, of molecules is possible in a gas than in a liquid than in a solid. In equation **A**, a solid is converted to a solid and a gas. More disorder can be present in the reaction system in the products, where a gas is produced, than in the reactants, where a solid is used. Disorder increases. In equation **B** a gas is converted to a liquid. Disorder decreases. In equation **C** two different gases are converted to a liquid. Disorder decreases. In equation **D** a liquid and a gas are converted to a solid. Disorder decreases.

109. Answer is **A**. Only a change in temperature can cause a change in the equilibrium constant of a reaction. An increase in temperature causes the reaction to shift towards the direction that absorbs heat, *i.e.* the endothermic reaction. A decrease in temperature causes the reaction to shift towards the direction that evolves heat, *i.e.* the exothermic reaction. Changes in either the volume, answer **B**, or concentration, answer **C**, of one of the components in the reaction system will cause a corresponding change in the volume or concentration of another component in the system to maintain a constant equilibrium constant. A catalyst, answer **D**, will cause a change in the mechanism and the activation energy of a reaction but has no effect upon the equilibrium constant.

110. Answer is **C**. Gamma rays have the highest energy of the three forms of radiation listed. Therefore, the gamma rays can penetrate shields which would stop the other two forms of radiation. Beta particles are the next most energetic, and hence dangerous. Alpha particles are the least energetic and the least dangerous.

EXPLANATORY ANSWERS FOR BIOLOGY

111. Answer is **D**. Mushrooms belong to the Fungi Kingdom. See Table below:

Kingdom	Cell Type	Cell Number	Feeding Mode	Kingdom Characteristics	Examples
Monera	Procaryotic	One (occasionally chains or mats)	Autotrophic or heterotrophic (absorptive)	Small, simple cell, surrounded by rigid cell wall; many motile; some photosynthesize (blue-green bacteria), many feed by absorbing organic molecules from the surroundings (nonphotosynthetic bacteria)	bacteria blue-green algae
Protista	Eucaryotic	Mostly unicellular	Autotrophic or heterotrophic (absorptive or ingestive)	Complex cell with or without cell wall; many motile; some photosynthetic, some ingestive	algae amoeba
Fungi	Eucaryotic	Multicellular	Heterotrophic (absorptive)	Multicellular body, often with distinctive, specialized cell types; secrete digestive enzymes outside of body to digest food in surroundings, then absorb organic molecules into cells	mushrooms molds yeast
Plantae	Eucaryotic	Multicellular	Autotrophic	Multicellular, autotrophic organisms; complex cells with cell walls; make their food with chlorophyll and sunlight	trees ferns
Animalia	Eucaryotic	Multicellular	Heterotrophic	Multicellular body with cell specialization; large, complex cells without cell wall	insects fish mammals

112. Answer is **A**. See Table above.

113. Answer is **D**. The plasma membrane controls exchange of materials between the inside and outside of cell, regulates cell's chemical composition, and is the outermost layer of animal cells. The mitochondrion is the power plant of the cell and it provides energy in the form of ATP through oxidative phosphorylation.

114. Answer is **B**. These are characteristic of chloroplast.

115. Answer is **A**. See Figure.

116. Answer is **D**. See Figure.

117. Answer is **B**. See Figure.

118. Answer is **C**. See Figure.

119. Answer is **A**. Solutions that are <u>hypertonic</u> have a greater salt (electrolyte) concentration than the blood cells, and osmosis will cause water to leave the cell, shriveling it up until the concentrations of water inside and outside the cell become equal. <u>Hypotonic</u> solutions cause water to enter the cell. As the water enters, the cell will swell up. <u>Isotonic</u> means that the concentrations inside are the same as those on the outside, so there is no tendency for water either to enter or leave the cell.

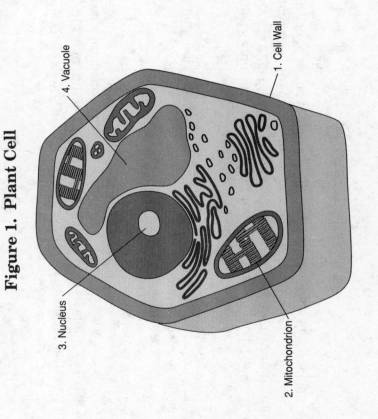

Figure 1. Plant Cell

120. Answer is **D**. See answer for 119.

121. Answer is **A**. The proper sequencing is prophase, metaphase, anaphase, and telophase. During prophase the chromosomes condense, the nuclear membrane deteriorates, and the spindle microtubules attach to the chromosomes. During metaphase the chromosomes move to the center of the cell. During anaphase each kinetochore divides and the chromosomes separate. During telophase the nuclear membrane reforms around each new daughter cell's nucleus.

122. Answer is **B**. Translation is a molecular event requiring close interaction among mRNA, tRNA, and a ribosome. Translation begins with a 'start' codon on the mRNA in the first position on the ribosome. A tRNA bearing the anticodon complementary to the start codon binds to the first tRNA site, and a second tRNA, bearing the anticodon complementary to the second codon, binds to the second tRNA site. The large ribosomal subunit catalyzes the formation of a peptide bond between the amino acids carried by the two tRNAs. The first tRNA then drops away, and the mRNA, still linked to the second tRNA, moves one codon over. This tRNA moves to the first tRNA binding site, thus vacating the second tRNA site. A new tRNA enters, a new peptide bond is formed, and the process repeats. The growing peptide chain is held to the ribosome by the latest tRNA, until a "stop" codon is encountered, freeing the newly completed protein from the ribosome.

123. Answer is **A**.

124. Answer is **D**. An endocrine gland has no ducts, releases its secretion into the surrounding interstitial fluid, and depends on the circulatory system to transport the secreted hormone to its target tissue.

125. Answer is **B**. Oxytocin is responsible for causing contractions of the uterus and ejecting milk from the mammary glands.

126. Answer is **D**. Iodine binds with the amino acid tyrosine to form the thyroid hormones (T3 and T4). The thyroid hormones are stored within the thyroid follicles as components of thyroglobulin. When released from the follicles, thyroid hormones are transported in the blood bound to thyroxin-binding globulin (TBG) or albumin.

127. **Answer is C.** Calcitonin causes blood calcium levels to decrease. It is produced by the parafollicular cells of the thyroid gland, and it increases in response to increased blood calcium level. Low blood calcium may result in weak bones and tetany.

128. **Answer is A.**

129. **Answer is D.** The medulla is a modified portion of the sympathetic nervous system. Its major secretory products are epinephrine and small amounts of norepinephrine, which are released during stress, exercise, injury, emotional excitement, or in response to low blood glucose.

130. **Answer is A.**

131. **Answer is D.**

132. **Answer is B.** The Tricuspid valve is the valve closing the orifice between the right atrium and the right ventricle of the heart. The Bicuspid valve is the valve closing the orifice between the left atrium and left ventricle of the heart. Choices C and D are not heart valves.

133. **Answer is B.** The red blood cell would enter the right atrium through the inferior vena cava and pass into the right ventricle. The red blood cell would exit the right ventricle through the pulmonary trunk, pass through the lungs, and return to the left atrium through the pulmonary vein. From the left atrium, the red blood cell would enter the left ventricle and leave the heart through the aorta.

134. **Answer is D.** About 97% of the oxygen transported in blood is bound to the heme portion of hemoglobin inside erythrocytes. About 3% is transported dissolved in plasma.

135. **Answer is D.** All of the structures listed increase the mucosal surface area of the small intestine.

136. **Answer is A.** Vitamins function as coenzymes, parts of coenzymes, or parts of enzymes. Most vitamins cannot be synthesized by the body, and they are not broken down before use. Vitamins A, D, E, and K are fat-soluble vitamins.

137. **Answer is D.** The kidney performs all of these functions.

138. Answer is <u>C</u>. A reaction in which the enzyme is the catalyst may be written as follows:

Enzyme + Substrate – Enzyme-Substrate complex – Enzyme + Product

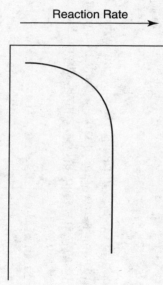

Substrate Concentration

The substrate binds to a specific site on the surface of the enzyme, known as the active site, after which product and enzyme are released. The enzyme is then available to bind another substrate. At low substrate concentration, the reaction rate increases sharply with increasing substrate concentration because there are abundant free enzyme molecules available to bind to an added substrate. At high substrate concentration, the reaction rate reaches a plateau as the enzyme active sites become saturated with substrate. The enzyme-substrate complex and no free enzymes are available to bind the added substrate.

139. Answer is <u>C</u>. In a heterozygous cross-height, for example, when T represents the dominant, tall, trait and t represents the recessive, short, trait. Tt represents both parents. A cross between Tt × Tt would produce an occurrence of the dominant trait 75 percent of the time.

	T	t
T	TT	Tt
t	Tt	tt

Tall: 3 (75%)   Short: 1 (25%)

140. Answer is <u>B</u>. The villi are specialized, finger-shaped structures in the lower intestine that are designed for absorption of digested nutrients. The alveoli are structures that allow the passage of carbon dioxide and oxygen into the lungs. Nephrons are the functional unit of the kidney. Bowman's capsule is where the filtration of the blood occurs in the nephrons of the kidney.

141. Answer is **A**. Choices B and C are learned behaviors. Caring for offspring seems to be one of those behaviors that is instinctual in most species.

142. Answer is **D**. Photosynthesis utilizes carbon dioxide and water from the atmosphere and light energy produced by the sun in the formation of chemical energy that is stored as glucose, starch, or other organic compounds in plant cells.

143. Answer is **C**. Fermentation allows for the production of ATP in the absence of oxygen. Certain fungi and bacteria (e.g., Brewer's yeast) produce alcohol as a result of fermentation, while human cells produce lactic acid.

144. Answer is **A**. One fourth of their offspring, on average, will have silver fur. Choices C and D are not a possibility because none of the parents have silver fur.

	B	b
B	BB	Bb
b	Bb	bb

145. Answer is **C**. The T-helper cells (T$_4$) cells are the most infected.

146. Answer is **A**. Digestion begins in the mouth and salivary amylase breaks down starches.

147. Answer is **B**. See below.

	B	b
b	Bb	bb
b	Bb	bb

148. Answer is **A**. Meiosis is a special process in cell division comprising two nuclear divisions in rapid succession that result in four gametocytes, each containing half the number of chromosomes found in somatic cells. When the two gametes unite in fertilization, the fusion reconstitutes the diploid number of chromosomes.

149. Answer is **D**. Messenger RNA (mRNA) carries the code for the amino acid sequences of proteins from the genes of DNA out of the nucleus and into the cytoplasm. Transfer RNA carries amino acids to the messenger RNA-ribosome complex during protein synthesis. Choices A and C are non-applicable.

150. Answer is **B**. Transfer RNA carries amino acids to the messenger RNA-ribosome complex during protein synthesis.

151. Answer is **B**. A major function of white blood cells (WBC) is to fight infections.

152. Answer is **A**. Because mitochondria use oxygen to produce ATP, the greater oxygen consumption indicates that tissue A has either a greater number of mitochondria, larger mitochondria, or more enzymatic activity then tissue B.

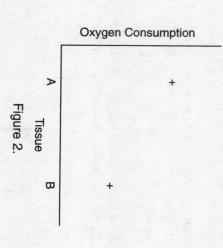

Figure 2.

153. Answer is **D**. A large sodium (Na$^+$) influx into the cell results in the resting potential becoming more positive. An action potential is produced when the charge difference across the plasma membrane reverses and then returns to the resting condition which requires the movement of sodium (Na$^+$) ions into the cell. There is generally a higher concentration of potassium (K$^+$) ions inside the cell than outside, and conversely a higher concentration of sodium (Na$^+$) ions outside the cell than inside. Following the action potential, the sodium-potassium exchange pump restores ion concentrations by moving sodium (Na$^+$) ions out of the cell and potassium (K$^+$) ions into the cell.

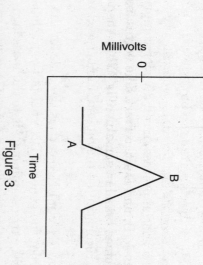

Figure 3.

154. Answer is **A**. See answer for Exercise 153.

155. Answer is **B**. Hormones are secreted in the blood from a specific gland and are distributed by the blood to a specific target site. Blood (answer B) plays a role in the general distribution of hormones.

156. Answer is **A**. In general, the smaller the animal, the farther to the right its curve will be. Therefore, small animals with high metabolic rates and correspondingly high oxygen requirements, tend to have hemoglobin that unloads more readily.

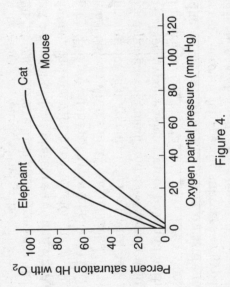

Figure 4.

157. Answer is **C**. Acetylcholine is the neurotransmitter by which vertebrate motor cells communicate with muscle cells.

158. Answer is **C**. Transmission across a synapse involves an influx of Ca+ ions into the terminal, followed by movement of transmitter vesicles, exocytosis, diffusion of the transmitter across the cleft, and finally the diffusion of ions through the postsynaptic channels.

159. Answer is **D**. Neurological drugs alter synaptic function by many different methods including: interfering with synthesis of the appropriate transmitter, blocking uptake of the transmitter into synaptic vesicles, preventing release of transmitter from vesicles into the cleft, or blocking the receptor sites on the postsynaptic membrane so that the transmitter has no effect even when released.

160. Answer is **C**. Statements A, B, and D are correct. The only false statement is C. The normal life span of red blood cells is approximately 120 days, not 30 days.

EXPLANATORY ANSWERS FOR READING COMPREHENSION

Passage 1:

As many as 50 million Americans have high blood pressure, defined as a systolic blood pressure ≥140 mm Hg and a diastolic blood pressure ≥90 mm Hg. Although blood pressure generally increases with age, the onset of hypertension most often occurs in the third, fourth, or fifth decade of life. The prevalence of hypertension in the elderly population (age ≥ 65 years) is approximately 63% in whites and 76% in blacks. In younger generations (35 to 45 years of age), the prevalence is markedly different with 44% among black men, 37% among black women, 26% among white men, and 17% among white women.

A specific cause of sustained hypertension cannot be found in the vast majority of individuals with high blood pressure. Genetic factors have been suggested to play a role in essential hypertension due to the fact that high blood pressure may be hereditary. Evidence that a single gene may account for specific subtypes of hypertension has also been suggested. Genetic traits include high angiotensin levels, increased aldosterone and other adrenal steroids, and high sodium-lithium counter-transport. More direct approaches for preventing or treating hypertension could be achieved by identifying individuals with these traits. Factors such as sodium excretion and transport rates, blood pressure response to plasma volume expansion, electrolyte homeostasis, and glomerular filtration rate help explain the predisposition for a person to develop hypertension.

Anti-hypertensive drug therapy should be individualized according to various patient characteristics and fundamental pathophysiologic circumstances. Dietary intake has been shown to be similar in all races but blacks ingest less potassium and calcium than whites. Supplemental potassium and calcium has shown to cause a modest reduction in blood pressure in some studies. Therefore, it would seem reasonable to ascertain the affects of increasing the amount of potassium and calcium in the diet as part of the non-pharmacologic regulation of hypertension. The initial treatment for hypertension is life-style unless target-organ damage is present. These changes include sodium reduction, weight reduction, increased physical activity, and ethanol reduction or abstinence. In terms of target-organ damage, diuretics and beta-blockers are first-line therapy. Control of blood pressure and prevention of cardiovascular morbidity and mortality are the goals of antihypertensive therapy. By maintaining arterial blood pressure below 140 mm Hg systolic and 90 mm Hg diastolic and by controlling other risk factors such as smoking, hyperlipidemia, and diabetes, morbidity and mortality may be averted.

161. Answer is B.

162. Answer is **B**. Although all choices may represent life-style changes, according to the passage life-style changes that are suggested to lower blood pressure include sodium restriction, weight reduction, increased physical activity, and ethanol reduction or abstinence. Weight gain and increased stress may increase blood pressure.

163. Answer is **D**.

164. Answer is **A**.

165. Answer is **C**.

Passage 2:

170. Non-adherence to medication therapy results in numerous adverse effects such as increased hospitalizations and even death. Additionally, it costs the U.S. healthcare system billions of dollars each year. It is important to assess patients adherence to medications.

168. Improper medication adherence encompasses an assortment of behaviors. These include not having a prescription filled, forgetting or intentionally not taking a medication, consuming an incorrect amount of a medication, taking a medication at the wrong time, ceasing therapy too soon, or continuing therapy after advised to discontinue. All forms of improper medication taking behavior may jeopardize health outcomes.

166. Measuring medication taking behavior is often difficult. The ideal method of measurement should be simultaneously unobtrusive (to avoid patient sensitization and maximize cooperation), objective (to produce discrete and reproducible data for each subject),

167. and practical (to maximize portability and minimize cost). Refill records, pill counts, electronic medication dispensers/caps, patient surveys (interviews), blood-drug level monitoring, and urine assay for drug metabolites can be used as clues to identify improper medication use.

169. Before altering therapy based on the assumption that a patient is taking a medication as prescribed, practitioners should ascertain patient's medication taking behavior. This becomes especially important when modifying dosages of medications. Due to the advantages and disadvantages of each measurement, it is important for practitioners to use a combination of methods to assess a patient's medication usage behavior and relate these findings to the patient's clinical presentation

166. Answer is **C**. The passage specifically states that the ideal method of measurement should be simultaneously unobtrusive (to avoid patient sensitization and maximize cooperation), objective (to produce discrete and reproducible data for each subject), and practical (to maximize portability and minimize cost).

167. Answer is **D**. According to the passage, half-life tables, nucleic acid levels, and patient examinations are not techniques for assessing patient's medication usage. Answer D lists techniques used to assess medication usage.

168. Answer is D. Choices A, B, and C are all forms of improper medication adherence.

169. Answer is A.

170. Answer is B. Medications may still work even if the patient does not take it as advised. Therefore, ruling-out A. C is not the answer because the passage specifically stated billions and not trillions, and no mention of lawsuits were made. Also, no mention of suicides were made. The first sentence of the passage discussed that non-adherence to medication therapy results in numerous adverse effects such as increased hospitalizations and even death. Therefore, the answer is B.

Passage 3:

Alzheimer's disease, first described by Alois Alzheimer in 1907, is a type of progressive dementia for which no cause is known, or no cure exists. People with Alzheimer's disease eventually lose their identity, memories, and all associated analytical, cognitive, and physical functions.

Several trials have been conducted to discover and evaluate drugs that may help Alzheimer's patients. One such trial of the drug memantine raised ethical and policy issues. Decline in cognitive and behavioral functioning was slower in trial participants with moderately severe disease receiving memantine than in those receiving placebo.

The benefits produced by this and other potential therapies for later-stage Alzheimer's must be carefully evaluated. There are many questions that need to be answered. Do patients receiving the investigational drug exhibit less personal distress or improved well-being during their last months? Does the drug improve patients' quality of life? Is the drug cost-effective?

These are hard questions with controversial moral dimensions. But they must be addressed if research is to offer meaningful help to patients and families coping with the effects of this awful disease. Currently, all treatments for Alzheimer's are palliative.

171. Answer is D.

172. Answer is B.

173. Answer is C. The passage clearly states that a decline in cognitive and behavioral functioning was slower in trial participants with moderately severe disease receiving memantine than in those receiving placebo, making choice C correct.

174. Answer is C.

175. Answer is B.

Passage 4:

179.   Imagine picking up a 10-kilogram piece of steak with your tongue. That's more or less what a chameleon can do with its so-called ballistic tongue. Its secret is suction, researchers reveal in the *Journal of Experimental Biology.*

   Scientists have determined that other lizards catch prey by using mainly surface tension—the stickiness created when a wet tongue contacts dry prey. But chameleons

177. consume creatures much too large for surface tension alone to handle. So evolutionary biologists at the University of Antwerp in Belgium and Northern Arizona University in Flagstaff decided to find out what else is going on. Dissecting tongues from several chameleon species, they found that two muscles form a pouch at the tip. Slow-motion film of chameleons capturing crickets, grasshoppers, and other lizards revealed that these muscles retract just before the tongue makes contact with the target.

177.
178.   The team suspected that the tongue pouch was behaving like a suction cup. So they anesthetized chameleons, inserted a glass tube into the pouch, and measured the force required to remove the tube as the pouch muscles were electrically stimulated. It took 10 times greater force to remove a sealed tube than a hollow (nonsuctionable) tube. The team also cut the nerve that controls the pouch muscles and found that although the animals

180. could still extend their tongues, they couldn't latch onto prey.

   Scientists seem to believe that these vacuum-generating tongues may be unique. A better understanding of this unusual mechanism should help scientists understand how it evolved.

Reprinted with permission from *Science*, Vol 290, October 2000. Page 79.

176. Answer is **C.** The main emphasis of the passage concerns how the chameleon tongue works and the great power of their tongues.

177. Answer is **C.** In order to answer this question correctly you may have to put together three parts of the passage. The first hint is that the passage states that the tongue pouch was behaving like a suction cup. The second hint is that the scientist believe that surface tension alone does not explain how the chameleons tongue works. The third hint, is when the scientist cut the nerve that controls the pouch muscles and found that the chameleons could not latch onto prey.

178. Answer is **D.**

179. Answer is **A.** The first two sentences of the passage describes that chameleons can pick-up approximately 10 kilograms which is equal to 22 pounds (1kg = 2.2 pounds; therefore 10kg = 22 pounds).

180. Answer is **D.**

Passage 5:

181. A dreaded disease is striking California's coast live oaks with the ferocity of an oak-tree Ebola virus, causing the trees to sprout sores, hemorrhage sap, and become infested with beetles and various fungi. The trees die within a few weeks of their first symptoms. Pathologists at the University of California, Davis, announced that his team had found

183. the cause of the disease dubbed "Sudden Oak Death." The tree-slayer is a new member of the genus Phytophthora, whose name means "plant destroyer". Its kin include pathogens responsible for the Irish potato famine and die-offs in Australian eucalyptus forests and European oak groves. "We don't know if (the new species) was just recently introduced, or if it has always been here and something else has changed that has allowed it to go crazy," one pathologist says.

182.-184 The first trees to succumb to the plague 5 years ago were tan oaks, which often grow in the under-story of redwood forests. Last year the disease began hitting large numbers of coast live oaks, the signature species in scenic coastal woodlands. Alarmingly, the pathogen has begun to blight another species, the black oak.

 Knowing the culprit doesn't make the outlook much brighter. Fungicides can save individual oaks, says one pathologist, but we can't go to Mount Tamalpais and spray 10,000 trees." And prevention is largely limited to warning people not to carry oak the firewood

185. to uninfected areas. The Sierra Nevada hosts black oaks, and pathologists fear deadly spores could strike groves in beloved Yosemite Valley.

Reprinted with permission from Science, Vol 289, August 2000. Page 859.

181. Answer is B.

182. Answer is A.

183. Answer is C.

184. Answer is A.

185. Answer is B.

Passage 6:

188. We humans sense old age through feeling those creaky joints or observing those gray-ing hairs but, according to Apfeld and Kenyon reporting in a recent issue of Nature, the nematode worm senses its age by smelling and tasting the environment. These investigators show that worms with defective olfactory organs (that would normally detect odor molecules in the environment) live longer than their comrades with a keener sense of smell. By comparing these worms with other mutant nematodes that live an unusually

189. long time, the researchers found clues to how a reduced ability to "smell the roses" might lengthen life-span.

187. The worm's olfactory sense organs—amphids on the head and plasmids on the tail—are composed of a cluster of nerve cells, the ends of which are modified into cilia. The cilia are encircled by a sheath and a socket cell that form a pore in the worm's skin through which the tips of the cilia protrude. Odor molecules and soluble compounds bind to G protein-coupled receptors (similar to the olfactory and taste receptors of mammals) located at the tip of each cilium. Worms with a poor sense of smell—because their olfactory organs have defective or absent cilia, blocked pores, or damaged sheaths—live much longer, yet are otherwise normal (for example, their feeding and reproductive behaviors are unchanged). Mutations in TAX-4—a channel regulated by cyclic GMP that sits under the G-protein-coupled receptor and transduces the sensory signals into electrical impulses—also imbue the worm with a longer life.

190. But mutations in the worms olfactory machinery are not the only defects that extend its life-span. In an earlier study, Kenyon's group found that defects in the reproductive 191. system could prolong life by decreasing the activity of DAF-2 (a receptor for an insulin-like molecule) and increasing the activity of DAF-16 (a transcription factor). By looking at 192. worms defective in both sensory perception and reproduction, Apfeld and Kenyon worked out a putative pathway through which smell might influence a worm's longevity.

An environmental signal, perhaps produced by bacteria (the worm's favorite food), binds to G protein-coupled olfactory receptors on sensory cilia activating TAX-4, which 193. then incites electrical activity in the sensory neurons. This activity triggers secretory vesicles in the neurons to release insulin-like molecules, which bind to DAF-2 and activate the insulin-like signaling pathway. This then switches on genes that will ensure the worm 186. dies at the usual age of 2 weeks. A reduced ability to sense olfactory cues would result in 195. a decrease in DAF-2 activation and an increase in life-span.

This chain of events is not proven, but insulin-like molecules that might bind to DAF-2 have been identified in the nematode. Such a pathway would also make physiological sense. After all, if food is scarce it may behoove the worm to live longer to ensure that it has the chance to produce its full quota of offspring. A scarcity of food also promotes 194. longevity in rodents and primates). But so far it seems that in these more complicated creatures a poor sense of smell is not a harbinger of a ripe old age.

Reprinted with permission from *Science*, Vol 287, January 2000. Page 54.

186. Answer is D.

187. Answer is A.

188. Answer is D.

189. Answer is C.

190. Answer is D.

191. Answer is **A**.

192. Answer is **B**.

193. Answer is **A**.

194. Answer is **D**.

195. Answer is **B**.

Passage 7:

Presidents of the United States are not like you and me. A new personality assessment presented this week at the American Psychological Association conference in Washington, D.C., shows that, compared to the public they serve, presidents are more likely to be extro-verted, assertive, and disagreeable. They're also less modest and straightforward.

Says who? Historians who have written book-length biographies of Oval Office occu-pants. Psychologist Steve Rubenzer of the Mental Health and Mental Retardation Authority of Harris County in Houston, Texas, and colleagues asked the biographers to fill out three standard personality inventories on their subjects, basing answers on the pres-idents' behavior during the 5 years preceding their reigns. The researchers compared the presidents' scores to population norms and compared the profiles of successful commanders-in-chief with those history hasn't smiled upon.

"Great" presidents, such as Jefferson and Lincoln, they find, "are attentive to their emotions, willing to question traditional values ... imaginative, and more interested in art and beauty than less successful Chief Executives." They're also more assertive, stubborn, and "tender-minded", which is a measure of concern for the less fortunate. Rubenzer hasn't analyzed the current presidential contenders yet—he prefers to have at least three "unbiased" historians fill out the forms for each president or presidential wanna-be.

Reprinted with permission from *Science*, Vol 289, August 2000. Page 859.

196. Answer is **C**.

197. Answer is **A**.

198. Answer is **B**.

199. Answer is **B**.

200. Answer is **A**.

Passage 8:

Drug interactions, a common type of drug-related problem, are categorized as pharmacokinetic, pharmacodynamic, or a combination of both. Pharmacokinetic drug interactions include changes in absorption, distribution, excretion, and metabolism; whereas, pharmacodynamic drug interactions may lead to antagonistic or synergistic effects. Not all drug interactions are undesirable, in fact, many drug interactions are used to produce desirable effects. Patients who take drugs with narrow therapeutic indices and drugs that interfere with the pharmacokinetic properties of other drugs are at increased risk of experiencing a drug interaction. Also, patients who take multiple medications per day or take multiple doses of medications per day are at increased risk. Because renal transplant patients take immunosuppressive agents that have narrow therapeutic indices and are subjected to multiple medications per day they are vulnerable to experiencing adverse drug events. To prevent adverse drug interactions, an alternative therapy should be considered when possible or the dose or schedule of the drugs should be adjusted to reduce the occurrence of an adverse experience. Additionally, adequate monitoring to prevent and detect adverse effects is an essential part of patient care.

A common pharmacokinetic interaction involves drugs that interfere with the absorption of other medications. Drugs that bind and decrease the gastrointestinal absorption of another drug, such as cholestyramine decreasing the absorption of tacrolimus, typically can be prevented by administering the agents two to three hours apart from each other. Prokinetic agents interfere with the rate of absorption. Since many transplant patients take prokinetic agents, such as metochlopromide, this may increase the bioavailability of other medications. This is of significant importance since immunosuppressive agents have narrow therapeutic indices and toxicity may result from this interaction. If the prokinetic agent cannot be avoided, careful monitoring (e.g., serum drug levels, clinical presentation of patient) and adjustments should be made to prevent immunosuppressant toxicity.

201. Answer is **C.**

202. Answer is **B.**

203. Answer is **D.**

204. Answer is **B.**

205. Answer is **C.**

EXPLANATORY ANSWERS FOR QUANTITATIVE ABILITY

206. <u>Answer is</u> <u>A</u>. **44,100**   A square has the same dimensions on all four sides. Area is calculated by multiplying two sides together. Thus, 210 feet $(\times)$ 210 feet = 44,100 square feet

Two other lessons should be learned from this question. (1) Since 210 $(\times)$ 210 means the right hand number will be a zero, any answer without a zero in the right hand position cannot be a correct answer. (2) Estimation can be a means of identifying possible answers. In this case, one can multiply 200 $(\times)$ 200 to get 40,000. Since 210 is greater than 200, the answer must be greater than 40,000. Any number smaller than that cannot be the correct answer.

207. <u>Answer is</u> <u>B</u>. **12**   Rearrangement changes the equation to $6x = 60 + 12$, which becomes $6x = 72$.

72 divided by 6 = 12

208. <u>Answer is</u> <u>A</u>. **4**   Rearrangement changes the equation to $x^2 = 66 - 50$, which becomes $x^2 = 16$

The square root of 16 is 4.

209. <u>Answer is</u> <u>B</u>. **8**   12 ounces times 30 mL per ounce = 360 mL total volume

15 mL $(\times)$ 3 doses per day = 45 mL per day; 360 mL divided by 45 mL = 8 days

An alternative solution: Since 30 mL = one ounce and 15 mL = one dose, then each ounce has two doses. Twelve ounces times two doses per ounce = 24 doses; divide by 3 doses per day to obtain 8 days.

210. <u>Answer is</u> <u>B</u>. $\dfrac{2}{3}$ Percent is parts per 100. Thus, 66% can also be written as $\dfrac{66}{100}$, which will reduce to approximately $\dfrac{2}{3}$.

211. <u>Answer is</u> <u>D</u>. **20**   Divide both sides of the equation by 2 to obtain $x^2 = 400$. The square root of 400 is 20

212. <u>Answer is</u> <u>D</u>. **250** $10^4 = 10 \times 10 \times 10 \times 10 = 10,000$ $10,000 \times 0.025 = 250$

213. <u>Answer is</u> <u>C</u>. **0.527** $0.3^3 = 0.3 \times 0.3 \times 0.3 = 0.027$ $\dfrac{1}{2} = 0.5$

$0.5 + 0.027 = 0.527$

214. <u>Answer is</u> **B**. **1%**   Percentage is parts per 100. To increase the 50 to 100, one would multiply by 2. 0.5 times 2 = 1. Thus, 0.5 per 50 is the same as 1 per 100 or 1 percent.

215. <u>Answer is</u> **C**. **1.81 × 10²**   Calculate each number separately such that $10^2 = 100$ and $9^2 = 81$. Added together they equal 181. 181 can also be expressed as $1.81 × 10^2$.

216. <u>Answer is</u> **C**. **10**   Any number raised to the zero power is one. $1 × 10 = 10$

217. <u>Answer is</u> **A**. **9.9 × 10⁴** $10^5 = 100,000$; $10^3 = 1,000$; so $100,000 - 1,000 = 99,000$

99,000 can also be expressed as $9.9 × 10^4$

NOTE: Subtraction of exponents is a mathematical method of doing division. Thus, $100,000 ÷ 1,000 = 100$ and 100 can be expressed as 10^2. Addition of exponents is a method of performing multiplication.

218. <u>Answer is</u> **C**. **33%** $\frac{11}{33}$ reduces to $\frac{1}{3}$. $1 ÷ 3 = 0.33$.

0.33 is converted to be percent when it is multiplied by 100. Thus, $0.33 × 100 = 33\%$

219. <u>Answer is</u> **D**. $\frac{1}{10}$ Division of fractions is performed by writing all elements as fractions.

Thus, $\frac{2}{5} ÷ 4$ becomes $\frac{2}{5} ÷ \frac{4}{1}$. The dividing number is then inverted, so the equation becomes $\frac{2}{5} ÷ \frac{1}{4}$. Inversion of division converts to operation to multiplication providing a final result of $\frac{2}{5} × \frac{1}{4} = \frac{2}{20} = \frac{1}{10}$

220. <u>Answer is</u> **D**. $1\frac{7}{15}$ To add fractions one must first find a common denominator. A simple method to do so is to multiply all denominators together; thus, 3 (×) 5 = 15.

Using 15 as the denominator, $\frac{2}{3}$ becomes $\frac{10}{15}$ [calculated by dividing 15 by 3 (=5) and multiplying 2 by 5 (= 10)]. The same type of steps are used to convert $\frac{4}{5}$ to $\frac{12}{15}$.

Adding $\frac{10}{15}$ and $\frac{12}{15} = \frac{22}{15}$ or $1\frac{7}{15}$

221. Answer is B. 250 Percent converts to a decimal value when the percent number is divided by 100. Thus, 25% divided by 100 = 0.25. Multiply 100 by 0.25 = 25 for 25% of 100.

To calculate the right side of the equation, divide 100% by 10% to get 10. Then multiply 25 (×) 10 = 250.

222. Answer is C. 60% One method to perform this is to increase $\frac{3}{5}$ to its equivalent value of $\frac{x}{100}$. Divide the denominator of the unknown fraction (100) by 5 (the denominator of the known fraction (5) to get 20. Multiply the numerator of the known fraction (3) by 20 to get the numerator of the unknown fraction (60). Thus, $\frac{3}{5}$ is the same as $\frac{60}{100}$, which is the same as 60%.

223. Answer is B. $\frac{33}{5}$ A whole number can become a fraction expressed as that number over 1 or, in this case, $\frac{6}{1}$. Addition is then accomplished using a common denominator which, in this case, would be 5. 30 + 3 = 33. The fraction is expressed as $\frac{33}{5}$.

224. Answer is C. 0.27 Solving $\frac{4}{5} \div 3$ required coverted 3 to the fraction $\frac{3}{1}$, the inverting the $\frac{3}{1}$ to obtain $\frac{4}{5}$ (×) $\frac{1}{3}$ which becomes $\frac{4}{15}$. Then 4 ÷ 15 = 0.26666, or 0.27.

225. Answer is C. 381 $5^3 = 5$ (×) 5 (×) 5 = 125. $4^4 = 4$ (×) 4 (×) 4 (×) 4 = 256. Then, 125 + 256 = 381

226. Answer is A. 120 The exclamation point after a number indicates that the number, and all numbers up to that number, are to be multiplied together. Thus, 5! represents: 1 (×) 2 (×) 3 (×) 4 (×) 5 = 120

227. Answer is C. 372 From 12 Noon to 6 PM is 6 hours. At a speed of 100 kilometers (km) per hour, the truck will travel 600 kilometers. Several conversions can be used to change kilometers to miles. One mile = 1.6 kilometers; one kilometer = 0.62 miles

For this problem 600 km (×) 0.62 miles per km = 372 miles

228. <u>Answer is **C**. **2**</u> The formula for slope (m) of a line is $m = \dfrac{y^2 - y^1}{x^2 - x^1}$

The points in a line (4,6) means that this point is $x = 4$, $y = 6$. Substituting the

values into the formula yields $m = \dfrac{6-2}{4-2} = \dfrac{4}{2} = 2$

229. <u>Answer is **B**. **5**</u> 1 inch = 2.54 cm; 1 foot = 12 inches

By ratio and proportion: $\dfrac{x \text{ inches}}{152.4 \text{ cm}} = \dfrac{1 \text{ inch}}{2.54 \text{ cm}}$ $x = 60$ inches

60 inches divided by 12 inches per foot = 5 feet

NOTE: There is more than one way of setting up ratio and proportion problems.
The method shown has advantages: (1) It mathematically expresses the question to
be solved—"How many inches will be in 152.4 cm if there is 1 inch in 2.54 cm?". (2)
The setup of the problem can be checked because the same units are used in the
numerators and again in the denominators. If the units are not kept together, the
problem has been set up incorrectly. (3) Only one mathematical step is necessary to
rearrange the problem for a final solution.

230. <u>Answer is **C**. **24**</u> one pound (lb) = 16 ounces (oz)

6 pounds (×) 16 oz per pound = 96 ounces

96 ounces divided by 4 ounces per lemon = 24 lemons

231. <u>Answer is **B**. **100**</u> 1 kilogram (kg) = 2.2 pounds (lb)

$$\dfrac{x \text{ kg}}{220 \text{ lb}} = \dfrac{1 \text{ lb}}{2.2 \text{ kg}} = 100 \text{ pounds}$$

232. <u>Answer is **A**. **0.5**</u> When a coin is tossed only two outcomes are possible, heads or
tails. No matter how many times a coin has been tossed, the probability on any one
toss is 50:50 or 1 chance out of 2 for either heads or tails. Thus, there is a 50%
chance for heads (or tails) on this toss.

233. <u>Answer is **C**. **4 hours**</u>

$$\dfrac{x \text{ minutes}}{2400 \text{ oranges}} = \dfrac{1 \text{ minute}}{10 \text{ oranges}} = 240 \text{ minutes}$$

1 hour (hr) = 60 minutes (min)   240 min ÷ 60 min/hour = 4 hours

234. Answer is D. 250 mph The number of hours from 10 AM to 4 PM is 6. Thus, the plane must travel 1500 miles in 6 hours.

$$\frac{1500 \text{ miles}}{6 \text{ hours}} = 250 \text{ miles per hour}$$

235. Answer is D. 10 The cube root of 1000 is written as $\sqrt[3]{1,000}$.

The cube root would be 10 $(\times)$ 10 $(\times)$ 10 = 1000

236. Answer is D. $\frac{1}{8}$ The expression $4x = \frac{1}{2}$ can be solved by dividing both sides of the

equation by four to provide the new equation $x = \frac{1}{2} \div 4$. The four can become $\frac{4}{1}$.

Now the equation is $x = \frac{1}{2} \div \frac{4}{1}$. This rearranges for the purpose of division to

become $x = \frac{1}{2} (x) \frac{1}{4}$. Solving yields $x = \frac{1}{8}$.

237. Answer is B. 4 8.8 pounds divided by 2.2 pounds per kilogram = 4 kilograms

238. Answer is C. 3.2 The $\sqrt{16}$ is 4. Expressed as a decimal, 80% = 0.8. 4 $(\times)$ 0.8 = 3.2

239. Answer is D. 7000 The $\sqrt{49}$ is 7. $10^3 = 10 (\times) 10 (\times) 10 = 1000$

$$7 (\times) 1000 = 7000$$

240. Answer is C. 1.0 mL 1 milligram (mg) = 1000 micrograms (mcg). You must convert either the concentration of the Digoxin Injection (500 mcg/2 ml = 0.5 mg/2 mL) or the dose desired (0.25 mg = 250 mcg) so that you are working with numbers that have the same dimension.

Thus, either $\dfrac{x \text{ mL}}{250 \text{ mcg}} = \dfrac{2 \text{ mL}}{500 \text{ mcg}}$ **-or-** $\dfrac{x \text{ mL}}{0.25 \text{ mg}} = \dfrac{2 \text{ mL}}{0.5 \text{ mg}}$ Both = 1 mL

241. Answer is B. 0.92 $\dfrac{2}{3} = \dfrac{8}{12}$; $\dfrac{1}{4} = \dfrac{3}{12}$. $\dfrac{8}{12} + \dfrac{3}{12} = \dfrac{11}{12}$

$$\frac{11}{12} = 0.92$$

242. Answer is A. 3   The formula for calculating the length of the sides of a right triangle is $a^2 + b^2 = c^2$. In the diagram shown, $BE = a$, $ED = b$, and $BD = c$. Substituting the known values into the formula gives us: $a^2 + 4^2 = 5^2$ which becomes: $a^2 + 16 = 25$.

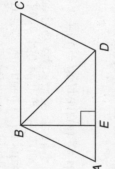

By rearrangement $a^2 = 25 - 16$ **-or-** $a^2 = 9$

Since the square root of 9 = 3, then $BE = 3$

243. Answer is B. 750 mg   There are two methods to solve this problem. (1) 2.5% equals 25 mg per gram. 25 mg/gram (×) 30 grams = 750 mg of active ingredient. (2) Convert 2.5% to a decimal. This is 0.025 (×) 30 grams = 0.750 grams. There are 1000 mg in 1 gram, so 0.750 grams = 750 mg.

244. Answer is D. $\dfrac{1}{8}$ Each coin toss has a $\dfrac{1}{2}$ chance of being tails (or heads). If a coin is tossed 3 times, then the chance of all three tosses being tails is

$$\frac{1}{2} \;(\times)\; \frac{1}{2} \;(\times)\; \frac{1}{2} = \frac{1}{8}$$

245. Answer is D. 1680 feet   Four contiguous acres that formed a perfect square would have the appearance shown in the diagram with each acre being a square. If one acre is 4900 square yards, each side of the acre would be 70 yards (70 squared is 4900). There are 3 feet in one yard, so 70 yards/side (×) 3 feet per yard = 210 feet per side. The four contiguous acres have the sides of two acres (420 feet) per side. Since there are four sides to form the perimeter, then 420 feet/side (×) four sides = 1680 feet.

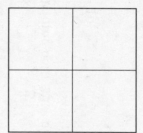

246. Answer is D. 0.45 grams   30 capsules (×) 15 mg of codeine per capsule = 450 mg needed

1 gram = 1000 mg, so 450 mg = 0.45 grams

NOTE: This problem illustrates the need to be sure of the units used for an answer since both the 450 mcg and the 450 grams are 1000 fold errors.

247. Answer is A. −4   To solve $x^2 + 50 = 66$, rearrange the equation to $x^2 = 66 − 50$ **or** $x^2 = 16$.

The square root of 16 is 4, but this is not an answer choice. Remember that squaring a number makes it a positive number so, when −4 is squared, it becomes 16.

248. Answer is B. 7   To solve $x^2 + 5 = 54$, rearrange the equation to $x^2 = 54 − 5$ **or** $x^2 = 49$.

The square root of 49 is 7. This answer choice is B.

249. Answer is B. 20   0.3 grams = 300 mg (1 gram = 1000 mg) 300 mg needed. Since 15 mg is in each tablet (300 mg ÷ 15 mg = 20), 20 tablets are needed.

250. Answer is C. 44,100   One yard = 3 feet. A square yard is then 3 feet on each side, so a square yard is 9 square feet (3^2 = 9) 4900 square yards (×) 9 square feet per square yard = 44,100 square feet.

NOTE: One acre actually contains 43,650 square feet which is equal to 4,840 square yards. A square plot of land 208.9 feet on a side = one acre.

251. Answer is B. 200   One teaspoonful (5 mL) four times a day = 20 mL per day [5 mL (×) 4 doses]

20 mL per day (×) 10 days = 200 mL needed for a ten day supply.

252. Answer is B. Pint   Sixteen fluid ounces equal one pint. One ounce = 30 mL; one pint = 480 mL. Both are approximations of the exact equivalents of 29.57 mL and 473 mL.

253. Answer is C. 10   Begin by dividing both sides of the equation by 3 to provide $x^2 = 100$.

Then the square root of 100 is 10.

254. Answer is **D**. $\dfrac{15}{25}$ Sixty percent (60%) expressed as a fraction would be $\dfrac{60}{100}$. To enlarge each of the other choices to $\underline{\ x\ }$, divide the denominator of the fraction into 100, then use that value to multiply times the numerator to obtain the fraction.

Thus, $\dfrac{1}{2} = \dfrac{50}{100}$, $\dfrac{2}{3} = \dfrac{67}{100}$, $\dfrac{8}{15} = \dfrac{53}{100}$ and $\dfrac{15}{25} = \dfrac{60}{100}$

255. Answer is **D**. $\log 6 + \log 4$ Since $\log(ab) = \log a + \log b$, then $\log(6 \times 4) = \log 6 + \log 4$

A second solution would be to multiply $(6 \times 4 = 24)$ to have $\log 24$.

256. Answer is **A**. $\dfrac{2}{5}$ Forty percent expressed as a fraction would be $\dfrac{40}{100}$.

To enlarge each of the other choices to $\underline{\ x\ }$, divide the denominator of the fraction into 100, then use that value to multiply times the numerator to obtain the fraction.

Thus, $\dfrac{2}{5} = \dfrac{40}{100}$, $\dfrac{1}{10} = \dfrac{10}{100}$, $\dfrac{1}{20} = \dfrac{5}{100}$ and $\dfrac{1}{2} = \dfrac{50}{100}$

257. Answer is **A**. 18.84 cm   The circumference of a circle is calculated by the formula $C = \pi d$, where $\pi = 3.14$ and d = the diameter of the circle. Thus, for a circle with a diameter of 6 cm:

$$C = 3.14 \ (\times) \ 6\,\text{cm} = 18.84\,\text{cm}$$

258. Answer is **B**. 5.08 cm   One inch = 2.54 centimeters (cm)

2.54 cm/inch $(\times)$ 2 inches = 5.08 cm

259. Answer is **D**. $7\sqrt{5}$ $\sqrt{45} = \sqrt{9(\times)5} = 3\sqrt{5}$

$\sqrt{80} = \sqrt{16(\times)5} = 4\sqrt{5}$

$3\sqrt{5} + 4\sqrt{5} = 7\sqrt{5}$

260. Answer is **A**. 1   The formula for slope (m) of a line is $m = \dfrac{y^2 - y^1}{x^2 - x^1}$

Substituting the values into the formula yields $m = \dfrac{5-1}{5-1} = 1$

261. Answer is C. 12.5   The area of the square is 25; then AB and BC must = 5(5 × 5 = 25). If BC = CE, then CE = 5. This means the area of the triangle is one-half the area of the square or 12.5. This could also be calculated from the formula for the area of a triangle: a = $\frac{1}{2}$ base (×) height. Since ABCD is a square, DC also equals 5. Therefore, 5 (×) 5 = 25; one-half of 25 = 12.5

262. Answer is C. 10   An average is calculated by totaling all the data points, then dividing the result by the number of data points. Since, 10 + 12 + 9 + 10 + 11 + 9 + 9 + 10 + 8 + 12 = 100, and there are 10 data points, 100 divided by 10 = 10.

263. Answer is B. 11   22% can be expressed as 0.22, which multiplied by 50 = 11

264. Answer is A. 3   Rearrange the equation to: $x^3 = 54 - 27$ **-or-** $x^3 = 27$

The cube root of 27 = 3

265. Answer is A. 150 |−100| = 100   100 + 50 = 150

266. Answer is D. 50.24   The formula for the area of a circle is A = πr^2

Since the diameter of the circle is 8, then the radius (one-half of the diameter) will be 4.

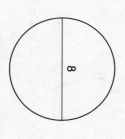

Thus, 4 (×) 4 (×) 3.14 = 50.24

267. Answer is B. 4   Rearrange the expression to 6x = 20 + 4 **-or-** 6x = 24 -or- x = 4

268. Answer is D. 9   This problem, without a calculator, requires some insight and a little trial and error. Look at the answer choices to see which numbers can be divided into 729 and then divided again into the result of the first division. Only 9 fits this requirement, as shown: 729 ÷ 9 = 81, then 81 ÷ 9 = 9. Thus, the cube root of 729 = 9. Because the value of a number increases rapidly when doing cube roots, it is usually best to start with a smaller number when doing problems by trial and error.

269. Answer is **B**. **32.13 square feet**   Calculating the area of the rectangle is simple:

6 feet ($\times$) 3 feet = 18 square feet.

The formula for the area of a circle is $A = \pi r^2$, but only one-half of a circle is involved. To get the radius of the circle, recognize that the six foot side of the rectangle is the diameter of the circle. Thus, the radius of the circle is three (3) feet. Therefore, the area of the half circle is: 3.14 ($\times$) 3^2 ($\times$) 0.5 = 14.13 square feet. Add the area of the rectangle to obtain a total area of 32.13 square feet.

270. Answer is **B**. $x = 2$ In order to form a line parallel to the Y axis, the value of X must remain constant, while the value of Y either increases or decreases.

Appendix:
Weights, Measures, and Conversions

LENGTH

1 inch (in.)	= 2.54 cm	
1 foot (ft.)	= 12 in.	= 0.3048 m
1 yard (yd.)	= 3 ft.	= 0.9144 m
1 mile (mi.)	= 1,760 yd.	= 1.6093 km
1 millimeter (mm)	= 0.0394 in.	
1 centimeter (cm)	= 10 mm	= 0.3937 in.
1 meter (m)	= 1,000 mm	= 1.0936 yd.
1 kilometer (km)	= 1,000 m	= 0.6214 mi.

AREA

1 square inch (in².)	= 6.4516 cm²	
1 square foot (ft².)	= 144 in².	= 0.093 m²
1 square yard (yd².)	= 9 ft².	= 0.8361 m²
1 acre	= 4840 yd².	= 4046.86 m²
1 square mile (mi²).	= 640 acres	= 2.59 km²
1 square centimeter (cm²)	= 100 mm²	= .155 in².
1 square meter (m²)	= 10,000 cm²	= 1.196 yd².
1 hectare (ha)	= 10,000 m²	= 2.4711 acres
1 square kilometer (km²)	= 100 ha	= .3861 mi².

WEIGHT

1 ounce (oz.)	= 437.5 grains	= 28.35 g
1 pound (lb.)	= 16 oz.	= 0.4536 kg
1 kg		= 2.2 lb.
1 short ton	= 2,000 lb.	= 0.9072 metric ton
1 long ton	= 2,240 lb.	= 1.0161 metric ton
1 milligram (mg)		= 0.0154 grain
1 gram (g)	= 1,000 mg	= 0.0353 oz.
1 kilogram (kg)	= 1,000 g	= 2.2046 lb.
1 tonne	= 1,000 g	= 1.1023 short tons
1 tonne	= 1,000 kg	= 0.9842 long ton

VOLUME

1 cubic inch (in³.)		= 16.387 cm³
1 cubic foot (ft³.)	= 1,728 in.³	= 0.028 m³
1 cubic yard (yd³.)	= 27 ft.³	= 0.7646 m³
1 cubic centimeter (cm³)		= 0.061 in.³
1 cubic decimeter (dm³)	= 1,000 cm³	= 0.0353 ft.³
1 cubic meter (m³)	= 1,000 dm³	= 1.3079 yd.³
1 liter (L)	= 1 dm³	= 0.2642 gal.
1 hectoliter (hL)	= 100 L	= 2.8378 bu.
1 fluid ounce (fl. oz.)		= 29.573 mL
1 liquid pint (pt.)	= 16 fl. oz.	= .4732 L
1 liquid quart (qt.)	= 2 pt.	= .946 L
1 gallon (gal.)	= 4 qt.	= 3.7853 L

TEMPERATURE

$$\text{Celsius}° = \frac{5}{9}(\text{F}° - 32°) \qquad \text{Fahrenheit}° = \frac{9}{5}(\text{C}°) + 32°$$